Benign focal epilepsies in infancy, childhood and adolescence

Benign focal epilepsies in infancy, childhood and adolescence

Editors:
Natalio Fejerman
Roberto H. Caraballo

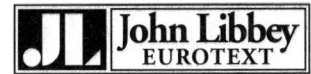

ISBN: 978-7-7420-0659-5
Current problems in epilepsy series: vol. 21
ISSN: 0950-4591

Éditions John Libbey Eurotext
127, avenue de la République
92120 Montrouge, France.
Tél. : 33 (0)1 46 73 06 60
e-mail : contact@jle.com
http://www.jle.com

Editor: Maud Thévenin

John Libbey Eurotext
42-46 High Street
Esher, Surrey
KT10 9KY
United Kingdom

© 2007 John Libbey Eurotext. All rights reserved.

It is prohibited to reproduce this work or any part of it without authorisation of the publisher or of the Centre Français d'Exploitation du Droit de Copie (CFC), 20, rue des Grands-Augustins, 75006 Paris.

Foreword

The history of the benign epilepsies in infancy and childhood began discreetly over 40 years ago with publications by French clinical electroencephysiologists who showed that localized epileptiform discharges could be recorded in the electroencephalogram of individuals with or without clinical epileptic manifestations, in the absence of any detectable brain lesion, suggesting that narrowly restricted cortical areas of hyperexcitability could be of purely "functional" origin. Over the following years, this type of electroencephalographic abnormality was found to be associated, in part of these cases, with certain clinical epileptic manifestations which were progressively better described and led to the delineation of the current concept of benign focal epilepsies and to the recognition that localized epileptic 'foci' were not necessarily associated with brain pathology. The concept has now been universally accepted in the following years and has become one of the most spectacular 'success stories' of modern epileptology. It established a new category of epilepsies due a localized dysfunction of a cortical area without any demonstrable lesion. This view represented a real breakthrough in the understanding of epilepsy, especially as it became evident that the new type of epilepsy was by no means a rarity but one of the commonest types especially among young persons. The associated benignity radically challenged the traditional thinking about epilepsy, a condition previously regarded as essentially chronic, often lifelong and of poor prognosis. The simultaneous development of the concept of epilepsy syndrome contributed to a completely new approach to the diagnosis, prognosis and therapeutic approaches of the epilepsies. It was of particular importance in child neurology as the epilepsies belonging to this category, occurred essentially in children and demonstrated a striking age dependency. This age dependency eventually was found to be a fundamental characteristic of the whole group with special age of appearance for specific types.

The senior author of this book was among the first to appreciate the importance of the benign focal epilepsies in child neurology and has greatly contributed, together with his co-authors, to the further delineation of this domain and its ramifications and remains a prominent member of the group of specialists who are still working to define the limits and explore the full implications of the new concept.

This book offers a timely and masterly description of the multifaceted clinical and electrophysiological aspects of the benign epilepsies of young age beginning with the first and best defined condition, childhood epilepsy with centrorolandic spikes that remains the best-known and most frequent form. Many other types have been added since and the reader will find an exhaustive and in-depth review of the multiple syndromes with extensive and up to date literature review of all their aspects. A special emphasis is placed on the benign type of occipital epilepsy as it is still less commonly recognized despite its relative frequency. A new feature is the inclusion of the benign early infantile syndromes of convulsions whose inclusion in the benign focal epilepsies is often rejected mainly on the basis of their short duration and great benignity, they certainly share most clinical and neurophysiological characteristics of the other benign epilepsies except for their duration and their exclusion is only explained by the fear still raised by the word epilepsy, which cannot be regarded as a scientific argument.

The descriptions of each syndrome are thorough and, for each syndrome, there is a systematic review of the clinical ictal and interictal features, the electroencephalographic findings, the required work-up, the differential diagnosis from other idiopathic epilepsies and from related syndromes. A large place is given to the unusual evolutions of some types of benign focal epilepsy such as atypical benign epilepsy, status epilepticus of benign centrotemporal epilepsy, Landau-Kleffner syndrome and the syndrome of continuous spike and wave during slow wave sleep. These syndromes clearly bear a relationship to the more typical forms and share with them many clinical and neurophysiological features but differ in their outcome: even though the evolution of the epilepsy remains ultimately benign despite frightening electrical and clinical features, neurodevelopmental disturbances are the rule and may be lasting. These disturbances might be the direct consequence of the epileptic process itself rather than indicate a progressive degenerative condition an important point for both diagnostic and therapeutic points of view, as control of the epileptic process could theoretically prevent developmental sequelae. These syndromes are part of the still poorly defined and understood group of the *epileptic encephalopathies* whose mechanisms remain to be worked out and may well be variable in different cases. Interestingly, the benign focal epilepsies may represent one possible clue to the understanding of this puzzling phenomenon as the epilepsy is the pure of any other pathology, the initial condition of the child at onset clearly normal and the final situation reasonably well defined. More recently, the benignity of even rolandic epilepsy has been questioned and various disturbances especially of language but also of other learning processes and of behaviour have been reported which might represent a minimal expression of epileptic encephalopathy and result from a similar mechanism. This view remains debated and I agree with the authors that these new findings do not put seriously into question the overall benignity of the syndrome although very long-term studies are needed.

The authors also discuss at length important points still debated such as definitions, limits of the domain, and classification. This has become a necessity as a result of the very success of the concept that might be in danger of losing its clinical significance if not clearly delimitated.

The authors have rightly used enough space to define the terms used. This is not always straightforward. The term 'benign' itself may be equivocal. The Webster dictionary defines it as "doing little or no harm" or when applied to disorders "not malignant". This is generally applicable to the benign epilepsies although not in all cases and some could contend that having epileptic seizures always does some harm at least psychologically. The term focal itself, replacing those of partial or 'localization-related' epilepsies previously used, may not be entirely satisfactory at least from a neurophysiological point of view as indicated in the chapter on cortical hyperexcitability in the book where the term regional areas of hyperexcitability is preferred although the EEG paroxysms are focal.

Classification and definition of the various syndromes is always an impossible task because biological reality does no respect clearcut borderlines that are a need of the human mind not of nature. The classification system used in this book is generally applicable and reasonable; Inevitably, some syndromes proposed by various authors are not accepted by others but this is no great concern so long as a clear description of the facts is given. Some syndromes that have been once regarded by some investigators as sufficiently characterized to qualify for inclusion in the group of the benign focal such as benign frontal epilepsy, benign affective epilepsy or benign partial epilepsy with somatosensory evoked potentials are no longer accepted as distinct syndromes but as variants or subtypes of other established syndromes.

Such difficulties often result from the lack or paucity of data as in the case of early infantile seizure syndromes. Whether these belong to several syndromes remains, in my opinion, debatable as the clinical manifestations are similar, the long-term course often unknown (e.g. a movement disorder may appear long after the end of follow-up), neurophysiological information is often fragmentary and certainly of very unequal completeness or quality in different works. I agree therefore that even though different genes can be involved, this should not detract from grouping such cases under a single syndrome as defined on a clinical/EEG basis as in the International League Classification. The same reservations may apply for a few rare syndromes and in general, I believe that, while even rare cases are of interest and deserve to be published, they need not be included into classification schemes too early.

The overwhelmingly important point from a clinical and practical point of view is the benign nature of the epilepsies studied in this book. Despite all the restrictions due to the existence of occasional not-so-benign or even of rare malignant cases, a phenomenon that always exists in medicine and does not detract from the general rule, benignity is clearly the one essential feature which sets the group apart from most other epilepsies and confers it its medical importance. This has been known for many years in the case of benign childhood epilepsies. It is of more recent knowledge for infantile cases whose frequency is still uncertain but probably higher than suspected. This new knowledge is essential to avoid prognostic errors of sometimes serious or even tragic consequences as I had unfortunately occasions to witness such as wrongly predicting the probability of serious cognitive difficulties for an infant with benign infantile seizures. It is also important to avoid unnecessary and often potentially dangerous or poorly tolerated treatments. It may also be of consequence for the indication of investigations especially imaging which may be considered as invasive in infants and young children. Clearly there are still divergent opinions about these indications because the degree of diagnosis and consequently of certainty about the benignity persists. A more precise knowledge of the possible outcomes and a better diagnostic capability are important before it can be decided more firmly whether these tools are really required or can be dispensed with.

The benign focal epilepsies will surely continue to represent a fruitful field of investigation as they have proved essential for the understanding of fundamental aspects of epilepsy and challenged respected received ideas on the nature, origin, mechanisms and consequences of epilepsy in general Many fundamental issues such as the effect of paroxysmal discharges, the mechanism of age limitation and relation to cerebral maturation, relationship of foci to generalized hyperexcitability, relation to sleep and cognition remain to be explored.

This book consequently will be of major importance for all those interested in epilepsy but especially for paediatricians and all physicians dealing with children. It will help them not only to understand better epilepsy but also to improve their insight into some problems of brain maturation and of learning.

Jean Aicardi MD, FRCP, FRCPCH
France

List of contributors

Eva Andermann, 3801 University Street Room 127, Montreal, Québec, H3A 2B4 Canada

Frederick Andermann, 3801 University Street Room 127, Montreal, Québec H3A 2B4 Canada

Giuliano Avanzini, Fondazione Istituto Nazionale Neurologico C.Besta, Via Celoria 11, 20133 Milano, Italy

Francesca Beccaria, Child Neuropsichiatry Dept, Epilepsy Center, C. Poma Hospital, Viale Albertoni 1, 46100 Mantova, Italy

Giuseppe Capovilla, Child Neuropsichiatry Dept, Epilepsy Center, C. Poma Hospital, Viale Albertoni 1, 46100 Mantova, Italy

Roberto Horacio Caraballo, Service of Neurology, "Prof. Dr Juan P. Garrahan" National Pediatric Hospital, Combate de los Pozos 1881, 1245 Buenos Aires, Argentina

Ricardo Cersósimo, Service of Neurology, "Prof. Dr Juan P. Garrahan" National Pediatric Hospital, Combate de los Pozos 1881, 1245 Buenos Aires, Argentina

Bernardo Dalla Bernardina, Servizio di Neuropsichiatria Infantile, Policlinico G.B. Rossi, P.le L.A. Scuro, 10, 37134 Verona, Italy

Francesca Darra, Servizio di Neuropsichiatria Infantile, Policlinico G.B. Rossi, P.le L.A. Scuro, 10, 37134 Verona, Italy

Natalio Fejerman, Service of Neurology, "Prof. Dr Juan P. Garrahan" National Pediatric Hospital, Combate de los Pozos 1881, 1245 Buenos Aires, Argentina

Elena Fontana, Servizio di Neuropsichiatria Infantile, Policlinico G.B. Rossi, P.le L.A. Scuro, 10, 37134 Verona, Italy

Silvana Franceschetti, Dept. Neurophysiopatology, Istituto Nazionale Neurologico C.Besta, Via Celoria 11, 20133 Milano, Italy

Eliane Kobayashi, Montreal Neurological Institute, McGill University, 3801 University Street, Montreal, Quebec, H3A 2B4 Canada

Ingrid Scheffer, Epilepsy Research Centre, Level 1, Neurosciences Building, Austin Health, Banksia Street, West Heidelberg VIC 3081, Australia

Pierre Szepetowski, Genetics of Human Epilepsies Group, INSERM U491, Faculté de Médecine de la Timone, 27 Bd Jean Moulin, 13385 Marseille Cedex 5, France

Contents

Foreword.. V
    Jean Aicardi

Part I. Introduction

- Definition of syndromes, seizure types and nosologic spectrum.   3
  Natalio Fejerman, Roberto H. Caraballo

- Cortical excitability in benign focal epilepsies............................. 15
  Giuliano Avanzini, Silvana Franceschetti

Part II. Familial and non-familial infantile seizures

- Benign familial and non-familial infantile seizures..................... 31
  Roberto H. Caraballo, Natalio Fejerman

- Benign familial infantile seizures and paroxysmal choreoathetosis 51
  Pierre Szepetowski

- Benign infantile focal epilepsy with midline spikes and waves during sleep 63
  Giuseppe Capovilla, Francesca Beccaria

Part III. Idiopathic focal epilepsies in childhood

- Benign childhood epilepsy with centrotemporal spikes............... 77
  Natalio Fejerman, Roberto H. Caraballo, Bernardo Dalla Bernardina

- Early onset benign childhood occipital epilepsy (Panayiotopoulos type) 115
  Natalio Fejerman, Roberto H. Caraballo

- Late onset childhood occipital epilepsy (Gastaut type) 145
  Roberto H. Caraballo, Natalio Fejerman

- Are there other types of benign focal epilepsies in childhood?... 169
  Bernardo Dalla Bernardina, Elena Fontana, Francesca Darra

- Atypical evolutions of benign focal epilepsies in childhood 179
  Natalio Fejerman, Roberto H. Caraballo, Bernardo Dalla Bernardina

- Symptomatic focal epilepsies imitating atypical evolutions of idiopathic focal epilepsies in childhood.. 221
  Roberto H. Caraballo, Ricardo Cersósimo, Natalio Fejerman

Part IV. Idiopathic focal epilepsies in adolescence

- Benign focal seizures of adolescence.. 243
  Roberto H. Caraballo, Ricardo Cersósimo, Giuseppe Capovilla, Natalio Fejerman

Part V. Autosomal dominant focal epilepsies

- Is there a subset of benign cases within the autosomal dominant focal epilepsies?.. 255
  Eliane Kobayashi, Eva Andermann, Frederick Andermann, Ingrid Scheffer

Part I
Introduction

Definition of syndromes, seizure types and nosologic spectrum

Natalio Fejerman, Roberto H. Caraballo
Buenos Aires, Argentina

The recognition of epilepsies in children associating focal clinical manifestations and unilateral electroencephalographic (EEG) discharges, with the features of functional epilepsies and with a natural trend towards a good outcome, which is to say towards the disappearance of seizures and EEG epileptiform abnormalities without neuropsychological deterioration, was one of the most interesting contributions to pediatric epileptology in the last 50 years.

The use of the term "benign" has been questioned and deserves clarifications. When we say that a condition is benign, what do we mean? That it is easily treatable? Or has a spontaneous good outcome even without treatment? Or it presents a short course before disappearance of electro-clinical features? Or there is absence of neuropsychological impairment? Can we call benign a condition implying the need of medication for many years? Can we denominate as benign an epilepsy syndrome in which some cases may not show at all a benign evolution?

In the last proposal of the Task Force on Classification of the International League Against Epilepsy (ILAE), five epilepsy syndromes (not counting neonatal epilepsies) included the term benign in their names, and four of them are considered focal (Engel, 2001): "Benign infantile seizures", "Benign familial infantile seizures", "Benign childhood epilepsy with centrotemporal spikes" (BCECTS) and "Early onset benign childhood occipital epilepsy (Panayiotopoulos type)". In the corresponding chapters, we'll explain the reasons why we are terming now the latter condition as "Panayiotopoulos syndrome" (PS) and why the "Late-onset childhood occipital epilepsy (Gastaut type)" does not include the word "benign" in its name. Incidentally, in the same report, it was proposed to use again the old term "focal" replacing the terms "partial" and "localization-related" which were used in previous ILAE's classifications. The reasons were: 1) previous criticism to the term "partial" because it implies part of a seizure, or part of a syndrome, rather than a seizure or syndrome that begins in part of one hemisphere; 2) *"the term localization-related has been cumbersome and is not consistently used [...], and in fact the older term focal remains in common use"* (Engel, 2001). Within the spectrum of idiopathic generalized epilepsies, a couple of syndromes were initially considered as benign. However, Juvenile myoclonic epilepsy does not meet criteria to be called benign, not only because control of seizures is not always easy, but because relapses upon discontinuing medication are quite frequent. Even the so called "Benign myoclonic epilepsy in infancy" (Engel, 2001) may now lose the term benign because it was acknowledged that a non-negligible percent of patients do show important learning difficulties (Fejerman, 2004; Engel, 2006).

We are using the terms benign and focal in the title of this book *(Benign focal epilepsies)* assuming that all the syndromes included in this category have focal electroclinical features and that in the vast majority of the patients presenting these syndromes, spontaneous cure is the usual outcome, with or without medication. Due to the real existence of a small minority of patients with not so benign features, the concept of a benign syndrome consistently remitting without sequelae has been challenged (Echenne *et al.*, 2001). In a recent paper, the definition of possible, probable and definite benign epilepsy syndromes was proposed, although the condition of definite implied long-term follow-up (Chahine and Mikati, 2006a).

Of course, the terms "absolute" or "100%" are quite rarely applied in biology, and the report of a number of cases within the most frequent benign focal epilepsy syndromes in childhood showing atypical evolutions with serious risks of neuropsychologic impairment has captured our interest in the last 20 years (Fejerman and Di Blasi, 1987; Fejerman, 1996; Fejerman *et al.*, 2000; Caraballo *et al.*, 2001).

In Chapter 10 we'll comment not only on several published series of patients showing different variants of learning difficulties, but also on our experience with patients who first presented with clear features of benign focal epilepsy (BFE) and years later showed electroclinical manifestations compatible with the diagnosis of Landau-Kleffner syndrome and Continuous spike and wave during slow sleep syndrome. We also include our follow-up of a series of patients with diagnosis of congenital unilateral polymicrogyria that clearly cannot be included among the BFE, but who do present a similar atypical evolution to the described here (see chapter 11). We intend to show that even in children with non-evolutive structural brain abnormalities as are the malformations of cortical development, a similar bilateral secondary synchrony causing aggravation of seizures may appear, perhaps related in some cases to antiepileptic drug (AED) treatment.

The term "idiopathic" has been applied to certain epilepsy syndromes in the 1989 ILAE classification and in the 2001 ILAE proposal, and most of the syndromes included in this text are in fact idiopathic, but not all. A good example as an exception is the growing number of babies recognized as having an autosomal dominant condition, the syndrome of Benign familial infantile seizures (Engel, 2001). We are also speculating that among the other familial (autosomal dominant) focal epilepsies which have been reported (Berkovic *et al.*, 1999; Andermann *et al.*, 2005) we might find a subset of children showing a benign evolution (see Chapter 13).

Definition of syndromes

Epilepsy syndrome has been briefly defined as a complex of signs and symptoms that define an unique epileptic condition (Engel, 2001). It should be made clear, however, that the concept of syndrome includes more elements to be detailed. The "signs and symptoms" may refer to visible seizures or symptomatic seizure manifestations, but the accompanying interictal and ictal EEG features, the age of prevalence, the neurologic status of the affected persons, eventual imaging findings, and even probable outcome have to be considered and included in the definition (Engel, 2006).

When a syndrome is "only epilepsy", with no underlying structural brain lesion or other neurological signs and symptoms, we denominate it idiopathic epilepsy syndrome (Engel, 2001). When we identify a syndrome in which the epileptic seizures are the result of one or more structural lesions or metabolic disturbances affecting the brain, we use the term "symptomatic epilepsy syndrome". In syndromes in which no aetiology has been identified, whether believed to be symptomatic or not fitting to known idiopathic syndromes, the terms "cryptogenic" or "probably symptomatic" have been applied (Commission on Classification, 1989; Engel, 2001; Engel, 2006). The recent ILAE Classification Core Group preferred the term "probably symptomatic" based on the statement that *"cryptogenic epilepsies are presumed to be symptomatic but the aetiology is not known"* (Engel, 2006).

Another important criterion in the definition of epilepsy syndrome is that more than one aetiology can cause the same clusters of signs and symptoms. Moreover, even in clearly idiopathic epilepsy syndromes assumed to be genetically determined, more than one gene are involved. In fact, if we were to find an epilepsy syndrome with only one specific aetiology, we would have to call it "disease" and not syndrome (Engel, 1998).

We think that the field of pediatric epileptology has been quite enriched after the first publication of the book *Epileptic Syndromes in Infancy, Childhood and Adolescence*, now friendly called "the blue guide" (Roger *et al.*, 1985). This valorization of the concept of epilepsy syndromes was later made official by the establishment of the International classification of epilepsies, epileptic syndromes and related disorders (Commission..., 1989). As member of the Task Force that elaborated the 2001 proposal of ILAE (Engel, 2001) and the ILAE Core Group report of 2006 (Engel, 2006), one of us (NF) wants to remind the readers that the 1989 classification is still valid and that the reports presented by the ILAE experts in 2001 and 2006 are proposals showing a way to keep working. An interesting discussion regarding criteria for classifications took place a few years ago (Wolf, 2003; Engel, 2003; Luders *et al.*, 2003; Berg and Blackstone; 2003; Avanzini, 2003). Besides the need to use appropriate methods to recognize each epileptic syndrome we must understand that classifications have to be practical schemes and that nothing is carved in stone (Engel & Fejerman, 2007).

Isolated questionings regarding the utility of the concept of syndromes and even the frequency of the diagnosis of definite epilepsy syndromes in epilepsy centers had been reported (Kellinghaus *et al.*, 2004; Luders *et al.*, 2006; Iinuma *et al.*, 2006), which lead to due responses (ILAE Classification Task Force Core Group..., 2006; Besag, 2006). Clear epidemiologic evidence exists showing that, especially in pediatric age, an epilepsy syndrome diagnosis is obtained in more than 90% of the cases attending epilepsy centers. Analyzing the clinical records of 645 consecutive outpatients followed at a children's epilepsy center, the 251 newly diagnosed cases were considered as a less biased sample of the epileptic population. A proper classification of epileptic syndromes was possible in 96% of them (Viani *et al.*, 1998). A cohort of 407 children with a first unprovoked seizure was prospectively recruited and followed-up for a mean of 9.4 years. Epilepsy syndromes were classified by using the ILAE guidelines in the 182 children with 2 or more seizures at last follow-up. The final syndrome diagnosis was different from the initial syndrome analysis in 33 (18%) cases (Shinnar *et al.*, 1999). However, the criteria of having a first seizure for inclusion created a bias because children with absences and myoclonic seizures did not enter the study. In one prospective follow-up study of 3469 patients aged 4-80 years aimed to achieve a more precise syndrome classification using the ILAE's 1989 guidelines, only 9% of the cases were considered as "uncertain" epilepsies (Osservatorio..., 1997). In a most comprehensive study of 1942 patients aged from 1 month to 95 years with newly diagnosed unprovoked epileptic seizures, 926 patients entered after a single seizure and 1016 with newly diagnosed epilepsy. Information was provided by 243 child or adult neurologists and 4 neurologists who classified each case according to the ILAE's criteria. The 1016 cases of newly diagnosed Epilepsia constituted the best sample to identify epileptic syndromes and only 14 of them were considered as "unclassified" (Jallon *et al.*, 2001).

We are reproducing in *Table I* the table 5 of the 2001 proposal of the ILAE Task Force *"an example of a classification of epilepsy syndromes"* (Engel, 2001), and in *Table II* the recent list of accepted epilepsy syndromes published as final report of the ILAE's Task Force (Engel, 2006). As can be seen in *Table I*, the two first groups [Idiopathic focal epilepsies of infancy and childhood and Familial (autosomal dominant) focal epilepsies] comprise all the benign focal epilepsies we are describing in this book. Some changes have been introduced in the Core Group report *(Table II)* where epilepsy syndromes are listed by age of onset. This time familial and non-familial benign infantile seizures are dealt together, and we'll explain later the reasons (see Chapter 4). Finally, we want to update the definition of epileptic encephalopathy: *"a condition in which the epileptiform abnormalities themselves are believed to contribute to the progressive disturbance in cerebral functions"* (Engel, 2001). We think now that the repetition of seizures without overt severe EEG discharges may also provoke an encephalopathic course of the condition (*e.g.* Dravet syndrome). Even when a book on benign epilepsies should apparently have nothing to do with epileptic encephalopathies, we will present evidence that at least some patients with typical benign focal epileptic syndromes may evolve into other syndromes included among the epileptic encephalopathies, such as the Landau-Kleffner syndrome and the syndrome of Continuous spikes and waves during slow sleep (see Chapter 10). Again, even when these two lists of epilepsy syndromes are still not officially incorporated by the ILAE, they constitute a good clue to envisage the new trends in the identification of epilepsy syndromes. It is interesting to know that experts not always agree 100% when the time for definitions comes. That is the reason why in the 2001 proposal some new syndromes were only partially accepted and named "in development", and it can be seen how some of those syndromes seem to have developed according to the most recent criteria of the core group.

Coming back to the subjects of our present interest, Fejerman proposed in the last meetings of the Core Group that Benign focal seizures in adolescence met the criteria to be considered a

Table I. An example of a classification of epilepsy syndromes*

Idiopathic focal epilepsies of infancy and childhood
    Benign infantile seizures (non-familial)
    Benign childhood epilepsy with centrotemporal spikes
    Early-onset benign childhood occipital epilepsy (Panayiotopoulos type)
    Late-onset childhood occipital epilepsy (Gastaut type)
Familial (autosomal dominant) focal epilepsies
    Benign familial neonatal seizures
    Benign familial infantile seizures
    Autosomal dominant nocturnal frontal lobe epilepsy
    Familial temporal lobe epilepsy
    Familial focal epilepsy with variable foci**
Symptomatic (or probably symptomatic) focal epilepsies
    Limbic epilepsies
        Mesial temporal lobe epilepsy with hippocampal sclerosis
        Mesial temporal lobe epilepsy defined by specific aetiologies
        Other types defined by location and aetiology
    Neocortical epilepsies
        Rasmussen syndrome
        Hemiconvulsion-hemiplegia-epilepsy syndrome
        Other types defined by location and aetiology
        *Migrating partial seizures of early infancy***
Idiopathic generalized epilepsies
    Benign myoclonic epilepsy in infancy
    Epilepsy with myoclonic astatic seizures
    Childhood absence epilepsy
    Epilepsy with myoclonic absences
    Idiopathic generalized epilepsies with variable phenotypes
        Juvenile absence epilepsy
        Juvenile myoclonic epilepsy
        Epilepsy with generalized tonic-clonic seizures only
    Generalized epilepsies with febrile seizures plus**
Reflex epilepsies
    Idiopathic photosensitive occipital lobe epilepsy
    Other visual sensitive epilepsies
    Primary reading epilepsy
    Startle epilepsy
Epileptic encephalopathies (in which the epileptiform abnormalities may contribute to progressive dysfunction)
    Early myoclonic encephalopathy
    Ohtahara syndrome
    West syndrome
    Dravet syndrome (previously known as severe myoclonic epilepsy in infancy)
    Myoclonic status in nonprogressive encephalopathies**
    Lennox-Gastaut syndrome
    Landau-Kleffner syndrome
    Epilepsy with continuous spike-waves during slow-wave sleep
Progressive myoclonus epilepsies
    See specific diseases
Seizures not necessarily requiring a diagnosis of epilepsy
    Benign neonatal seizures
    Febrile seizures
    Reflex seizures
    Alcohol-withdrawal seizures
    Drug or other chemically induced seizures
    Immediate and early posttraumatic seizures
    Single seizures or isolated clusters of seizures
    Rarely repeated seizures (oligo-epilepsy)

* *Reproduced with permission from Engel, 2001.*

** *Syndromes in development.*

syndrome, but a majority of the members thought that more evidence was needed. Therefore, we feel free to include in this book a chapter on this subject gathering reported evidences in the literature and our present series of followed-up cases (see Chapter 12).

We are presenting here the state of the art regarding benign focal epilepsies in infancy, childhood and adolescence, and we decided to include all the reported syndromes. Therefore, there is room here not only for the officially accepted syndromes, but also for some new more rare conditions which may be considered intermediate forms of already well-known syndromes, *e.g.* the new variant between neonatal and infantile familial seizures, and the proposed syndrome with spikes in vertex (see Chapters 3 and 5). A few other examples of reported benign focal epilepsies in childhood are also discussed, even when there is now consensus that their independent existence was not ratified in the experience of pediatric epileptologists (see Chapter 9).

Table II. Epilepsy syndromes by age of onset and related conditions*

Neonatal period
Benign familial neonatal seizures (BFNS)
Early myoclonic encephalopathy (EME)
Ohtahara syndrome
Infancy
Migrating partial seizures of infancy
West syndrome
Myoclonic epilepsy in infancy (MEI)
Benign infantile seizures
Dravet syndrome
Myoclonic encephalopathy in nonprogressive disorders
Childhood
Early onset benign childhood occipital epilepsy (Panayiotopoulos type)
Epilepsy with myoclonic astatic seizures
Benign childhood epilepsy with centrotemporal spikes (BECTS)
Late onset childhood occipital epilepsy (Gastaut type)
Epilepsy with myoclonic absences
Lennox-Gastaut syndrome
Epileptic encephalopathy with continuous spike-and-wave during sleep (CSWS) including
Landau-Kleffner syndrome (LKS)
Childhood absence epilepsy (CAE)
Adolescence
Juvenile absence epilepsy (JAE)
Juvenile myoclonic epilepsy (JME)
Progressive myoclonus epilepsies (PME)
Less Specific Age Relationship
Autosomal-dominant nocturnal frontal lobe epilepsy (ADNFLE)
Familial temporal lobe epilepsies
Mesial temporal lobe epilepsy with hippocampal sclerosis (MTLE with HS)
Rasmussen syndrome
Gelastic seizures with hypothalamic hamartoma
Special Epilepsy Conditions
Symptomatic focal epilepsies not otherwise specified
Epilepsy with generalized tonic-clonic seizures only
Reflex epilepsies
Febrile seizures plus (FS +)
Familial focal epilepsy with variable foci
Conditions with epileptic seizures that do not require a diagnosis of epilepsy
Benign neonatal seizures (BNS)
Febrile seizures (FS)

* *Reproduced with permission from Engel, 2006.*

Seizure types

Having said that we prioritize the identification of epileptic syndromes, we cannot ignore the importance of recognizing the different types of seizures comprised within the syndromes, because as clinical manifestations, the seizures are the initial visible expression of an epileptic illness. In *Table III* we reproduce the list of "self-limited epileptic seizure types which have focal onset" as recently published (Engel, 2006). Incidentally, in the section of the last mentioned report devoted to status epilepticus, no mention to autonomic status epilepticus is present and we'll see later how frequent this phenomenon is in children with PS (Ferrie *et al.*, 2007). It is stated that a number of factors will need to be investigated in order to develop more definitive criteria for distinguishing between different types of seizures, which include:

- Factors that might distinguish between focal seizures due to discretely localized lesions, as occur with focal symptomatic epilepsy, and focal seizures due to more distributed network disturbances, as might occur with some focal idiopathic epilepsies (*e.g.*, those responsible for the transverse dipole of BCECTS), or even in idiopathic generalized epilepsies;
- Maturational factors;
- Modes of precipitation, as in reflex seizures;
- Pathology;
- Pathophysiologic mechanisms;
- Location;
- Factors influencing seizure-induced progressive disturbances in neuronal function and structure at the site of, and downstream from, ictal onset.

It is beyond the scope of this text to discuss the differential diagnosis between epileptic and non-epileptic paroxysmal phenomena. However, there are some particularities among the seizure types seen in the BFE that we want to show with emphasis in this introductory chapter.

1) By definition, seizures in BFE are focal and in the majority of the cases conscience is therefore preserved during attacks.

2) Nevertheless, the so called complex partial seizures have been reported in babies with benign familial and non-familial infantile seizures. In children with the Benign childhood occipital epilepsy Panayiotopoulos type, consciousness is also frequently affected.

3) Again, almost by definition, any focal seizure may follow a course towards a secondary generalized seizure. This fact has been registered in ictal EEG recordings, which are of special aid when the first focal phase of the event is not witnessed.

4) Focal unilateral or bilateral inhibitory seizures are not part of the presenting features of BFE, but constitute a characteristic finding in certain atypical evolutions associated with secondary bilateral synchronies in the EEG. Moreover, in unilateral inhibitory motor seizures the phenomenon of negative myoclonus has been clearly demonstrated (Tassinari *et al.*, 1995). These types of seizures, causing falls with risk of injuries, clearly imply a change in the character of the disorder which obviously cannot then be described as benign.

5) Besides the mentioned focal inhibitory seizures, another epileptic phenomenon as an inherent risk of prolonged focal seizures, the post-ictal Todd's paresis, has been occasionally reported in BFE cases (Dai & Weinstock, 2005).

6) Again, as it may happen in any epileptic seizure type, status epilepticus (SE) may also occur in BFE. We reported the first two cases of SE in BCECTS (Fejerman & Di Blasi, 1987). Of course, these are exceptions that confirm the rule of benignity, but in the last years evidence was presented showing that SE (seizures lasting more than 30 minutes) is quite frequent in patients with the early onset Benign childhood occipital epilepsy or PS (Caraballo et al., 2000). Curiously enough, in this particular case, the occurrence of SE has no influence on the benign outcome of the condition.

7) There is something new regarding seizure types in BFE. Even when we are going to describe all details in Chapter 9, we cannot avoid mentioning here that in the syndrome first described by Panayiotopoulos, ictal vomiting constitutes one of the core manifestations (Panayiotopoulos, 1989; Caraballo et al., 2000; Fejerman & Panayiotopoulos, 2007). This may be considered a revolutionary finding because pediatricians and neurologists never thought before that vomiting might be a substantial part of the seizures in children, instead of being a mechanical complication within a seizure.

Moreover, other autonomic manifestations are non-rarely part of the seizures in PS. Again, autonomic SE is more frequently seen in children with PS than in any other epileptic seizures or syndromes in childhood or adults (Panayiotopoulos, 2005; Ferrie et al., 2006, 2007).

Table III. Seizure Types. Self-limited epileptic seizures*

II. Focal onset (partial)
A. Local
1. Neocortical
a. Without local spread
1) Focal clonic seizures
2) Focal myoclonic seizures
3) Inhibitory motor seizures
4) Focal sensory seizures with elementary symptoms
5) Aphasic seizures
b. With local spread
1) Jacksonian march seizures
2) Focal (asymmetrical) tonic seizures
3) Focal sensory seizures with experiential symptoms
2. Hippocampal and parahippocampal
B. With ipsilateral propagation to:
1. Neocortical areas (includes hemiclonic seizures)
2. Limbic areas (includes gelastic seizures)
C. With contralateral spread to:
1. Neocortical areas (hyperkinetic seizures)
2. Limbic areas (dyscognitive seizures with or without automatisms {psychomotor])
D. Secondarily generalized
1. Tonic-clonic seizures
2. Absence seizures
3. Epileptic spasms (unverified)

Partially reproduced with permission from Engel, 2006.

Nosologic spectrum

As can be seen, the nosologic spectrum of BFE in infancy, childhood and adolescence is quite wide. The age span is broad and there are no clear-cut boundaries between some of the described syndromes, even if we also consider the benign neonatal epilepsies. The age sequence of recognized epilepsy syndromes which may show some blurry boundaries between them is: Benign familial neonatal seizures – A new variant between neonatal and infantile familial seizures – Benign infantile seizures (familial and non-familial) – A new proposed syndrome with spikes in vertex – Early onset benign childhood occipital epilepsy (Panayiotopoulos type) – Benign childhood epilepsy with centrotemporal spikes – Late onset childhood occipital epilepsy (Gastaut type). Benign convulsions in adolescence do not seem to link to any other close aged-related BFE syndrome.

One might even speculate that the concept of idiopathic generalized epilepsies with variable phenotypes introduced in the 2001 proposed scheme of the ILAE Task Force on Classification (Engel, 2001) could be applied to the BFE (Lundborg and Eeg Olofsson, 2003) and perhaps a couple of groups of BFE with variable phenotypes might be recognized, such as Benign familial neonatal seizures – New variant between neonatal and infantile familial seizures – Benign infantile seizures (familial and non-familial) on one side, and the Syndrome with spikes in vertex – Early onset benign childhood occipital epilepsy (Panayiotopoulos type) or Panayiotopoulos syndrome (PS) – Benign childhood epilepsy with centrotemporal spikes (BCECTS) – as a second group. There is evidence that PS and BECTS can coexist in the same child, either at the same time or one after the other (Caraballo *et al.*, 1998; Covanis *et al.*, 2003). Curiously enough, three patients with absence epilepsy appearing 1-4 years after recovering of an electroclinical picture typical of benign childhood partial epilepsy were reported (Gambardella et al., 1996). We also reported cases of PS and the Gastaut type of childhood occipital epilepsy evolving to an idiopathic generalized epilepsy syndrome such as childhood absence epilepsy (Caraballo *et al.*, 2004, 2005).

References

- Andermann F, Kobayashi E, Andermann E. Genetic focal epilepsies: state of the art and path to the future. *Epilepsia* 2005; 46 (Suppl. 10): 61-7.

- Avanzini G. Of cabbages and kings: Do we really need a systematic classification of epilepsies? *Epilepsia* 2003; 44: 12-3.

- Berg AT, Blackstone NW. Of cabbages and kings: Perspectives on classification from the field of systematics. *Epilepsia* 2003; 44: 8-12.

- Berkovic SF, Genton P, Hirsch E, Picard F (Eds). *Genetics of focal epilepsies*. London: John Libbey, 1999.

- Besag FMC. Epilepsy syndromes still survive. Letter to the Editor. *Epileptic disorders* 2006; 8 (2): 161-2.

- Caraballo RH, Astorino F, Cersosimo R, Soprano AM, Fejerman N. Atypical evolution in childhood epilepsy with occipital paroxysms (Panayiotopoulos type). *Epileptic Disord* 2001; 3 (3): 157-62.

- Caraballo R, Cersosimo R, Espeche A, Fejerman N. Benign familial and non-familial infantile seizures: a study of 64 patients. *Epileptic Disorders* 2003; 5 (1): 45-9.

- Caraballo RH, Sologuestua A, Granana N, *et al*. Idiopathic occipital and absence epilepsies appearing in the same children. *Pediatr Neurol* 2004; 30 (1): 24-8.

- Caraballo RH, Cersosimo RO, Fejerman N. Late-onset, "Gastaut type", childhood occipital epilepsy: an unusual evolution. *Epileptic Disord* 2005; 7 (4): 341-6.

- Chahine LM, Mikati MA. Benign pediatric localization-related epilepsies. Part I. Syndromes in infancy. *Epileptic Disord* 2006; 8 (3): 169-83.

- Commission on Classification and Terminology of the International League against Epilepsy. Proposal for revised classification of epilepsies and epileptic syndromes. *Epilepsia* 1989; 30: 389-99.

- Dai AI, Weinstock A. Postictal paresis in children with benign rolandic epilepsy. *J Child Neurol* 2005; 20 (10): 834-6.

- Echenne B, Cheminal R, Roubertie A, Rivier F. Are idiopathic generalized epilepsies of childhood really benign? *Epileptic Disord* 2001; 3 (Spec No 2): SI67-SI72. French.

- Engel J Jr. Classifications of the International League Against Epilepsy: time for reappraisal. *Epilepsia* 1998; 39 (9): 1014-7.

- Engel J Jr. A proposed diagnostic scheme for people with epileptic seizures and with epilepsy: Report of the ILAE Task Force on Classification and Terminology. *Epilepsia* 2001; 42: 796-803.

- Engel J Jr. Reply to "Of cabbages and kings: Some considerations on classifications, diagnostic schemes, semiology, and concepts". *Epilepsia* 2003; 44: 4-6.

- Engel J. Report of the ILAE classification core group. *Epilepsia* 2006; 47 (9): 1558-68.

- Engel J Jr, Fejerman N. International Classification of the Epilepsies. In: Engel J Jr, Pedley TA (Eds). *Epilepsy: A Comprehensive Textbook* (2nd Ed). Philadelphia: Lippincott Williams & Wilkins, 2007, Chapter 68 (In Press).

- Fejerman N, Di Blasi AM. Status epilepticus of benign partial epilepsies in children: report of two cases. *Epilepsia* 1987; 28 (4): 351-55.

- Fejerman N. Atypical evolution of benign partial epilepsy in children. *Rev Neurol* 1996; 24 (135): 1415-20. Spanish.

- Fejerman N, Caraballo R, Tenembaum SN. Atypical evolutions of benign partial epilepsy of infancy with centrotemporal spikes. *Rev Neurol* 2000; 31 (4): 389-96. Spanish.

- Fejerman N. Benign Myoclonic Epilepsy in Infancy. In: Wallace S, Farrell K. (Eds). Epilepsy in Children. London: Arnold Publishers, 2004, pp. 153-56.

- Ferrie CD, Caraballo RH, Covanis A, *et al*. Panayiotopoulos syndrome: a consensus view. *Develop Med Child Neurol* 2006; 48 (3): 236-40.

- Ferrie CD, Caraballo R, Covanis A, *et al*. Autonomic status epilepticus in Panayiotopoulos syndrome and other childhood and adult epilepsies: a consensus view. *Epilepsia* 2007; In Press.

- Gambardella A, Aguglia U, Guerrini R, *et al*. Sequential occurrence of benign partial epilepsy and childhood absence epilepsy in three patients. *Brain Dev* 1996; 18 (3): 212-5.

- Iinuma K, Morimoto K, Akiyama T, *et al*. Proposed diagnostic scheme for the classification of epileptic seizures and epilepsies (ILAE, 2001): proposal from Japan Epilepsy Society. *Epilepsia* 2006; 47 (9): 1588-9.

- ILAE Classification Task Force Core Group and ILAE Classification Commission. Are epilepsy classifications based on epileptic syndromes and seizure types outdated? Letter to the Editor. *Epileptic Disorders* 2006; 8 (2): 159-61.

- Jallon P, Loiseau P, Loiseau J. Newly diagnosed unprovoked epileptic seizures: presentation at diagnosis in CAROLE study. *Epilepsia* 2001; 42: 464-75.

- Kellinghaus C, Loddenkemper T, Najm IM, *et al*. Specific epileptic syndromes are rare even in tertiary epilepsy centers: a patient-oriented approach to epilepsy classification. *Epilepsia* 2004; 45 (3): 268-75.

- Lüders H, Najm I, Wyllie E. Reply to "Of cabbages and kings: Some considerations on classifications, diagnostic schemes, semiology, and concepts". *Epilepsia* 2003; 44: 6-8.

- Luders HO, Acharya J, Alexopoulos A. Are epilepsy classifications based on epileptic syndromes and seizure types outdated? *Epileptic Disord* 2006; 8 (1): 81-5.

- Lundborg S, Eeg-Olofsson O. Rolandic epilepsy: a challenge in terminology and classification. *European Journal of Pediatric Neurology* 2003; 7: 239-41.

- Osservatorio Regionale per l'Epilessia (OREp), Lombardy. The contribution of tertiary centers to the quality of the diagnosis and treatment of epilepsy. *Epilepsia* 1997; 38 (12): 1338-43.

- Panayiotopoulos CP. Vomiting as an ictal manifestation of epileptic seizures and syndromes. *J Neurol Neurosurg Psychiatr* 1988; 51: 1448-51.

- Panayiotopoulos CP. Benign nocturnal childhood occipital epilepsy: a new syndrome with nocturnal seizures, tonic deviation of the eyes, and vomiting. *J Child Neurol* 1989; 4: 43-9.

- Panayiotopoulos CP. *Panayiotopoulos syndrome: A common and benign childhood epileptic syndrome*. London: John Libbey, 2002.

- Panayiotopoulos CP. Benign childhood focal seizures and related epileptic syndromes. In: Panayiotopoulos CP (ed.) *The epilepsies: Seizures, syndromes and management*. Oxford: Bladon Medical Publishing, 2005, pp. 223-69.

- Shinnar S, O'Dell C, Berg AT. Distribution of epilepsy syndromes in a cohort of children prospectively monitored from the time of their first unprovoked seizure. *Epilepsia* 1999; 40 (10): 1378-83.

- Tassinari CA, Rubboli G, Parmeggiani L, *et al*. Epileptic negative myoclonus. In: Fahn S, *et al*. (Eds). Negative motor phenomena. *Adv Neurol*. Philadelphia: Lippincot-Raven, 1995; vol. 67: 181-97.

- Viani F, Beghi E, Atza MG, Gulotta MP. Classifications of epileptic syndromes: advantages and limitations for evaluation of childhood epileptic syndromes in clinical practice. *Epilepsia* 1988; 29: 440-5.

- Wolf P. Of cabbages and kings: Some considerations on classifications, diagnostic schemes, semiology, and concepts. *Epilepsia* 2003; 44: 1-4.

Cortical excitability in benign focal epilepsies

Giuliano Avanzini, Silvana Franceschetti
Milano, Italy

The emergence of the concept of benign focal epilepsies (BFEs) in the late 1950s and early 1960s (Bancaud et al., 1958; Nayrac & Beaussard, 1958; Faure & Loiseau, 1960) offered a novel view of the pathophysiological concepts introduced by John Hughlings Jackson (Jackson, 1873), and further elaborated by Penfield and Jasper (1954). In addition to epilepsies due to focal epileptogenic lesions and "functional" epilepsies due to misfunctioning diffusely projecting ("centrencephalic") structures, it established a new category of epilepsies due to a misfunction affecting a cortical area with no demonstrable sign of a lesion. These localisation-related epilepsies were not attributable to an epileptic focus in an anatomical sense but rather to an age-related hyperexcitable condition in a given cortical region (most frequently, the sensory-motor or visual region), with no detectable structural alteration. This definition implies the assumption that any type of brain pathology found in a patient with typical picture of BFE should be considered merely coincidental and devoid of any pathogenetic relevance to his epilepsy.

This chapter will review the findings that can shed some light on the mechanisms involved in generating the epileptic discharges underlying BFE. As no experimental models of these epilepsies exist, the discussion will be based on the analysis of the human electroclinical data.

Electroencephalographic features of benign focal epilepsy

Background electroencephalographic (EEG) activity is normal by definition. Typical interictal discharges of high voltage spikes, spike waves or sharp waves occur over the involved region, which are consistently activated by sleep (see Chapter 6).

Kellaway's (2000) detailed analysis of the surface negative spikes characterising the interictal discharge of benign epilepsy with centrotemporal spikes (BECTS) showed an average duration of ~74 ms (which fits the definition of a sharp wave rather than a spike). The average sharpness or degree of curvature of the peak was 0.022 pV/ms/8 ms, indicating a relatively blunt character; the average amplitude was about 160 µV, but some individual spikes exceeded 300 µV. The predominantly negative spikes can be preceded by a low-amplitude sharper surface positive spike.

After the large negative spike, there is a trough followed by a slow wave *(Figs. 1A & B)*. In the study of Berroya *et al.* (2005) of a population of 60 children with BECTS, maximal negativity was recorded at T3-T4 in 63%, C3-C4 in 30% and P3-P4 in 3% of the records. According to Kellaway, there are two distinct types of potential field: a stationary pattern with negativity in the inferior rolandic region and simultaneous positivity in the frontal region, and a nonstationary pattern consisting of an initial sharp spike, that reaches peak negativity in the frontal region before the onset of the ascending arm of the rolandic spike, and shows simultaneous positivity in the rolandic region *(Fig. 1C)*.

The findings of dipole analyses made by Kellaway (1985), Frost *et al.* (1986), Gutierrez *et al.* (1990), Gregory and Wong (1984), Baumgartner *et al.* (1996) and Berroya *et al.* (2005) indicate that the sources of the small positive spike, the large rolandic spike, the trough and the slow wave are very close to each other, but the rolandic spike dipole vector is pointed in the direction of the temporal area (T6), whereas the spike source vector of the preceding spike is pointed in the direction of the frontal region (F4). This suggests that the rolandic cortical discharges are generated by a propagated process between simultaneously active and differently oriented neuronal populations (Baumgartner *et al.*, 1996).

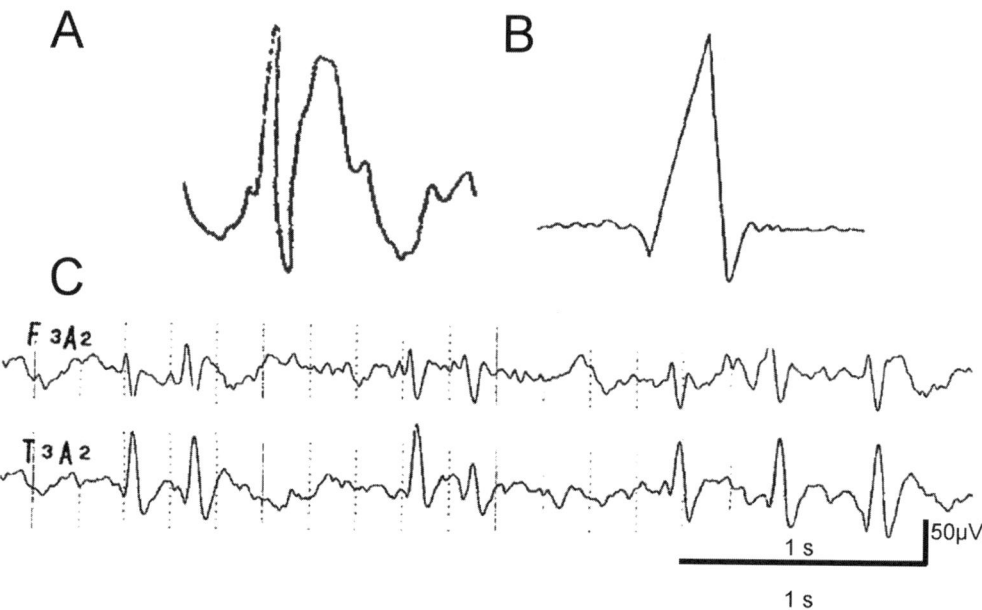

Figure 1. EEG features of BECTS. **A:** Typical rolandic spike composed by a high amplitude surface-negative spike preceded by a low amplitude positive spike and followed by a trough that is in turn followed by an aftergoing slow wave. **B:** Schematic representation of the three positive-negative-positive components. **C:** Time relationship between BECTS interictal discharges recorded simultaneously from F3 and T3 leads. For explanation see text. (Modified from Kellaway, 2000).

Benign focal epilepsy and sensory systems

The two main types of BFE, BECTS and benign occipital epilepsies (BOEs) of either the Gastaut (1982) or Panayotopoulos (1989) type, are respectively related to areas of representation of somato-sensory and visual systems, and a number of studies have investigated whether this has any pathophysiological implications.

The effect of sensory input on EEG discharges and seizures was first demonstrated in BOE. In his original description, Gastaut (1982) emphasised the fact that typical occipital paroxysms occur only when the eyes are closed and are suppressed by eye opening; and one year before, Panayotopoulos (1981) had pointed out that the posterior discharges in occipital lobe seizures are sensitive to darkness. He also showed that the effect of darkness was due to the abolition of central vision, and that the paroxysms were inhibited by fixation even in darkness.

The finding of parietal focal spikes evoked by contralateral foot tapping observed by De Marco and Negrini in 1973 in a group of children without overt neurological pathology is particularly interesting. Later, De Marco and Tassinari (1981) found that tapping-evoked spikes could forecast the occurrence of seizures and proposed a special type of BPE called "Benign Partial Epilepsy with Extreme Somato-Sensory Evoked Potentials" (Tassinari & De Marco, 1985), later renamed "Somato-sensory Evoked Spikes Epilepsy" (De Marco and Calzolari in 1999). More recently, Fonseca and Tedrus (2000) found evoked spikes to be associated with localisation-related idiopathic epilepsies in 73.6% of a group of patients with epilepsy. Manganotti *et al.* (1998) found the spikes evoked by either tapping or electrical stimulation of the fingers of one hand in a group of patients with *Benign Partial Epilepsy with Extreme Somato-Sensory Evoked Potentials* has a similar morphology and scalp distribution to the spontaneously occurring spikes *(Fig. 2)*. After first digital nerve stimulation, the somato-sensory evoked potentials (SEPs) were characterised by a late, high-amplitude positive-negative-positive complex that was similar in latency, morphology and scalp distribution to the single spike elicited by 3 Hz stimulation. According to Manganotti *et al.* (1998), this late SEP component is simply the average of the evoked spikes elicited by electrical stimulation, and can be differentiated from the late negative component (N60) of normal SEPs on the basis of its dipole configuration and dynamic range.

Manganotti and Zanette (2000) have demonstrated that motor evoked potentials (MEPs) induced by transcranial magnetic stimulation in patients with BECTS are consistently facilitated by a conditioning electrical stimulation of the thumb at inter-stimulus intervals of 50-80 msec. A similar time-course of MEP facilitation has been reported by Canafoglia *et al.* (2004) in *Lafora disease* but not *Unwerricht-Lundborg disease* in which MEP facilitation occurs at shorter intervals *(Fig. 3)* that are in line with the definition of cortical reflex myoclonus.

Overall, the results of somato-sensory stimulations are consistent with the hypothesis that the initial source of evoked spikes is in the sensory cortex and that there is subsequent involvement of the motor and secondary sensory areas (Manganotti *et al.*, 1998), which would also account for the observation that the clinical seizures in some patients are heralded by paresthesias of the mouth and hand preceding the clonic jerk in the face and arm (Lombroso, 1967; Luders *et al.*, 1987; Holmes, 1993).

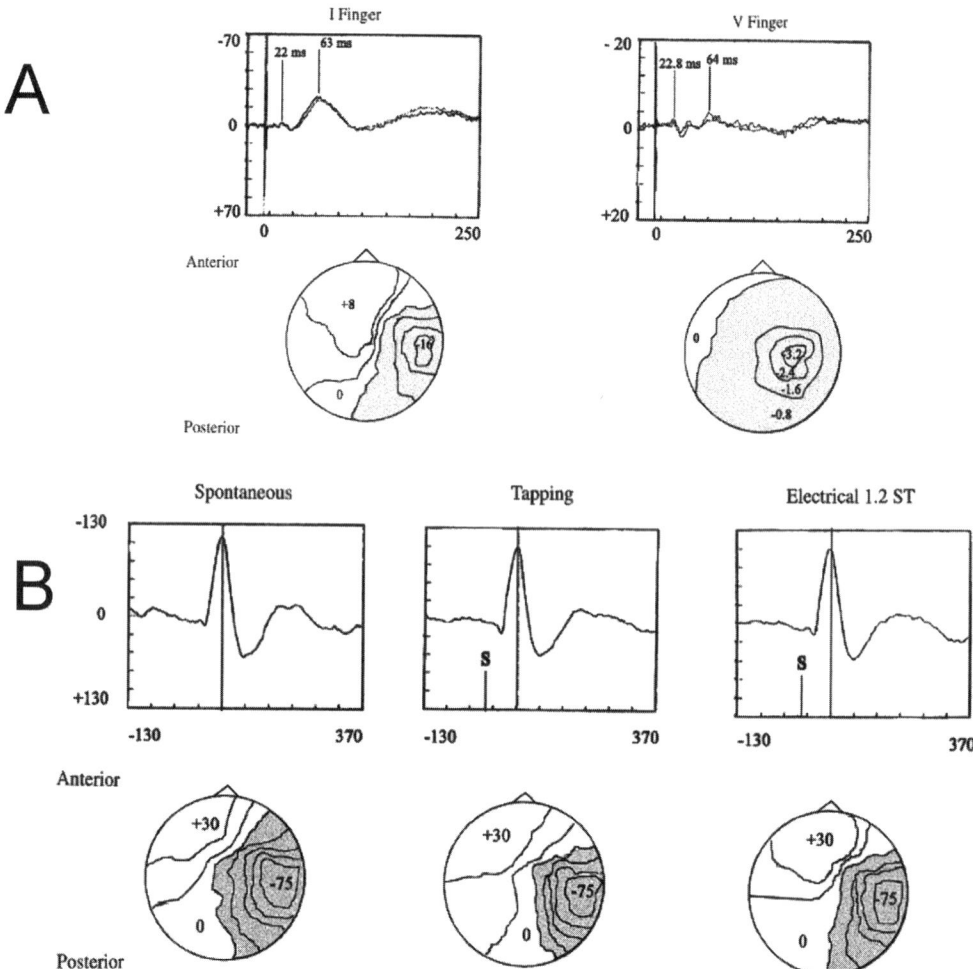

Figure 2. Topographic representation of negativity peak of SEPs, spontaneous and evoked spikes in a child with BECTS. **A:** SEPs following 1st finger stimulation shows a large positive-negative-positive complex with maximal amplitude over the central, parietal and temporal electrodes, which is not evident on SEPs obtained by stimulation of 5st finger, showing morphology and radial distribution similar to those observed in normal subjects. **B:** spontaneous and evoked spikes, elicited by tapping and electrical stimulation, showing similar morphology distribution. The vertical cursors denote the time of the voltage maps, grey is negative and white positive. For the evoked spikes S indicates the stimulus. For further explanations see text. (Modified from Manganotti et al., 1998).

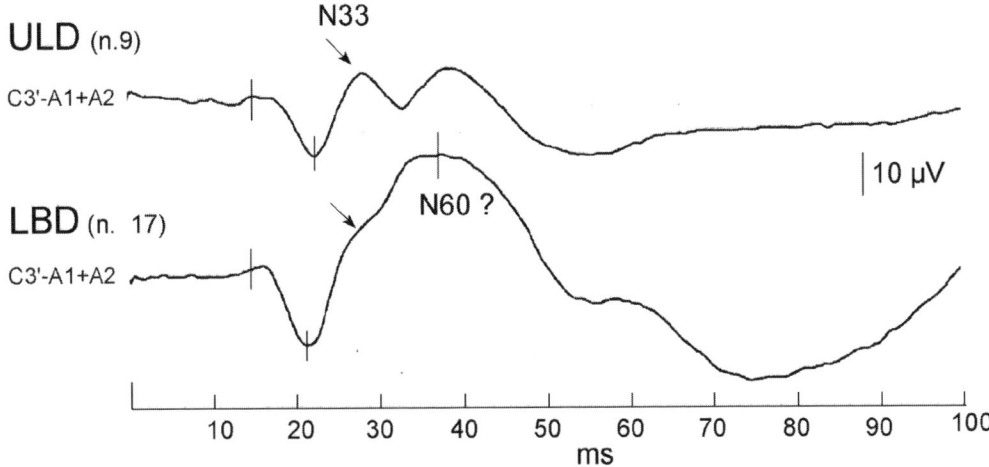

Figure 3. SEPs of representative patients with Unverricht-Lundborg disease (ULD) **(A)** and Lafora body disease (LBD) **(B)** (right median nerve stimulation; N33 is hardly detectable in patients with LBD (arrowhead), merging in a subsequent very large negative (N60) component (arrows) on C3' derivation). (From Canafoglia et al., 2004).

Age dependency of benign focal epilepsy-associated cortical hyperexcitability

Despite the putative importance of genetic factors in the pathogenesis of BECTS and BOEs (which implies that their causal mechanism is present from birth), their clinical onset and remission is time limited. This suggests that there may be a developmental window during which permissive conditions occur that they may be related to some maturational changes in the sensory-motor or visual systems. However, evidence in favour of this hypothesis is scarce and largely limited to the age-dependent phenomenon of tactile evoked spikes that were serendipitously discovered by De Marco, and then systematically characterised by him in a population of non-epileptic children without overt neurological pathology (De Marco & Negrini, 1973). Tactile evoked spikes are high-voltage (up to 400 µV) EEG potentials that are best evoked by tapping the soles of the feet with a reflex hammer and by asking the subject to tap the fingertips of the right hand against the fingertips of the left hand.

The relationship of tactile evoked spikes with SEPs and the centrotemporal spikes that spontaneously occur in BECTS has been discussed in the previous section. We will here discuss their age dependence, whether or not they are associated with the special subtype of BECTS that Tassinari and De Marco christened "Benign Partial Epilepsy with Extreme Somato-Sensory Evoked Potentials" (De Marco & Tassinari, 1981; Tassinari & De Marco 1985), and which is now referred to as *Somato-sensory Evoked Spikes Epilepsy* (De Marco & Calzolari in 1999).

The most comprehensive study (published by De Marco & Calzolari in 1999) was based on a review of data relating to 32,800 children aged 3-14 years who underwent a first EEG recording between 1970 and 1996. Tactile spikes were evoked in 566 (1.72%), 215 (38%) of whom were referred because of epileptic seizures or febrile convulsions, 76 (12.5%) because of headache, 51 (9.5%) because of a history of head trauma, and 224 (40%) for various other reasons (behavioural abnormalities, learning disabilities, language impairment, poor school performance, certification for sport activities, etc.). The 215 children with seizure disorders included 86 cases with somato-sensory evoked spikes epilepsy, 68 with febrile convulsions, 53 with BECTS, two with juvenile myoclonic epilepsy, two with grand mal, one with childhood absence epilepsy, one with multifocal cryptogenic epilepsy, and one with symptomatic partial motor epilepsy.

In the 86 children with somato-sensory evoked spikes epilepsy, the evoked spikes were parietal in 38, centrotemporal in 26, and both parietal and centrotemporal in 22 cases. In all of the other children, except those with febrile convulsions, the tactile evoked spikes were similarly distribution, being parietal in 42%, centrotemporal in 32%, and both parietal and centrotemporal in 26%. A parietal localisation was predominant among children aged 3-8 years, whereas a centrotemporal localisation was mainly observed in older children (6-11 years); the simultaneous presence of tactile evoked spikes in both areas was typical of the intermediate age group (6-8 years), and probably reflects a transition between the two localisation patterns. In agreement with these findings, the tactile evoked spikes in the children with febrile convulsions (who were usually younger) were mainly localised in the parietal area. In 25% of the children, the evoked spikes were only present on one side.

The tactile evoked spikes in 136 children were discovered at an early age and were followed-up for more than 10 years (mean 13 ± 2.5 years). They showed a typical course in 73.6% of the children: they could be elicited only at the feet at 4-5 years of age, and also by finger tapping at 6-7 years; by 10-11 years, they could no longer be elicited from the feet and, by 13-14 years of age, they could not be evoked from any site *(Fig. 4)*. In children with somato-sensory evoked spikes epilepsy, both the tactile evoked spikes and giant SEPs had a greater amplitude, shorter refractory period and persisted longer (in a few cases up to 18 years of age) than in the subjects who had tactile evoked spikes without *somato-sensory evoked spikes epilepsy*.

The developmental window during which tactile spikes could be evoked corresponds rather precisely to a post-natal phase of considerable cerebral cortex functional activity, as defined on the basis of regional cerebral blood flow (Chiron *et al.*, 1992, 1997) and local cerebral metabolic rates (Chugani *et al.*, 1997; Chugani, 1998).

At birth, cortical regional cerebral blood flow is lower than in adults; after birth, it increases until 5 or 6 years of age to values that are 50%-85% higher than those observed in adults and then decreases, reaching adult levels between the ages of 5 and 19 years *(Fig. 5)*. The time needed to reach normal adult values differs for each cortical region, the shortest being found in the primary cortex and the longest inn the associative cortex.

The profile of metabolic maturation (measured as glucose utilization) is almost superimposable: low at birth, it increases until the age of about 4 years, when a child's cerebral cortex uses more than twice as much glucose as that of an adult; these very high rates of glucose consumption are maintained between the ages of 4 and 10 years, when they begin to decline until reaching

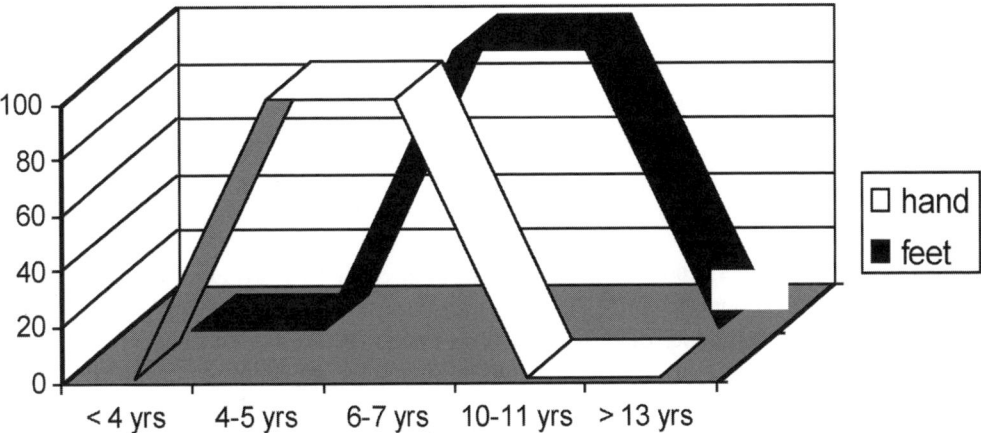

Figure 4. Tactile evoked spikes following feet and hand stimulation recorded from 136 children followed-up for more than 10 years (mean 13 ± 2.5 years). For explanation see text. (Graphic representation based on De Marco & Calzolari's 1999 data).

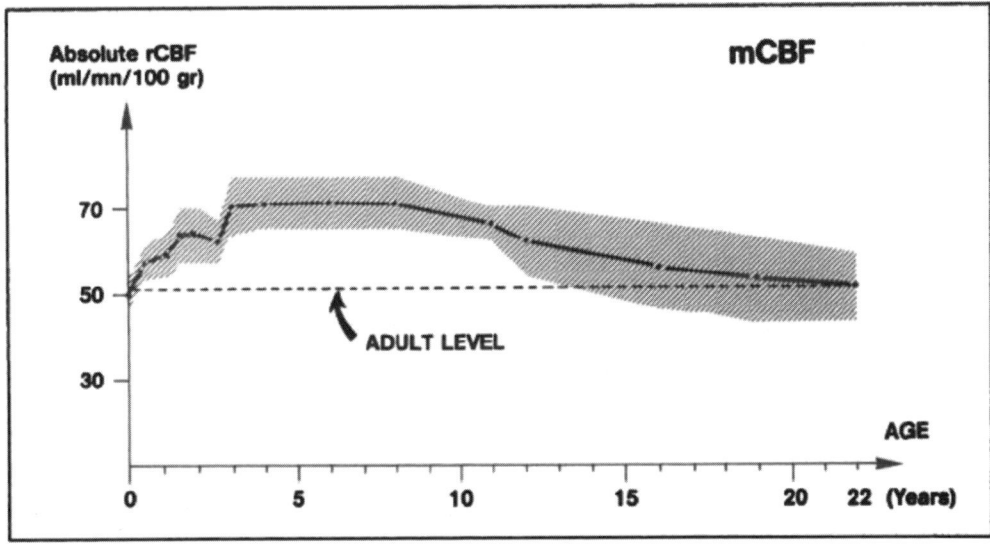

Figure 5. Global blood-flow from birth to adulthood in 42 neurologically normal subjects. The solid line represents the reference values; the hatched area corresponds to the interval defined by the reference values plus or minus one standard deviation. The broken line indicates the adult level (From Chiron et al., 1992).

adult values by the age of 16-18 years. The highest metabolic increases over adult values occur in the cerebral cortical structures; smaller increases are observed in the subcortical structures and cerebellum (Chugani et al., 1997; Chugani, 1998).

This time-course of regional blood flow and glucose consumption changes matches that describing the process of the initial overproduction and subsequent elimination of excessive neurons, synapses and dendritic spines known to occur in the developing brain.

Sleep and benign focal epilepsies

A striking finding common to all BFEs is a significant increase in interictal discharges during drowsiness through slow wave sleep *(Fig. 6)*, and so it is conceivable that a better understanding of the basic mechanisms underlying BFE/sleep interactions may shed some light on the pathophysiology of BFE.

It has been known that sleep has a powerful activating effect on epileptic discharges since the pioneering works of Gloor *et al.* (1958), Cadillhac and Passouant (1964), Gastaut *et al.* (1964) and Perria *et al.* (1966). A number of subsequent investigations have demonstrated that epileptic events are generally activated during high-voltage, slow-wave synchronised EEG activity (non-REM sleep) and deactivated during low-voltage EEG activity with rapid eye movements (REM sleep), although occasional seizures during REM sleep may occur because of arousal shifts during the REM stage (Halasz, 1991).

Distinct components of non-REM sleep have been identified, such as the K-complex, sleep spindles and the cyclic alternating patterns (CAPs) upon which the description of non-REM sleep microstructure is based. CAPs are rhythmic changes occurring in physiological non-REM sleep that were first identified by Terzano *et al.* (1985, 1988), who coined the name. CAP sequences consist of transient repetitive patterns lasting 8 ± 15 s (phase A) separated by intervals of 15 ± 20 s (phase B); the A phases consist of stage-related arousal complexes (bursts of K-complexes or delta waves, arousals), whereas the B phases consist of stage-related background activities. During CAPs, the EEG rhythms of sleep oscillate with periodic excitatory (phase A) and inhibitory swings (phase B). Non-CAP periods (NCAP) essentially consist of a rhythmic and stable EEG background, and are scored whenever arousal complexes are absent for 60 consecutive seconds.

Parrino *et al.* (2000) found clear-cut differences between cryptogenic and idiopathic partial epilepsies in a study aimed at correlating the time-course of interictal activities with the microstructure of slow-wave sleep. In primary generalised epilepsy and lesional epilepsies with a fronto-temporal focus, the activation of interictal discharges is high during CAPs, reaching a climax during phase A and the greatest inhibition during phase B. In BECTS, on the other hand, a lack of modulation has been observed.

Nobili *et al.* (1999) analysed the time-course of *BECTS* discharges during sleep with respect to two spectral EEG components corresponding to slow wave activity (0.5-4.0 Hz) and sigma activity (12.0-16.0 Hz), a frequency band that is of particular interest because it includes organised spindle bursts. A spike index (the number of spikes in a given stage or time spent in that stage) has been calculated for total sleep time, individual sleep stages, and the first four consecutive non-REM cycles (Feinberg and Floyd, 1979). There is a high, positive correlation for all subjects with BECTS, and for both delta and sigma bands, during total sleep time, with the correlation coefficient being much higher for the sigma than the delta band.

A similar distribution of interictal discharges has been found in five children with benign epilepsy with occipital paroxysms (Beelke *et al.*, 2000). These results agree and complement the

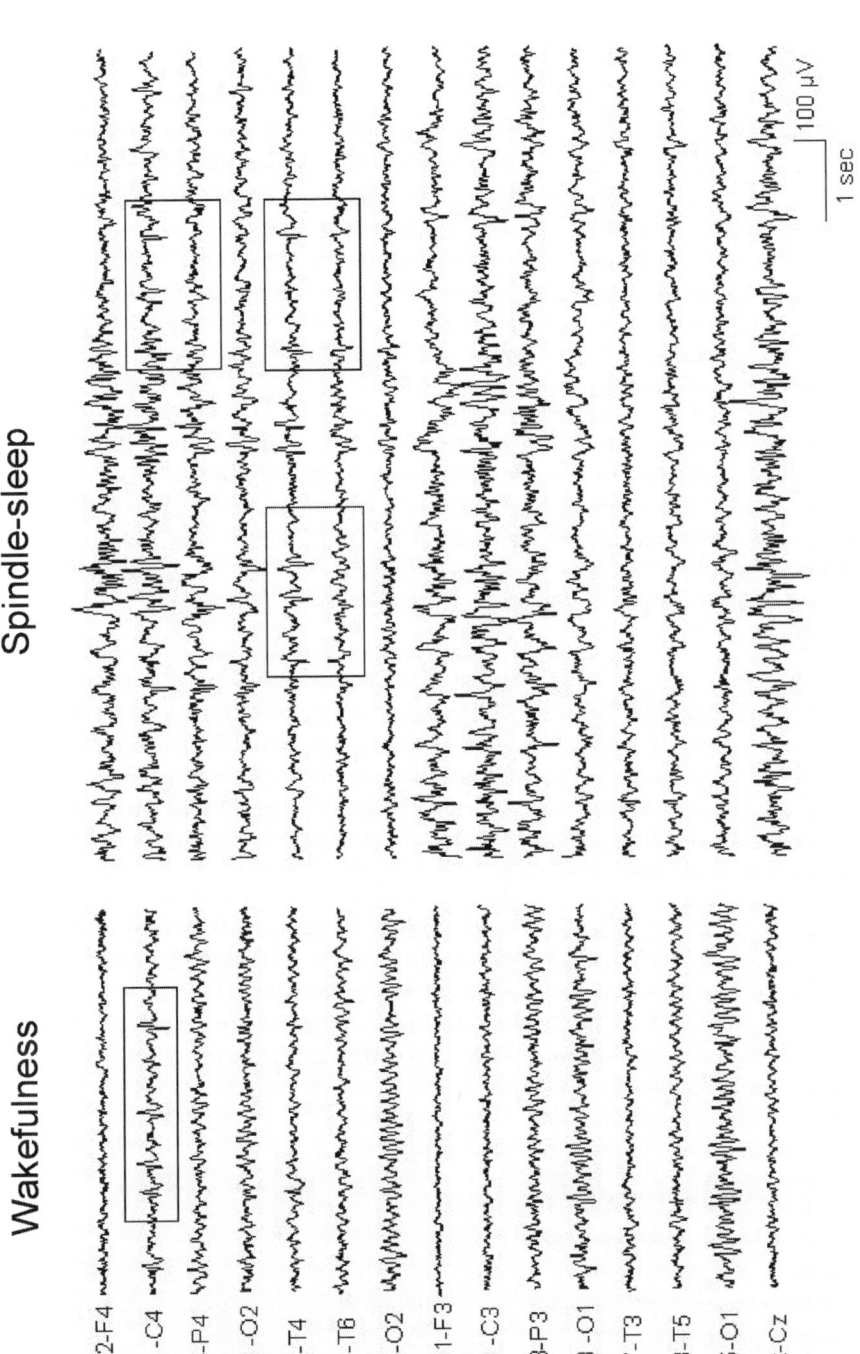

Figure 6. Activation of BECTS interictal discharges during non-REM sleep with spindles. Note that interictal spikes, limited to right central region during wakefulness, involve also the midtemporal derivation during spindle-sleep, preserving a quite invariable morphology.

observations of Parrino *et al.* (2000) showing that BFE has distinct behaviour, with the discharges being activated by sleep spindles that are generally separate from CAP activity. However, a further analysis of seven children with cryptogenic or symptomatic epilepsies by Nobili *et al.* (1999) showed a positive correlation between interictal discharges and the sigma band, and they concluded that the mechanisms involved in the generation of sleep-spindles in childhood are particularly effective in facilitating the interictal discharges of partial epilepsies, whether they are idiopathic or cryptogenic/symptomatic. They also hypothesised that, during developmental ages, the thalamic volley that normally induces sleep spindles by impinging on a hyperexcitable cortex may facilitate the generation of interictal epileptic activities, whereas the lower level of cortical excitability in adult patients requires stronger synchronising inputs to induce the delta waves necessary to produce spike activation.

It is worth making one last point about the interference focal interictal discharges of BFE during non-REM sleep with cognitive processes (See chapters 6 and 10). It is well known that severe cognitive and behavioural disturbances occur in children with *Electrical Status Epilepticus during Sleep* (Patry *et al.*, 1971; Tassinari *et al.*, 1985), and it has been postulated that many childhood developmental or acquired language defects (such as *acquired epileptic aphasia* or *Landau-Kleffner syndrome*) or behavioural defects (such as autism) are a consequence of apparently subclinical spikes interfering with specific cerebral processes. Various observations concur in demonstrating a close correlation between disturbances of the higher cortical functions (working memory and executive functions) and the rate of interictal discharges during slow-wave sleep in children with BECTS (Tassinari and Rubboli, 2006). Executive functions, which are mainly under frontal lobe control, seem to be particularly vulnerable to epileptic EEG activity during maturational age, and their disruption possibly interferes with the normal development of learning processes (Metz-Lutz *et al.*, 1999; Deonna *et al.*, 2000; Riva *et al.*, 2005, 2007).

Huber *et al.* (2004) have recently demonstrated that a local increase in slow wave activity during sleep after a learning task involving a specific brain region is correlated with a significant improvement in task performance, and so it can be hypothesised that the disruption of cognitive-related slow wave activity by local interictal discharges may explain cognitive disturbances occurring in children with BECTS whose focal activity is particularly activated during slow-wave sleep (Tassinari and Rubboli, 2006).

Conclusions

Most of the data reviewed above come from studies of BECTS, and so the following points may only partially apply to other BFEs.
1. BFEs are age-related epilepsies presenting with ictal focal symptoms that are not associated with any other neurological sign or symptom. It is thought that they depend on alterations in neural excitability that cannot be attributed to any *"underlying cause other than a possible hereditary predisposition"* (ILAE Classification 1989).

2. BFEs are characterised by normal background activity overlaid by typical focal paroxysmal abnormalities. On the basis of their electroclinical features, BFEs cannot be attributed to an epileptic focus in an anatomical sense, but rather to regional cortical hyperexcitability.
3. The most common types of BFE (BECTS and BOEs) relate to the cortical representation of sensory systems whose effects on epileptic discharges provide some insight into their pathophysiology.
4. The time-course of some cerebral cortex maturational events may account for the age-dependency of BFE.
5. A further contribution to our understanding of the generation of BFE discharges is provided by studies of sleep/BFE interactions, which highlight the role of spindle generating mechanisms.

According to analyses of BECTS discharge generators, the positive-negative-positive pattern arises in the somato-sensory cortex, and is then transmitted to motor cortex. The finding of changing focal discharge sites in the ipsilateral or contralateral hemisphere suggest that the cortical dysfunction is widely distributed throughout the cortex.

The identification of a subgroup of children with BECTS in whom rolandic spikes can be evoked by tactile and electrical stimulation raises the question of the pathophysiological role of somato-sensory inputs. On the basis of the results of a number well-designed studies, the late high-amplitude component called "extreme somato-sensory evoked potentials" (De Marco & Tassinari, 1981) is simply a cortically generated spike elicited by the peripheral stimulus. It therefore cannot be assimilated to the giant somato-sensory evoked potentials described in patients with pure cortical reflex myoclonus (Shibasaki et al., 1985) or, specifically, myoclonus Unwerricht-Lundborg disease (Canafoglia et al., 2004). The potential significance of the modulation of cortical spikes by afferent sensory inputs in the pathogenesis of *Somato-sensory Evoked Spikes Epilepsy* is still unclear.

Interesting information from the longitudinal study of tactile evoked spikes concerns the age span (3-14 years) of its expression, which corresponds quite precisely to the developmental window during which functional activity of the cerebral cortex (as defined by regional cerebral blood flow and local cerebral metabolic rates) is significantly increased in comparison with early infancy and adulthood. In more general terms, this developmental window corresponds to the phase of BFE expression, and may account for their age dependency.

Finally, the studies of BFE epileptic discharges during sleep support the facilitating effect of spindle-generating mechanisms on BFE discharges. Various data demonstrate the role of thalamo-cortical circuitry involving the reticular thalamic nucleus in the generation of sleep spindles (Mulle et al., 1986) and generalised 3/sec spike wave discharges (Avoli & Gloor, 1981; Avanzini et al., 1989). The finding of a highly significant correlation between BECTS interictal discharges and the EEG sigma band (which include sleep spindles) suggests that regional thalamo-cortical mechanisms also play a role in BFE. This hypothesis is indirectly supported by the occasional occurrence of generalised spike-wave discharges in children with BFE. According to the study by Nobili et al. (1999) of cryptogenic and symptomatic childhood epilepsy, the facilitating effect of spindle-generating mechanisms on discharge expression is particularly pronounced in childhood, when it is not limited to generalised or focal idiopathic epilepsies.

References

• Avanzini G, de Curtis M, Panzica F, Spreafico R. Intrinsic properties of nucleus reticularis thalami neurones of the rat studied *in vitro*. *Journal of Physiology* 1989; 416: 111-22.

• Avoli M, Gloor P. The effects of transient functional depression of the thalamus on spindles and on bilateral synchronous epileptic discharges of feline generalized penicillin epilepsy. *Epilepsia* 1981; 22: 443-52.

• Bancaud J, Collomb J, Dell MB. Les pointes rolandiques : un symptôme EEG propre à l'enfant. *Revue Neurologique* (Paris) 1958; 99: 206-9.

• Baumgartner C, Graf M, Doppelbauer A, *et al*. The functional organization of the interictal spike complex in benign rolandic epilepsy. *Epilepsia* 1996; 37 (1) 164-74.

• Beelke M, Nobili L, Baglietto MG, *et al*. Relationship of sigma activity to sleep interictal epileptic discharges: a study in children affected by Benign Epilepsy with Occipital Paroxysms. *Epilepsy Research* 2000; 40: 179-86.

• Berroya AM, Bleasel AF, Stevermuer TL, Lawson J, Bye AME. Spike morphology, location and frequency in benign epilepsy with centrotemporal spikes. *Journal of Child Neurology* 2005; 20 (3): 188-94.

• Buchthal F, Rosenfalck A. Evoked action potentials and conduction velocity in human sensory nerves. *Brain Research* 1966; 3: 1-122.

• Cadillhac J, Passouant P. Influence of various phases of night sleep on the epileptic discharges in man. *Electroencephalography & Clinical Neurophysiology* 1964; 17: 441-2.

• Canafoglia L, Ciano C, Panzica F, *et al*. Sensorimotor cortex excitability in Unverricht-Lundborg disease and Lafora body disease. *Neurology* 2004; 63 (12): 2309-15.

• Chiron C, Jambaque I, Nabbout R, Lounes R, Syrota A, Dulac O The right brain hemisphere is dominant in human infants. *Brain* 1997; 120 (Pt 6): 1057-65.

• Chiron C, Raynaud C, Maziere B, *et al*. Changes in regional cerebral blood flow during brain maturation in children and adolescents. *Journal of Nuclear Medicine* 1992; 33 (5): 696-703.

• Chugani HT. A critical period of brain development: studies of cerebral glucose utilization whit PET. *Preventive Medicine* 1998; 27 (2): 184-8.

• Chugani HT, Phelps ME, Mazziotta JC. Position emission tomography study of human brain functional development. *Annals of Neurology* 1987; 22 (4): 487-97.

• De Marco P, Negrini P. Parietal focal spikes evoked by contralateral tactile somatotopic stimulations in four non-epileptic subjects. *Electroencephalography and Clinical Neurophysiology* 1973; 34: 308-12.

• De Marco P, Tassinari CA. Extreme somatosensory evoked potential (ESEP): an EEG sign forecasting the possible occurrence of seizures in children. *Epilepsia* 1981; 22: 569-75.

• De Marco P, Calzolari S. Tactile evoked spikes in children. *Epileptic Disorders* 1999; 1 (2): 113-9.

• Deonna T, Zisiger P, Davidoff V, *et al*. Benign partial epilepsy of childhood: a longitudinal neuropsychological and EEG study of cognitive function. *Developmental Medicine Child Neurology* 2000; 42: 595-603.

• Faure J, Loiseau P. Une corrélation clinique particulière des pointes-ondes sans signification locale. *Revue Neurologique* (Paris) 1960 ; 102: 399-406.

• Feinberg I, Floyd TC. Systematic trends across the night in human sleep cycles. *Psychophysiology* 1979; 16: 282-91.

• Fonseca LC, Tedrus G. Somatosensory evoked spikes and epileptic seizures: a study of 385 cases. *Clinical Electroencephalography* 2000; 31 (2): 71-5.

• Frost JD, Kellaway P, Hrachovy RA, Glaze DG, Mirrahi EM. Changes in epileptic spike configuration associated with attainment of seizure control. *Annals of Neurology* 1986; 20: 723-6.

- Gastaut H, Batini C, Fressy J, Broughton R, Tassinari CA. Étude électroencéphalographique du sommeil nocturne chez les épileptiques. *Revue Neurologique* 1964 ; 110: 311-3.

- Gastaut H. A new type of epilepsy: benign partial epilepsy of childhood with occipital spike-waves. *Clinical Electroencephalography* 1982; 12: 13-22.

- Gloor P, Tsai C, Haddad F. An assessment of the value of sleep-electroencephalography for the diagnosis of temporal lobe epilepsy. *Electroencephalography & Clinical Neurophysiology* 1958; 10: 633-48.

- Gregory DL, Wong PK. Topographical analysis of the centrotemporal discharges in benign rolandic epilepsy of childhood. *Epilepsia* 1984; 25 (6): 705-11.

- Gutierrez AR, Brick JF, Bodensteiner J. Dipole reversal: an ictal feature of benign partial epilepsy with centrotemporal spikes. *Epilepsia* 1990; 3 (1): 544-8.

- Halasz P. Sleep arousal and electroclinical manifestations of generalized epilepsy with spike wave pattern. In: Degen R, Rodin EA (Eds) Epilepsy, sleep and sleep deprivation. 2nd ed. *Epilepsy Research* (suppl. 2) Elsevier, Amsterdam, 1991: 43-8.

- Holmes GL. Benign focal epilepsies of childhood. [Review]. *Epilepsia* 1993; 34 (suppl. 3): 49-61.

- Huber R, Ghilardi MF, Massimini M, Tononi G. Local sleep and learning. *Nature* 2004; 430: 78-81.

- Jackson JH. On the anatomical and physiological localization in the brain. *The Lancet* 1873; 1: 84-5.

- Kellaway P. Sleep and epilepsy. *Epilepsia* 1985; 26 (suppl. 1): S15-S30.

- Kellaway P. The electroencephalographic features of benign centrotemporal (rolandic) epilepsy of childhood. *Epilepsia* 2000; 41 (8): 1053-6.

- Lesser RP, Koehle R, Luders R. Effect of stimulus intensity on short latency somatosensory evoked potentials. *Electroencephalography & Clinical Neurophysiology* 1979; 47: 377-82.

- Lombroso CT. Sylvian seizures and midtemporal spike foci in children. *Archives of Neurology* 1967; 17: 52-9.

- Luders H, Lesser RP, Dinner DS, Morris HH. Benign focal epilepsy of childhood. In: Luders H, Lesser RP (Eds). Springer, London, 1987: 303-46.

- Manganotti P, Miniussi C, Santorum E, *et al*. Influence of somatosensory input on paroxysmal activity in benign rolandic epilepsy with "extreme somatosensory evoked potentials". *Brain* 1998, 121: 647-58.

- Manganotti P, Zanette G. Contribution of motor cortex in generation of evoked spikes in patients with benign rolandic epilepsy. *Clinical Neurophysiology* 2000; 111: 964-74.

- Metz-Lutz MN, Kleitz C, de Saint Martin, *et al*. Cognitive development in benign focal epilepsies of childhood. *Developmental Neuropsychology* 1999; 21: 182-90.

- Mulle C, Madariaga A, Deschenes M. Morphology and electrophysiologycal properties of reticularis thalami neurons in cat: *in vivo* study of a thalamic pacemaker. *Journal of Neurosciences* 1986; 6: 2134-45.

- Nayrac P, Beaussard M. Les pointes-ondes prérolandiques : expression EEG très particulière. *Revue Neurologique* (Paris) 1958 ; 99: 201-6.

- Nobili L, Ferrillo F, Baglietto MG, *et al*. Modulation sleep interictal epileptiform discharges in partial epilepsy of childhood. *Clinical Neurophysiology* 1999; 110: 839-45.

- Panayiotopoulos CP. Benign childhood epilepsy with occipital paroxysms: a 15-year prospectice study. *Annals of Neurology* 1989; 26: 51-6.

- Panayiotopoulos CP. Inhibitory effect of central vision on occipital lobe seizure. *Neurology* 1981; 31: 1331-3.

- Parrino L, Smerieri A, Spaggiari MC, Terzano MG. Cyclic alternating pattern (CAP) and epilepsy during sleep: how a physiological rhythm modulates a pathological event. *Clinical Neurophysiology* 2000; 111 (suppl. 2): 39-46.

- Patry G, Lyagouby S, Tassinari CA. Sublinical "electrical status epilepticus" induced by sleep in children. *Archives of Neurology* 1971; 24: 242-52.

- Penfield W and Jasper W. *Epilepsy and the functional anatomy of the human brain.* Boston: Little Brown & C, 1954.

- Perria L, Rosadini G, Rossi GF, Gentilomo A. Neurosurgical aspects of epilepsy: physiological sleep as a means for focalizing EEG epileptic discharges. *Acta Neurochirurgica* (Wien) 1966; 14 (1): 1-9.

- Proposal for revised classification of epilepsies and epileptic syndromes. Commission on Classification and Terminology of the International League Against Epilepsy. *Epilepsia* 1989; 30 (4): 389-99.

- Riva D, Avanzini G, Franceschetti S, *et al*. Unilateral frontal lobe epilepsy affects executive functions in children. *Neurological Sciences* 2005; 26 (4): 263-70.

- Riva D, Vago C, Franceschetti S, *et al*. Intellectual and language findings and their relationship to EEG characteristics in benign childhood epilepsy with centrotemporal spikes. *Epilepsy & Behavior* 2007; 10 (2) : 278-85.

- Shibasaki H, Yamashita Y, Neshige R, Tobimatsu S, Fukui R. Pathogenesis of giant somatosensory evoked potentials in progressive myoclonic epilepsy. *Brain* 1985; 108: 225-40.

- Tassinari CA, DeMarco P. Benign partial epilepsy with extreme somato-sensory evoked potentials. In: Roger J, Dravet C, Bureau M, Dreifuss FE, Wolf P (Eds) *Epileptic syndromes in infancy, childhood and adolescence*. London: John Libbey Eutotext, 1985: 176-80.

- Tassinari CA, Bureau M, Dravet C, Dalla Bernardina B, Roger J. Epilepsy with continuous spikes and waves during slow sleep. In: Roger J, Dravet C, Bureau M, Dreifuss FE, Wolf P (Eds). *Epileptic syndromes in infancy, childhood and adolescence*. London: John Libbey Eurotext, 1985: 194-204.

- Tassinari CA, Rubboli G. Cognition and paroxysmal EEG activities: from a single spike to electrical status epilepticus during sleep. *Epilepsia* 2006; 47 (suppl. 2): 40-3.

- Terzano MG, Mancia D, Salati MR, Costani G, Decembrino A, Parrino L. The cyclic alternating pattern as a physiologic component of normal NREM sleep. *Sleep* 1985; 8: 137-45.

- Terzano MG, Parrino L, Spaggiari MC. The cyclic alternating pattern sequences in the dynamic organization of sleep. *Electroencephalography & Clinical Neurophysiology* 1988; 69: 437-7.

Part II
Familial and non-familial infantile seizures

Benign familial and non-familial infantile seizures

Roberto H. Caraballo, Natalio Fejerman
Buenos Aires, Argentina

The 2001 proposal of ILAE's Task Force on Classification recognized among epileptic syndromes the Benign familial infantile seizures and the Benign (non-familial) infantile seizures (Engel, 2001). However, the most recent report of the ILAE classification core group categorized both groups, familial and non-familial forms as benign infantile seizures (BIS) because both groups have similar age at onset, electroclinical features and evolution (Engel, 2006). Thus, the sporadic form cannot be considered a separate syndrome, and both should be combined into a single syndrome, unless subsequent information indicates otherwise. Our group has contributed in demonstrating that both familial and non-familial BIS have similar features (Caraballo et al., 2003a; Caraballo, 2005a). Over the last few years, variants of these two forms and other similar entities have been described (Bureau and Maton, 1998; Bureau et al., 2002; Capovilla and Beccaria, 2000; Heron et al., 2002; Berkovic et al., 2004).

Neonatal epilepsy syndromes are now well known, specially the Benign familial neonatal seizures, for which the gene KCNQ2 linked to chromosome 20q13.3 and the gene KCNQ3 linked to chromosome 8q24 have been recognized (Leppert et al., 1989; Singh et al., 1998), but we are not discussing syndromes with neonatal onset in this book.

What we are now talking about is in contrast with the overcome concept that focal seizures, single or in clusters, with onset during the first months of life, had a bad prognosis and a symptomatic aetiology. The history of these idiopathic epilepsies of infancy with a benign course started in 1963, when Fukuyama reported a series of infants with apparently generalized seizures, absence of aetiologic factors, and a benign evolution. Later, other authors from Japan were able to register ictal EEGs in similar cases, demonstrating focal onset and secondary generalization of seizures (Watanabe et al., 1987, 1990, 1993). Some of the patients had a family history of epilepsy.

Vigevano and co-workers (1992) described five patients exhibiting a family history of seizures with benign outcome during infancy, and autosomal dominant inheritance, and they proposed to call the syndrome benign infantile familial convulsions. Subsequently, reports of other series of familial patients appeared in many different countries (Lee et al., 1993; Luovigsson et al., 1993;

Echenne *et al.*, 1994, Caraballo *et al.*, 1997a; Giordano *et al.*, 1999; Mc Callenbach *et al.*, 2002), confirming a new epileptic syndrome. The ILAE Task Force on Classification and Terminology replaced the term "convulsion" by "seizure" (Engel, 2001).

Malafosse and co-workers (1994) reported that benign familial infantile seizures (BFIS) are not allelic forms of the benign neonatal familial seizures gene. Guipponi *et al.* (1997) mapped the benign familial infantile seizures gene to chromosome 19 in five Italian families. In other genetic studies, chromosome 19 was excluded; therefore, more genes may be involved in its aetiology (Terwindt *et al.*, 1997; Giordano *et al.*, 1999; Gennaro *et al.*, 1999; Baralle *et al.*, 2000). Malacarne *et al.* (2001) found pure forms of BFIS linked to chromosome2q24 in eight Italian families. In 1997, Szepetowski *et al.* (1997) described a syndrome of autosomal dominant infantile convulsions and paroxysmal dystonic choreoathetosis appearing later in life (ICCA) linked to chromosome 16 in six French families. Caraballo and co-workers (2001) reported four Argentine and three French families with members affected with pure forms of BFIS linked to chromosome 16. Incidentally, a member of one of the French families developed paroxysmal choreoathetosis years later.

This entity has also been confirmed by other authors (Lee *et al.*, 1998; Tomita *et al.*, 1999; Bennet *et al.*, 2000; Swoboda *et al.*, 2000; Hattori *et al.*, 2000). However, co-occurrence of epilepsy and paroxysmal dyskinesia in the same individual or their relatives was already described by Pryles and co-workers in 1952.

In 2002 Heron *et al.*, and later Berkovic *et al.* (2004), described families with onset in an intermediate age between neonatal and infantile forms. They found a missense mutation in SCN2A gene and reinforced the existence of the entity "benign familial neonatal-infantile seizures" (BFNIS).

Recently, a novel heterozygous mutation c.3003 T > A in the SCN2A gene was found in a family with three affected individuals over three generations with typical electroclinical features of BFIS (Striano *et al.*, 2006).

BIS is then an epileptic syndrome characterized by onset during the first two years of life in normal children. It comprises a group with autosomal dominant inheritance and a typical onset around 6 months of age, and a non-familial group of patients with seizures starting a few months later. Seizures are focal with or without secondarily generalization and typically occur in clusters of many per day. In most of cases interictal EEGs are normal. Outcome is always excellent with a normal psychomotor development after the seizures.

Epidemiology

Studies on prevalence and incidence are lacking up to now, but many cases with familial BIS of different ethnic origin have been reported (Vigevano *et al.*, 1992; Vigevano, 2005; Lee *et al.*, 1993; Luovigsson *et al.*, 1993; Echenne *et al.*, 1994; Caraballo *et al.*, 1997b; Giordano *et al.*, 1999; Mc Callenbach *et al.*, 2002; Weber *et al.*, 2004). Considering both familial and non-familial cases and not including the long lasting experience of Japanese authors, several series of patients, which may give an idea of frequency of BIS, have been reported. In a prospective study of 63 babies who developed epilepsy in the first year of life and were followed for more than 5 years, 19 were diagnosed as "definite" BIS (Okumura et al., 2000). Sixteen of 150 patients with new onset of epilepsy younger than two years were identified as BIS in another study (Kaleyias et al., 2006). In Chapter 5 the experience regarding BIS and the focal epilepsy with midline spikes and waves during sleep in an Italian center is reported. In our two studies, benign infantile seizures have been listed as the third most common type of epilepsy in the first two years of life. The first and second most frequent types were West syndrome and symptomatic focal epilepsies respectively (Caraballo et al., 2003; Caraballo, 2005b). In developed countries, however, BIS may be even more frequent.

Clinical features

Watanabe et al. (1987) described nine infants with complex focal seizures and a benign evolution, diagnosed by simultaneous electroencephalogram and video recording. The majority of these cases were not familial. The onset was in the first year of life, at the age of 3 to 10 months, and most of these patients had seizures in clusters characterized by motion arrest, decreased responsiveness, staring, simple automatisms, and mild convulsions, associated with focal paroxysmal discharges most frequently in the temporal area. All patients responded well to classic antiepileptic drugs (AEDs) and they remained seizure free during a follow-up more than 3 years. All infants showed normal interictal EEGs, and psychomotor development. In 1993, the same authors described seven infants with benign idiopathic focal epilepsy with seizures that often occurred in clusters characterized by motor focal seizures evolving to secondarily generalized tonic-clonic seizures, associated with focal ictal EEG abnormalities most frequently in the centroparietal region (Watanabe et al., 1993). The authors named these two types of entities "benign partial epilepsy in infancy".

Later, other series of patients with similar electroclinical features and evolution were described by Berger and co-workers (1997) and Capovilla and co-workers (1998). Our group published a series of familial and non-familial cases with a mix of both types of electroclinical features described by Watanabe et al. (1987, 1990, 1993, 2000). Evolution in our cases was similar as well (Caraballo et al., 2002, 2003a; Caraballo 2005a). Both these variants of benign focal seizures in infants with or without direct familial cases currently constitute the BIS syndrome.

The five familial cases, three girls and two boys, described by Vigevano and co-workers (1992) showed seizures characterized by psychomotor arrest, slow deviation of the head and eyes to one side, diffuse hypertonia, cyanosis, and unilateral limb jerks, which became bilateral and synchronous or asynchronous. The bilateral and asynchronous limb jerks are characteristic of this syndrome. The seizures were stereotyped, but the direction of the head and eye deviation sometimes changed from seizure to seizure in the same patient.

As mentioned previously, the clinical features are the same in both children with familial and non-familial BIS. Psychomotor development of all children with BIS is normal before the onset of seizures. A common finding in a half of cases is the occurrence of seizures in clusters of brief, repeated seizures, with a maximum of 10 to 12 a day. Seizures may be longer in the beginning, lasting 3 to 5 minutes approximately. The cluster may last 1 to 4 days. The seizures do not reach a status epilepticus. The median age at onset is slightly younger in familial cases than in non-familial cases; 6.5 months (range: 3-22 months) and 9 months (range 2-23) in familial and in non-familial cases, respectively *(Table I)*. The affected parents and relatives in familial cases have had similar types of seizures and a similar age of onset of 6 months (range: 4 to 13 months). All the cases with a novel heterozygous mutation c.3003 T > A in the SCN2A gene in a family with three affected individuals over three generations described by Striano *et al.* (2006) experienced clusters of focal seizures with or without secondary generalization, and onset between 4 and 12 months of life. They were diagnosed with BFIS. None of the infants developed other seizures later in life and all of them had normal developmental outcomes.

We described two particular infantile familial cases that started with simple and/or complex focal seizures with or without secondary generalization in the first year of life, but continued having sporadic seizures for several years. At the last control, at 4 and 6 years of age, respectively, neurological examinations and neuropsychological development were normal in both of them. The subsequent interictal EEG recordings and the neuroradiological imaging were normal as well. Their mothers have presented similar types of seizures when they had the same age and they continue with sporadic seizures and have a normal IQ (Caraballo *et al.*, 2005a). These two families may represent a type of BFIS with variable expression or a different familial infantile syndrome.

The electroclinical features and evolution in infants with the syndrome described by Szepetowski *et al.* (1997) are the same as in classic BIS, while paroxysmal choreoathetosis appears many years later. (See chapter 4).

Familial hemiplegic migraine (FHM) is a rare, severe autosomal dominant subtype of migraine with aura associated with hemiparesis (Ducros *et al.*, 2001). In a Dutch-Canadian family, FHM was found to be associated with BFIS (Terwindt *et al.*, 1997; Mc Callenbach *et al.*, 2002). In this family, BFISs were followed at an older age by FHM and concurred to co-segregate to chromosome 1q23 (Vanmolkot *et al.*, 2003).

Table I. Electroclinical features and evolution of familial and non-familial BIS

- Nonsignificant personal history
- Normal development and neurological examination before onset
- Family history of similar type of seizures and age at onset (familial cases).
- Autosomal dominant inheritance (familial cases).
- Age at onset: 6.5 months (median) in familial cases and 9.5 months (median) in non-familial patients
- Complex and simple focal seizures with or without secondary generalization
- Often in a cluster
- Normal interictal EEG
- Normal developmental prognosis
- Benign evolution

Benign familial neonatal-infantile seizures

In 1983, Kaplan and Lacey described familial seizures with an onset occurring between neonatal and infantile ages. The finding was ratified by Zonana et al. (1984). The onset of seizures varied from 2 days to 3.5 months and the authors proposed the term "benign familial neonatal-infantile seizures" (BFNIS).

The patients in the two families described by Heron *et al.* (2002) presented focal seizures with secondary generalization occurring between 1.9 and 3.8 months of life and an autosomal dominant mode of inheritance. They had a missense mutation in SCN2A, the gene coding for the alpha 2 subunit of the voltage-gated sodium channel. Subsequently, the same group reported the SCN2A mutation in five other families (Berkovic *et al.*, 2004). Seizures are characterized by a predominant focal motor manifestation, with head and eye deviation followed by tonic and clonic convulsions. Most of the seizures lasted up to 4 minutes. Some patients had only few seizures per day while others had clusters of seizures. Interictal EEGs were normal, or showed unspecific discharges in the posterior regions. When ictal EEGs were recorded, they showed a focal posterior onset of discharges. All patients had a normal development before and after the seizure occurrence.

Again, the genetic findings in the families described by Striano *et al.* (2006) not only provide new evidence that BFN-IS and BFIS may show some overlapping of their clinical manifestations but also of their genetic characteristics.

Benign Infantile seizures associated with Mild Gastroenteritis

The first patients with an association of BIS and mild gastroenteritis (MG) were described by Morooka in Japan in 1982. The previously healthy infants between 6 months and 3 years of age presented with non-febrile generalized seizures. Seizures often occurred in a cluster, and laboratory examination results, including blood and CSF glucose, were normal. Interictal EEGs were normal in all patients, and all of them had an excellent outcome.

After this first report, more than 60 other reports of Japanese patients with BIS and MG were published in Japan (Nakai and Soda, 1982; Kajiyama and Fukuyama, 1984; Ito *et al.*, 1988; Komori *et al.*, 1995; Shikano *et al.*, 1998; Kobayashi *et al.*, 1999; Omata *et al.*, 2002; Uemura *et al.*, 2002; Fukuyama and Sakauchi, 2006). Thereafter, nine series of patients with similar features of different ethnic origins were described (Gomez-Lado *et al.*, 2005; Iglesias Escalera *et al.*, 2005; Lionetti *et al.*, 2005; Narchi, 2004; Posner, 2003; Wong, 2001; Lynch *et al.*, 2001; Contino *et al.*, 1994). We evaluated 12 patients with BIS associated with gastroenteritis. In five, positive rotavirus antigen was found. Prophylactic antiepileptic treatment was not given, and all the patients remained seizure free in a 1 to 6-years follow-up.

BIS with MG are characterized by brief focal seizures that may evolve to secondary generalization *(Table II)*. The seizures often occur in clusters during the first two years of life within the first 5 days of the episode of gastroenteritis (Imai *et al.*, 1999). The ictal recording of cases with BIS and MG revealed that all seizures had partial onset (Imai *et al.*, 1999; Capovilla and Vigevano, 2001; Maruyama *et al.*, 2007). Imai *et al.* (1999) described a patient in whom three different seizures originated from three different cerebral regions (right occipital, right centroparietal-occipital, and left occipital). This feature is very similar to cases of BFIS. They hypothesized that immaturity of brain functions may play an important role in the genesis of this type of seizures. Seizures rarely recur, even without prophylactic antiepileptic treatment or when an infant has repeated episodes of gastroenteritis (Fukuyama and Sakauchi, 2006). In a study by Okumura *et al.* (2004) on the efficacy of antiepileptic drugs in BIS with MG, lidocaine was found to be the most effective drug to control the seizures during a cluster, although it seems to us excessive to use lidocaine in these infants. At least we didn't need to use other than the usual AED drugs in our twelve patients. In more than half of the patients, screening for the rotavirus antigen was positive (Uemura *et al.*, 2002).

The hypothesis that factors such as dehydration, hypoglycemia, and electrolyte disturbance may cause seizures during gastroenteritis episodes has been excluded by Morooka *et al.* (1982). Komori and co-workers (1995) reported infants in whom seizures preceded the onset of diarrhoea.

BIS associated with MG may be categorized within the situation-related seizures, although it has not been described in the 2001 ILAE's proposal (Engel, 2001).

EEG features of BIS

The interictal EEGs are normal in both familial and non-familial cases. Vigevano and co-workers (1992) found lateralized slow waves and spikes in the occipito-parietal areas on the interictal EEGs recorded between seizures during a cluster of seizures in familial cases, although we did not find those focal discharges between seizures in a cluster in our patients.

The ictal EEG recording shows a focal discharge characterized by a recruiting rhythm of increasing amplitude with onset in the occipito-parietal regions, spreading over the hemisphere and involving the entire brain (Vigevano *et al.*, 1994, 2007). The ictal event in the same patients shows onset of the seizures either in one or the other hemisphere. This alternating clinical pattern may

Table II. Electroclinical features of Benign infantile seizures associated with mild gastroenteritis

- Normal neurological state
- Age at onset between 8 and 24 months
- Focal seizures with or without secondary generalization
- Often seizures in a cluster
- Normal interictal EEG
- Clinical features of gastroenteritis
- Associated with Rotavirus in more than 50% of the cases
- Recurrence of seizures during new episodes of gastroenteritis is rare
- Benign prognosis

be explained by the immature cerebral cortex (Vigevano *et al.*, 2007). In non-familial cases with complex partial seizures, the temporal area is the site of origin (Watanabe *et al.*, 1987; Capovilla *et al.*, 1998; Capovilla & Vigevano, 2001), whereas in cases with secondary generalized seizures the site of onset varies (Watanabe *et al.*, 1993). In *figures 1 & 2* ictal EEGs with temporal lobe onset discharges are shown.

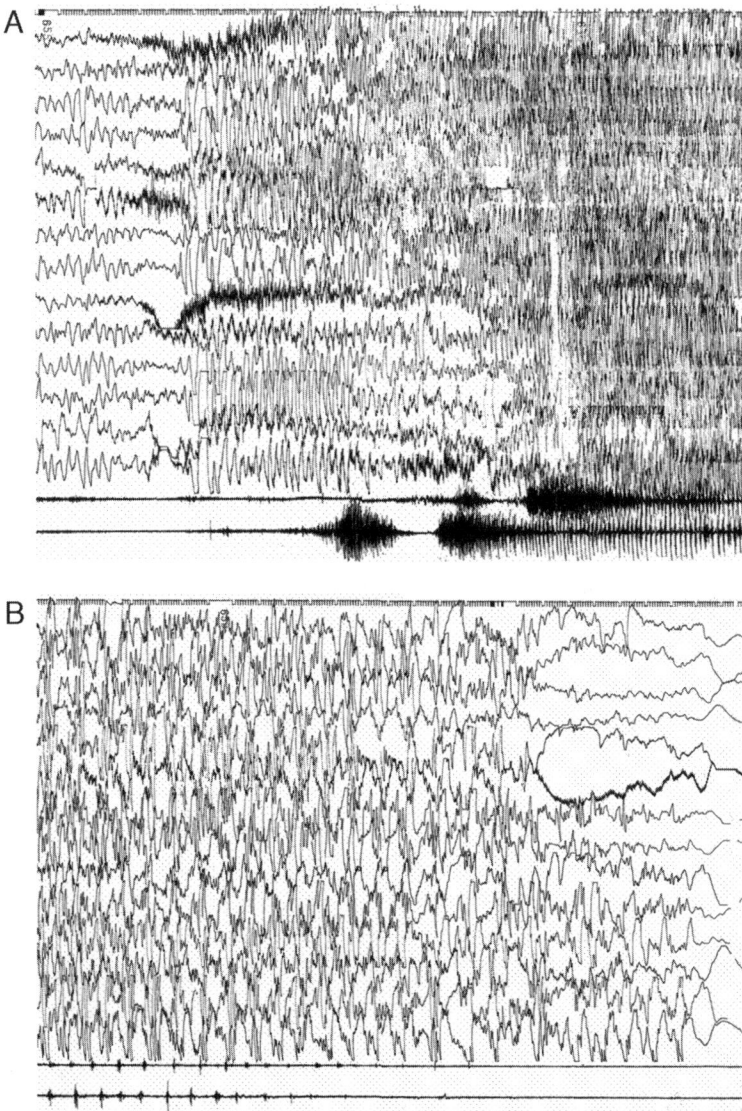

Figure 1. Six month old boy who had seizures characterized by motion arrest followed by loss of consciousness, right head and eye deviation, mild cyanosis and arrhythmic clonic movement of limbs. A: ictal EEG shows focal activity of delta-slow waves in left temporal and parietal regions rapidly followed by generalized discharges of slow wave interspersed with spikes. B: one minute later, the seizure finishes in left hemisphere. Courtesy of Dr Giuseppe Capovilla.

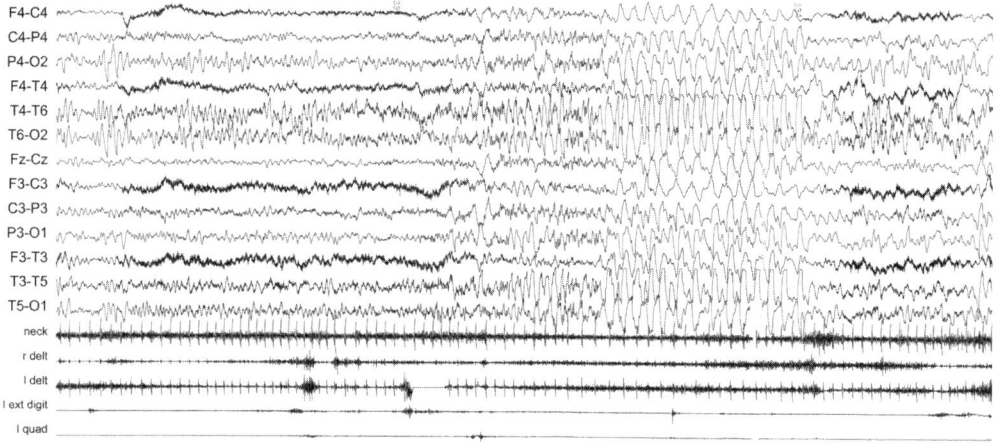

Figure 2. Ten months old normal infant with seizures characterized by staring, loss of consciousness and oral automatisms of sucking. Ictal EEG shows focal discharges of fast waves beginning in the right posterior temporal lobe and spreading to central and contralateral homologous regions. Critical discharge rapidly increases in amplitude and decreases in frequency, with a duration of 17 seconds. Courtesy of Dr Giuseppe Capovilla.

Aetiology

In familial cases an autosomal dominant mode of inheritance was evident. In infants with familial BIS, the researchers first tried to find the chromosome markers described in benign familial neonatal seizures (BFNS) (Leppert et al., 1989; Ryan et al., 1991; Singh et al., 1998). However, Malafosse et al. (1994) demonstrated that BFIS are not allelic forms of the BFNS gene and the authors excluded the marker on chromosome 20. In 1997, Guipponi et al. (1997) mapped a locus on chromosome 19q12-13.1 between markers D19S49 and D19245 in five Italian BFIS families. Gennaro et al. (1999) demonstrated the presence of linkage to chromosome 19q in a single family, suggesting genetic heterogeneity within the seven examined families.

Studies on familial cases with ICCA demonstrated a linkage to the pericentromeric region of chromosome 16 in six French families with this syndrome (Szepetowski et al., 1997). These findings were confirmed by Lee et al. (1998) in a Chinese family. We found linkage on chromosome 16p12-q12, the same region as ICCA, in four Argentine families and three French families with a pure form of BFIS suggesting that chromosome 16p12-q12 is a major genetic locus underlying both benign familial infantile seizures and paroxysmal dyskinesia (Caraballo et al., 2001). Similar results in 14 families with pure forms of BFIS have been reported (Weber et al., 2004). Malacarne and co-workers (2001) found pure forms of BFIS linked to chromosome 2q24 in eight Italian families, demonstrating thus a genetic heterogeneity, as in other autosomal dominant idiopathic epilepsies.

As mentioned before a new mutation has been found in SCN2A gene in cases described as having benign familial neonatal-infantile seizures, considered as an intermediate form between BFIS and benign familial neonatal seizures (Heron et al. 2002; Berkovic et al., 2004). For the first time a mutation of the same gene has recently been described in a family with clinical features typical of BFIS (Striano et al., 2006). Considering the different chromosomic loci already identified for BFIS we might expect other mutations to be found in the future. Findings of genetic heterogeneity are not going to be surprising at all. However, the main advance in aetiology of all these variants of benign neonatal and infantile seizures are linked to the fact that this function in ion channel underlay the causes of several epilepsy syndromes. Channelopathies have been already reported in a significant number of epilepsies. On account of the high proportion of babies presenting identical electroclinical features but we no familial antecedent, we believe that they might be interpreted as either the novo mutation or as sporadic cases of the same condition.

The rotavirus may be the aetiological factor in infantile seizures associated with mild gastroenteritis (Morooka, 1982, Uemura et al., 2002). A small round-structured virus, called Norwalk virus, was observed in similar infants (Abe et al., 2002).

Pathophysiology

The pathophysiology remains unclear. The different clinical phenotypes of BIS may be age-dependent manifestations of genetically determined cerebral cortex hyperexcitability.

Diagnostic work-up

The interictal EEG is normal or fails to show any diagnostic elements in all forms of BIS. As a general rule, in these forms of epilepsy it is not required to perform extensive and aggressive diagnostic investigations, except for prolonged wake and sleep EEGs. All of these children have a normal psychomotor development, and sometimes a clear familial recurrence; these findings at onset, could lead clinicians towards a diagnosis of idiopathic epilepsy. The follow-up and EEG studies of these patients confirm the diagnosis of benign forms. The brain MRI is always normal, as are all other diagnostic studies. In the presence of mild gastroenteritis, it is necessary to screen for rotavirus antigen, which is found in half of cases.

Even though these children have normal MRIs, it is necessary to perform such studies to rule out symptomatic types of epilepsy. However, in cases with a clear autosomal dominant pattern of inheritance and clear clinical features of benignity, it is possible to postpone the study. Specific indications for the laboratory assessment do not exist, but cardiovascular and respiratory function parameters have to be carefully studied in children with BFIS or BNFIS during the cluster. Of course, the more common metabolic disturbances such as hypoglycemia, hypocalcemia, hypomagnesemia, hyponatremia and other, should be looked for when the patient is admitted. An ictal single photon emission computed tomography performed in an infant with BFIS revealed that the epileptic discharge arose in the left frontal area (Nagase et al., 2002)

In cases with BIS and MG, electrolytes in serum and general clinical condition of the patient should also be evaluated.

It may be useful to collect familial cases for linkage studies. Genetic studies may confirm the mutations already identified, and are important for genetic counselling. In addition, the possibility of new genetic mutations causing BIS should be considered.

Differential diagnosis and relation with other epilepsy syndromes

Benign epilepsies in infancy have recently been recognized by the ILAE in the proposal of classification (Engel, 2001, 2006), but their nosologic definition and place still present some problems and we agree to use the term "seizures" instead "epilepsy" in these conditions (Engel, 2001).

Focal epilepsies in infancy had long been considered as being symptomatic and having a poor prognosis. Moreover, some authors doubted about the existence of focal idiopathic epilepsy in early infancy (Dulac *et al.*, 1989). We shall consider differential diagnosis of BIS with other idiopathic epileptic conditions and with cryptogenic or symptomatic epilepsy syndromes with onset in the same age period. Of course, non-epileptic paroxysmal events should also be considered (Fejerman, 2007).

Differential diagnosis between BIS and other idiopathic epileptic syndromes

1 – The distinction between BIS and benign familial neonatal seizures (BFNS) is clearly the age of onset and obviously, if it were possible, the existence of one of the two genes, KCNQ2 and KCNQ3 demonstrated in BFNS.

2 – The differential diagnosis between BIS and the intermediate form between BFNS and BIS (BFN-IS) is only a question of considering age of onset because the electroclinical features are quite similar. On the other side, search of the identified gene mutation is not still common practice.

3 – The distinction between BIS and the group of patients associating BIS with paroxysmal choreoathetosis (ICCA) is impossible at onset, unless older relatives with paroxysmal choreoathetosis are already identified in the family. We know one locus for ICCA but the gene or genes have not been discovered yet (see chapter 4). Therefore, we should be alert to follow the patients and their families to see if the episodes of choreoathetosis appear in any age.

4 – Differently from previously discussed entities, benign infantile seizures associated with mild gastroenteritis (BIS with MG) are more likely to be considered as situation-related seizures than as epilepsy. This syndrome can be misdiagnosed as epilepsy because the seizures are non-febrile, and may occur in clusters. It would be important to study this condition more thoroughly in the future.

5 – Our two familial cases with refractory seizures whose mothers continue with seizures in adult life may be an atypical variant of BIS or another familial entity (Caraballo, 2005a).

6 – Familial hemiplegic migraine (FHM) is a severe autosomal dominant subtype of migraine with aura associated with hemiparesis and BFIS (Terwindt *et al.*, 1997; Mc Callenbach *et al.*, 2002). In the reported Dutch-Canadian family, BFISs were followed by FHM at an older age and a novel mutation in the Na+, K+-ATPase pump gene ATP1A2 was found (Vanmolkot *et al.*, 2003).

7 – Benign infantile focal epilepsy with midline spikes and waves during sleep (BIMSE) has been distinguished from familial and non-familial BIS. Clinical and EEG features of this condition are detailed in chapter 5, and differential diagnosis between BIMSE, BIS, Benign childhood epilepsy with centrotemporal spikes and Panayiotopoulos syndrome (PS) are described in *table I* of that chapter (Caraballo *et al.*, 2000, Dalla Bernardina *et al.*, 2005). However, the interictal EEG recording in cases with BIS, particularly those with a later onset, needs to be more extensively investigated. Future studies will be useful to define if BIMSE is a new epileptic syndrome or an electroclinical variant of BIS or early onset benign focal epilepsies in childhood. *Table III* shows familial and non-familial BIS and related syndromes and *table IV* the differential diagnosis between BIS and other epileptic syndromes.

Differential diagnosis of BIS with cryptogenic or symptomatic epilepsies in infancy

1 – In cryptogenic cases with occipital lobe seizures, the ictal events start predominantly in the first months of life, while the frontal lobe seizures start in the last months of the first year of

Table III. Familial and non-familial BIS and related syndromes

– Benign familial neonatal-infantile seizures
– Benign infantile seizures with mild gastroenteritis
– Benign familial infantile seizures and paroxysmal choreoathetosis
– Benign familial infantile seizures and familial hemiplegic migraine
– Benign infantile focal epilepsy with midline spikes and waves during sleep

Table IV. Differential diagnosis of familial and non-familial BIS with other epileptic syndromes

• With idiopathic epileptic syndromes.
– Idiopathic West syndrome
– Panayiotopoulos syndrome
– Early onset cases of BECTS
• With cryptogenic or symptomatic epilepsies.
– Infantile spasms in clusters without hypsarrhythmia
– Probably symptomatic focal epilepsies
– Epilepsies due to structural brain lesion
– Seizures due to inborn error to metabolism
Pyridoxine dependency
Others
– Seizures associated with common metabolic disturbances

life. This finding may be related with cerebral maturational factors, since a sequence of maturation from occipital to frontal regions during the first year of life has been demonstrated through metabolic imaging studies (Chiron, 2007).

We prefer to consider the so called cryptogenic cases as probably symptomatic, because there are even age limitations in the power of MRI. As in other age periods, not visible cortical dysplasias are frequently present as a cause of seizures, and we should rest on the clinical judgment about the types and repetition of seizures to consider this diagnostic possibility. It is well known that MRI may show a variety of structural brain lesion which might not have produced overt clinical signs and may be responsible for local onset seizures in babies.

2 – Epileptic spasms in a cluster without hypsarrhythmia in previously normal infants may be another differential diagnosis (Caraballo *et al.*, 2003b). We have been studying 12 cases with epileptic spasms in cluster without hypsarrhythmia; eight cases are cryptogenic, one idiopathic and three symptomatic. In cryptogenic cases, the interictal EEG recordings may be normal at onset, but in the evolution focal abnormalities appear. In these cases, the epileptic spasms are frequently refractory to AEDs *(Table IV)*.

3 – Among seizures symptomatic of metabolic disturbances, the first condition to think about is Pyridoxine deficiency or dependency. Pyridoxine dependency is an uncommon familial disease transmitted as an autosomal recessive trait, characterized by seizures, usually refractory to AEDs occurring soon after birth or even *in utero*. However, the seizures may also occur in the two first years of life. The natural evolution is not benign (Baxter, 2001; Caraballo *et al.*, 2004). Oral administration of 50-150 mg/day is necessary to control the seizures. A trial of withdrawal is the only method of confirming pyridoxine dependency (Baxter, 2001). There is a large list of inborn errors of metabolism that may present focal or generalized seizures as first manifestation, but it is up to the clinician to decide if these specific studies are needed. We already mentioned in relation to diagnostic work-up about differential diagnosis with seizures provoked by common metabolic disturbances.

Differential diagnosis between BIS and paroxysmal non-epileptic events

The list of non-epileptic episodic events in infancy is large, and altogether those conditions are seen with a significant frequency (Fejerman, 2007). Differential diagnosis is mandatory and sometimes not so easy. Common thought of paediatricians would be that if EEG is normal in a baby who had brief motor seizures or other atypical episodes, the patient does not have epilepsy. This is true for the examples included in *table V*, but we should not forget about the wide spectrum of benign focal seizures in infants that we are considering in this chapter, as seen in *table V*.

Treatment

Seizures in these forms of BIS do not need to be treated, but in the clinical practice this is not always an easy decision. The early recognition of these syndromes is also relevant to define

Table V. Differential diagnosis of familial and non-familial BIS with non-epileptic episodic events in infancy

- Benign neonatal sleep myoclonus
- Hyperekplexia
- Increased Moro reflex and attacks of opisthotonos
- Reflex tonic episodes in infancy
- Sandifer syndrome
- Benign myoclonus of early infancy (including shuddering attacks)
- Benign paroxysmal tonic upward gaze
- Adverse reactions or intolerance to exogenous agents
- Paroxysmal dystonia and choreoathetosis (paroxysmal torticollis, benign infantile dystonia)
- Self-gratification or masturbation-like episodes

pharmacological treatment. It is difficult not to treat these epilepsies at the onset, as these infants have clusters of seizures, but avoiding or reducing the time of the pharmacological treatment may be a strong possibility. After the acute phase, many infants continue to follow a chronic therapy. In familial cases we may interrupt the therapy as early as possible, and in non-familial cases, should the benign diagnosis be confirmed, it will be possible to interrupt the treatment between 12 and 24 months after the last seizure.

Early in the syndrome, these children often present with seizures in clusters which sometimes require an emergency intervention with AEDs (Okumura *et al.*, 2006a). Patients who are not treated after the first cluster may repeat other seizures or clusters. At the emergency department, these patients are often managed by pediatricians who should be well informed about the syndrome in order to avoid aggressive treatment. All drugs seem to be effective in benign infantile seizures (valproate, carbamazepine, phenobarbital and phenytoin), with no apparent differences. Recently, Japanese authors (Matsufuji *et al.*, 2005) reported the efficacy of low doses of carbamazepine in a series of patients with benign infantile seizures. In this study, carbamazepine was administered at a once-daily dose of 5 mg/kg; seizures did not recur in any of the patients.

The treatment can be withdrawn one year after onset. Two brothers of our series of patients with infantile seizures did not respond well to phenobarbital, but were sensitive to carbamazepine.

Prognosis and long-term evolution

Currently, there are no data on the long-term prognosis of benign infantile seizures. All of the children followed up at the department of Neurology of the Garrahan Children's Hospital for a period of 16 years remained seizure free after discontinuation of medication. Neuropsychological development was normal in all. A study revealed that 33 of 39 patients diagnosed with possible non-familial BIS at age 2 years did not have a recurrence of unprovoked seizures beyond age 8 years. Neuropsychological development was normal in all cases (Okumura *et al.*, 2006b). Similar prognosis has been found by Vigevano *et al.* (2006).

During the follow-up of our 40 cases with familial BIS and 62 patients with non-familial BIS, control EEGs failed to show any abnormalities, except in two of the children who presented asymptomatic centrotemporal spikes and other three who developed clinical and EEG features of BECTS. The father of one of these patients and a cousin of another patient had isolated seizures compatible with benign focal seizures of adolescence. Three of our patients with familial BIS presented paroxysmal dyskinesia during the first or second decades of life as has been clearly reported (Szepetowki *et al.*, 1997; Lee *et al.*, 1998; Tomita *et al.*, 1999; Bennet *et al.*, 2000; Swoboda *et al.*, 2000; Caraballo *et al.*, 2001; Hattori *et al.*, 2000; Okumura *et al.*, 2006b). This association, the ICCA syndrome, is described in detail in chapter 4.

Data about our familial and non-familial BIS series of patients

In our series of 40 and 62 patients with familial and non-familial BIS, respectively, both groups presented similar electroclinical features and evolution. These characteristics are carefully described and compared in the *table VI*.

Table VI. Clinical features and follow-up in 105 patients

Epileptic Syndrome		BFIS	BNFIS
Number of patients		40	65
Age at onset (months)	Median	6.5	9
	Range	3-22	2-23
Types of seizures	Partial	20	31
	Apparently generalized	10	16
	Secondarily generalized	10	18
	In "clusters"	21	30
EEG	Normal	24	37
	Abnormal	1	2
Family history of infantile seizures	Mother or Father Others (Uncle)	39 1	0 0
Family history of other type of epilepsy		3	9
Paroxysmal Choreoathetosis	Patients	3	0
	In family members	5	0
	Age at onset (years) Range	11-18	0

References

- Abe T, Kobayashi M, Araki K et al. Infantile convulsions with mild gastroenteritis. *Brain Dev* 2002; 22: 301-6.

- Baralle D, Dearlove AM, Beach RF et al. Benign familial infantile convulsions: report of a UK family and confirmation of genetic heterogeneity. *J Med Genet* 2000 (abstract); 17: 31.

- Baxter P. *Vitamin Responsive Conditions in Pediatric Neurology*. Mac Keith Press for the International Child Neurology Association. England, 2001.

- Bennett LB, Roach ES, Bowcock AM. A locus for paroxysmal kinesigenic dyskinesia maps to human chromosome 16. *Neurology* 2000; 54: 125-30.

- Berger A, Diener W, Stephani E, Schaechtele M, Rating D. Benigne fruekindliche partialepilepsie nach Watanabe. *Epilepsie Blaetter* 1997; 10, 76-81.

- Berkovic SF, Heron SE, Giordano L, et al. Benign familial neonatal-infantile seizures: characterization of a new sodium channelopathy. *Ann Neurol* 2004; 55: 550-7.

- Bureau M, Maton B. Valeur de l'EEG dans le pronostic précoce des épilepsies partielles non idiopathiques de l'enfant. In: Bureau M, Kahane P, Munari C (Eds). *Épilepsies partielles graves pharmacorésistantes de l'enfant : stratégies diagnostiques et traitements chirurgicaux*. Montrouge: John Libbey Eurotext, 1998: 67-78.

- Capovilla G, Giordano L, Tiberti S, Valseriati D, Menegati E. Benign partial epilepsy in infancy with complex partial seizures (Watanabe's syndrome): 12 non-Japanese new cases. *Brain Dev* 1998; 20: 105-11.

- Capovilla G, Beccaria F. Benign partial epilepsy in infancy and early childhood with vertex spikes and waves during sleep: a new epileptic form. *Brain Dev* 2000; 22, 93-9.

- Capovilla G, Vigevano F. Benign idiopathic partial epilepsies in infancy. *J Child Neurol* 2001; 16: 874-1.

- Caraballo R, Cersósimo R, Galicchio S, Fejerman N. (1997a) Convulsiones familiares benignas de la infancia. *Rev Neurol* (Barc) 1997; 25 (141): 682-4.

- Caraballo R, Cersósimo R, Galicchio S, Fejerman N. (1997b) Epilepsias en el primer año de vida. *Rev Neurol* (Barc) 1997; 25 (146): 1521-4.

- Caraballo R, Cersósimo R, Medina C, Fejerman N. Panayiotopoulos-type benign childhood occipital epilepsy: A prospective study. *Neurology* 2000; 55: 1096-100.

- Caraballo R, Pavek S, Lemainque A, et al. Linkage of benign familial infantile convulsions to chromosome 16p12-q12 suggests allelism to the infantile convulsions and choreoathetosis syndrome. *Am J Hum Genet* 2001; 68: 788-94.

- Caraballo R, Cersósimo R, Amartino H, Szepetowski P, Fejerman N. Benign familial infantile seizures: further delineation of the syndrome. *Journal of child neurology* 2002; 17 (9): 696-9.

- Caraballo R, Cersósimo R, Espeche A, Fejerman N. (2003a) Benign familial and non-familial infantile seizures: a study of 64 patients. *Epileptic Disord* 2003; 5: 45-9.

- Caraballo R, Fejerman N, Dalla Bernardina et al. (2003b) Epileptic spasms in cluster without hypsarrythmia in infancy. *Epileptic Disorder* 2003; 5 (2): 109-13.

- Caraballo R, Garro F, Cersósimo R, Buompadre C, Gañez L, Fejerman N. Dependencia de Piridoxina: valor del diagnóstico clínico y del tratamiento precoz. *Rev neurol* (Barc) 2004; 38 (1): 49-52.

- Caraballo R. (2005a) Convulsiones familiares y no-familiares benignas del lactante. In: Ruggieri V, Caraballo R, Arroyo H (Eds). *Temas de Neuropediatría. Homenaje al Dr. Natalio Fejerman*. Buenos Aires: Editorial Médica Panamericana, 2005: 53-68.

- Caraballo R. (2005b) Epilepsias del lactante. *Medicina Infantil* 2005; XII: 158-63.

- Chiron C. Tomografia computarizada por emisión de fotones aislados. In: Fejerman N, Fernandez Alvarez E (Eds). *Neurología Pediátrica* (3rd edition). Buenos Aires: Panamericana, 2007: 106-10.

- Contino MF, Lebby T, Arcinue EL. Rotaviral gastrointestinal infection causing afebrile seizures in infancy and childhood. *Am J Emerg Med* 1994; 12: 94-5.

- Dalla Bernardina B, Sgrò V, Fejerman N. Epilepsy with centrotemporal spikes and related syndromes. In: Roger J, Bureau M, Dravet C, Genton P, Tassinari CA, Wolf P (Eds). *Epileptic Syndromes in Infancy, Childhood and Adolescence* (4th edition). Montrouge: John Libbey Eurotext, 2005: 203-25.

- Ducros A, Denier C, Joutel A, *et al*. The clinical spectrum of familial hemiplegic migraine associated with mutations in a neuronal calcium channel. *N Engl J Med* 2001; 345: 17-24.

- Dulac O, Cusmai, R, de Oliveira K. Is there a partial benign epilepsy in infancy? *Epilepsia* 1989; 30: 798-801.

- Echenne B, Humbertclaude V, Rivier F, Malafosse A, Cheminal R. Benign infantile epilepsy with autosomal dominant inheritance. *Brain Dev* 1994; 16: 108-11.

- Engel J. A proposed diagnostic scheme for people with epileptic seizures and with epilepsy: report of the ILAE Task Force on classification and terminology. *Epilepsia* 2001; 42: 796-803.

- Engel J. Report of the ILAE Classification Core Group. *Epilepsia* 2006; 47 (9): 1558-68.

- Fejerman N. Non-epileptic neurologic paroxysmal disorders and episodic symptoms in infants. In: Engel J, Pedley TA (Eds). *Epilepsy: A comprehensive textbook*. Philadelphia: Lippincott Williams & Wilkins, 2007 (in press).

- Fukuyama Y. Borderland of epilepsy with special reference to febrile convulsions and so-called infantile convulsions. *Seishin-Igaku* (Clin Psychiatry) 1963; 5: 211-23.

- Fukuyama Y, Sakauchi M. Benign infantile seizure syndromes complex. From classic to recent advances. *Epilepsies* 2006; 18 (1): 8-23.

- Gennaro E, Malacarne M, Carbone I, *et al*. No evidence of a major locus for benign familial infantile convulsions on chromosome 19q12-q13.1. *Epilepsia* 1999; 40: 1799-803.

- Giordano L, Accorsi P, Valseriati D, *et al*. Benign infantile familial convulsions: natural history of a case and clinical characteristics of a large Italian family. *Neuropediatrics* 1999; 30: 99-101.

- Guipponi M, Rivier F, Vigevano F, *et al*. Linkage mapping of benign familial infantile convulsions (BFIC) to chromosome 19. *Hum Mol Genet* 1997; 6, 473-7.

- Gomez-Lado C, Garcia-Reboredo M, Monasterio-Corral L, Bravo-Mat M, Eiris-Punal J, Castro-Cago M. Benign seizures associated with mild gastroenteritis: Apropos of two cases. *An Pediatr* 2005; 63: 558-60.

- Hattori H, Fujii T, Nigami H, Higuchi Y, Tsuji M, Hamada Y. Co-segregation of benign infantile convulsions and paroxysmal kinesigenic choreoathetosis. *Brain Dev* 2000; 22: 432-5.

- Heron SE, Crossland KM, Andermann E, *et al*. Sodium-channel defects in benign familial neonatal infantile seizures. *Lancet* 2002; 360: 851-2.

- Iglesias Escalera G, Usano Carrasco AI, Cueto Calvo E, Martinez Badas I, Guardia Nieto L, Sarrion Cano M. Benign afebrile convulsion due to rotavirus gastroenteritis. *An Pediatr* 2005; 63: 82-3.

- Imai K, Otani K, Yanagihara K, *et al*. Ictal video-EEG recording of three partial seizures in a patient with the benign infantile convulsions associated with mild gastroenteritis. *Epilepsia* 1999; 40: 1455-8.

- Ito J, Takahashi Y, Kusunoki Y, Oki J, Chou K. Convulsions associated with mild acute diarrhoea. *Shonika Rinsho* (Jpn J Pediatr) 1988; 41: 2011-5.

- Kaplan RE, Lacey DJ. Benign familial neonatal-infantile seizures. *Am J Med Genet* 1983; 16: 595-9.

- Kajiyama M, Fukuyama Y. Infantile convulsions associated with mild diarrhoea (in Japanese). *Nihon Shonika Gakkai Zasshi* (Tokyo) 1984; 88: 883-9.

- Kobayashi K, Araki K, Kobayashi S, Abe T. Infantile afebrile clustered convulsions associated small round structured virus infection (in Japanese). *Shonika Rinsho* (Tokyo) 1999; 52: 56-62.

- Kaleyias J, Khurana DS, Valencia I, et al. Benign partial epilepsy in infancy: Myth or reality? *Epilepsia* 2006; 47 (6): 1043-9.

- Komori H, Wada M, Eto M, Oki H, Aida K, Fujimoto T. Benign convulsions with mild gastroenteritis: a report of 10 recent cases detailing clinical varieties. *Brain Dev* 1995; 17: 334-7.

- Lee WL, Low PS, Rajan U. Benign familial infantile epilepsy. *J Pediatr* 1993; 123: 588-90.

- Lee WL, Tay A, Ong HT, Goh LM, Monaco AP, Szepetowski P. Association of infantile convulsions with paroxysmal dyskinesias (ICCA syndrome): confirmation of linkage to human chromosome 16p12-q12 in a Chinese family. *Hum Genet* 1998; 103: 608-12.

- Leppert M, Anderson VE, Quattlebaum T, et al. Benign familial neonatal convulsions linked to genetic markers on chromosome 20. *Nature* 1989; 337: 647-8.

- Lionetti P, Salvestrini C, Trapani S, de Martino M, Messineo A. An 18-month-old child with seizures and bloody diarrhoea. *Inflamm Bowel Dis* 2005; 11: 209-10.

- Luovigsson P, Olafsson E, Rich SS, Johannesson G, Anderson VE. Benign infantile familial epilepsy: three families with multiple affected members in three generations. *Epilepsia* 1993; 34: 18 (abstract).

- Lynch M, Lee B, Azimi P, et al. Rotavirus and central nervous system symptoms: cause or concomitant? Case reports and review. *Clin Infect Dis* 2001; 33: 932-8.

- Mc Callenbach P, De Coo RFM, Vein AA, et al. Benign familial infantile convulsions: a clinical study of seven Dutch families. *Eur J Paediatr Neurol* 2002; 6: 269-83.

- Malacarne M, Gennaro E, Madia F, et al. Benign familial infantile convulsions: mapping of a novel locus on chromosome 2q24 and evidence for genetic heterogeneity. *Am J Hum Genet* 2001; 68: 1521-6.

- Malaffose A, Beck C, Bellet H, et al. Benign infantile familial convulsions are not allelic form of the benign familial neonatal convulsion gene. *Ann Neurol* 1994; 35: 479-82.

- Maruyama K, Okumura A, Sofue A, et al. Ictal EEG in patients with convulsions with mild gastroenteritis. *Brain & Dev* 2007; 29 (1): 43-6.

- Matsufuji H, Ichiyama T, Isumi H, Furukawa S. Low-dose carbamazepine therapy for benign infantile convulsions. *Brain Dev* 2005; 27: 554-7.

- Morooka K. Convulsions and mild diarrhoea. *Shonika* (Tokyo) 1982; 23: 131-37 (in Japanese).

- Nagase T, Takahashi Y, Iida S, Masue M, Okamoto H, Kondo N. Ictal and interictal single photon emission computed tomography in a patient with benign familial infantile convulsions. *J Neuroimaging* 2002; 12: 75-7.

- Nakai M., Soda M. Benign convulsions with mild diarrhoea (in Japanese). *Shonika Rinsho* (Tokyo) 1982; 35: 2855-9.

- Narchi H. Benign afebrile cluster convulsion with gastroenteritis: an observational study. *BMC Pediatr* 2004; 4: 2.

- Okumura A, Hayakawa F, Kato T, Kuno K, Negoro T, Watanabe K. Early recognition of benign partila epilepsy in infancy. *Epilepsia* 2000; 41: 714-7.

- Okumura A, Uemura N, Negoro T, Watanabe K. Efficacy of antiepileptic drugs in patients with benign convulsions with mild gastroenteritis. *Brain Dev* 2004; 26: 164-7.

- Okumura A, Kato T, Hayakawa F, *et al.* (2006a) Antiepileptic treatment against clustered seizures in benign partial epilepsy in infancy. *Brain & Dev* 2006; 28 (9): 582-5.

- Okumura A, Watanabe K, Negoro T, *et al.* (2006b) Long-term follow-up of patients with benign partial epilepsy in infancy. *Epilepsia* 2006; 47: 181-5.

- Omata T, Tamai K, Kurosaki T, Nakada S, Furusima W, Motoyoshi Y. Clinical study of convulsions with mild gastroenteritis (in Japanese). *Nihon Shonika Gakkai Zasshi* (Tokyo) 2002; 106: 368-71.

- Pryles CV, Livingston S, Ford FR. Familial paroxysmal choreoathetosis of Mount and Reback: study of a second family in which this condition is found in association with epilepsy. *Pediatrics* 1952; 9: 44-7.

- Posner E. "Benign convulsion with mild gastroenteritis" a worldwide clinical entity. *Brain Dev* 2003; 25: 529.

- Ryan SG, Wiznitger M, Hollman C, Torres MC, Szekeresova M, Schneider S. Benign familial neonatal convulsions: evidence for clinical and genetic heterogeneity. *Ann Neurol* 1991; 29: 469-73.

- Shikano T, Kikukawa H, Kato M, Anakura M. Clinical findings of infants with afebrile seizures associated with mild diarrhoea (in Japanese). *Shonika Rinsho* (Tokyo) 1998; 51: 1074-8.

- Singh NA, Charlier C, Stauffer D, *et al.* A novel potassium channel gene, KCNQ2, is mutated in an inherited epilepsy of newborns. *Nat Genet* 1998; 18: 25-9.

- Striano P, Bordo L, Lispi ML, *et al.* A novel SCN2A mutation in family with benign familial infantile seizures. *Epilepsia* 2006; 47: 218-20.

- Swoboda KJ, Soong BW, McKenna C, *et al.* Paroxysmal kinesigenic dyskinesia and infantile convulsions. Clinical and linkage studies. *Neurology* 2000; 55: 224-30.

- Szepetowski P, Rochette J, Berquin P, Piussan C, Lathrop GM, Monaco AP. Familial infantile convulsions and paroxysmal choreoathetosis: a new neurological syndrome linked to the pericentromeric region of human chromosome 16. *Am J Hum Genet* 1997; 61: 889-98.

- Terwindt GM, Ophoff RA, Lindhout D, *et al.* Partial cosegregation of familial hemiplegic migraine and a benign familial infantile epileptic syndrome. *Epilepsia* 1997; 38: 915-21.

- Tomita H, Nagamitsu S, Wakui K, *et al.* Paroxysmal kinesigenic choreoathetosis locus maps to chromosome 16p11.2-q12.1. *Am J Hum Genet* 1999; 65: 1688-97.

- Uemura N, Okumura A, Negoro T, Watanabe K. Clinical features of benign convulsions with mild gastroenteritis. *Brain Dev* 2002; 24: 745-9.

- Vanmolkot KR, Kors EE., Hottenga JJ, *et al.* Novel mutations in the Na+, K+-ATPase pump gene ATP1A2 associated with familial hemiplegic migraine and benign familial infantile convulsions. *Ann Neurol* 2003; 54: 360-6.

- Vigevano F, Fusco L, Di Capua M, Ricci, S, Sebastianelli R, Lucchini P. Benign infantile familial convulsions. *Eur J Pediatr* 1992; 151: 608-12.

- Vigevano F, Sebastianelli R, Fusco L, Di Capua M, Ricci S, Lucchini P. Benign infantile familial convulsions. In: Malafosse A, Genton P, Hirsch E, Marescaux C, Broglin D, Bernasconi R (Eds). *Idiopathic Generalized Epilepsies: Clinical, Experimental and Genetic Aspects.* London: John Libbey, 1994: 45-9.

- Vigevano F. Benign familial infantile seizures. *Brain Dev* 2005 ; 27: 172-7.

- Vigevano F, Specchio N, Caraballo R, Watanabe K. Benign familial and non-familial infantile seizures. In: Engel J, Pedley TA (Eds). *Epilepsy: a comprehensive textbook.* Philadelphia: Lippincott, 2007 (in press).

- Watanabe K, Yamamoto N, Negoro T, *et al.* Benign complex partial epilepsies in infancy. *Pediatr Neurol* 1987; 3: 208-11.

- Watanabe K, Yamamoto N, Negoro T, Takahashi I, Aso K, Maehara M. Benign infantile epilepsy with complex partial seizures. *J Clin Neurophysiol* 1990; 7: 409-16.

- Watanabe K, Negoro T, Aso K. Benign partial epilepsy with secondarily generalized seizures in infancy. *Epilepsia* 1993; 34: 635-8.

- Watanabe K, Okumura A. Benign partial epilepsies in infancy. *Brain Dev* 2000; 22: 296-300.

- Weber YG, Berger A, Bebek N, *et al*. Benign familial infantile convulsions: linkage to chromosome 16p12-q12 in 14 families. *Epilepsia* 2004; 45: 601-9.

- Wong V. Acute gastroenteritis – related encephalopathy. *J Child Neurol* 2001; 16: 906-10.

- Zonana J, Silvey K, Strimling B. Familial neonatal and infantile seizures: an autosomal dominant disorder. *Am J Med Genet* 1984; 18 (3): 455-9.

Benign familial infantile seizures and paroxysmal choreoathetosis

Pierre Szepetowski
Marseille, France

The relationship between the epilepsies on the one hand and various non-epileptic cerebral disorders on the other hand, is well established. The epilepsies and non-paroxysmal brain disorders such as autism (Tuchman & Rapin, 2002) and language impairment (Roll et al., 2006) have obvious links. At the clinical, epidemiological, therapeutic, and genetic levels, several features are also shared in common between epilepsy and paroxysmal albeit non-epileptic disorders of the brain (Kullmann, 2002): migraine (Bigal et al., 2003), episodic ataxia, paroxysmal dyskinesia (PD) (see below) (Guerrini, 2001).

Benign infantile seizures (BIS) (see Chapter 3) correspond to non-febrile convulsions with the first seizure at age 3-12 months and a favourable outcome. Familial and non-familial forms have been described.

PD are rare disorders characterized by episodes of involuntary abnormal movements. These correspond to attacks of choreoathetosis or dystonia. PD have been classified into two broad categories: paroxysmal kinesigenic dystonia/choreoathetosis on the one hand, and non-kinesigenic paroxysmal dystonic choreoathetosis on the other hand. However, whether the hyperkinetic movements are of the dystonic, ballistic, choreic, or choreoathetoid type, has sometimes proved difficult to determine. Consequently, another classification has been proposed (Demirkiran & Jankovic, 1995; Jankovic & Demirkiran, 2002) that distinguishes between kinesigenic PD (PKD) (attacks usually last < 5 min.), exercice-induced PD (PED) (attacks usually last > 5 min.), and non-kinesigenic PD (PNKD) (attacks usually last several hours).

First descriptions of BIS were made in the 60's (see Chapter 3). PD was also reported a long time ago (Mount & Reback, 1940; Fukuyama & Okada, 1967; Richards & Barnett, 1968). Much earlier descriptions of movement-triggered attacks of choreoathetosis or dystonia have even been reported (for a recent update: Kato et al., 2006). Paroxysmal choreoathetosis has long been suspected to be related to epileptic seizures (Stevens, 1966). Historically, the relationship of infantile convulsions with PD has been debated for a long time. Indeed, there are similarities between PD and epilepsy and the motor manifestations may sometimes be difficult to distinguish. Attacks of PD share several characteristics in common with epileptic seizures: crises are paroxysmal, there is tendency towards spontaneous remission, and the response to anticonvulsants may be good in a subset of the PD. EEG abnormalities consistent with an epileptogenic basis have even been reported (Hirata *et al.*, 1991; Lombroso, 1995). The epileptic origin of PD has long been a matter of debate (Hudgins & Corbin, 1966; Stevens, 1966; Kinast *et al.*, 1980; Beaumanoir *et al.*, 1996) and PD have been considered a reflex epilepsy (Stevens, 1966). Paroxysmal choreoathetosis and epileptic seizures have been described in the same patients (Pryles *et al.*, 1952) and in the same families (Hudgins & Corbin, 1966). In 1997, description of the ICCA (Infantile Convulsions and ChoreoAthetosis) syndrome and linkage to chromosome 16 provided the first genetic evidence for common mechanisms shared by PD and BIS (Szepetowski *et al.*, 1997).

Epidemiology

Although their relative prevalence is not known with precision, BIS usually are considered quite rare. However, many cases with familial and non-familial BIS have been described, and it may be one of the most common epilepsy in the two first years of life (see Chapter 3). Similarly, PD represent a rare heterogeneous group of neurological movement disorders. Familial cases in which PKD is inherited as an autosomal dominant trait are more common than sporadic or secondary cases (Boel and Casaer 1984), and there is higher prevalence of PKD in males. Generally, most cases of PD are primary, whether inherited or sporadic. The association of BIS with PD obviously is not that infrequent, although only a few families show unambiguous monogenic inheritance of epilepsy and PD as a definite and single entity.

Clinical findings

The association of BIS with PD is inherently composed of two distinct clinical entities that can also exist separately. Describing the clinical aspects of pure BIS and pure PD is beyond the scope of this chapter. However, one important question is whether the BIS and the PD that associate with each other in patients or families, are identical to their respective pure isolated forms, or show differences. Generally, there is no clear clinical discrepancy between those BIS and PD that present separately, and those that are associated in the same patients or that are co-inherited in the same families. In the idiopathic PKD, BIS are more frequent in the familial than in the sporadic forms (Bruno *et al.*, 2004).

Clearly there is inter- and intrafamilial variability in the ICCA and ICCA-related patients. This variability is largely sustained by the type of PD (kinesigenic, exercice-induced, or non-kinesigenic) but can also be due to variability in the BIS. These latter looked quite homogeneous in the former ICCA families (Szepetowski *et al.*, 1997) and consisted in partial seizures with motor characteristics and typical age of onset. However, BIS were generalized in an additional family of Chinese origin (Lee *et al.*, 1998) where seizures showed recurrence at later age in some patients. BIS have also been described in the context of other ICCA and ICCA-like families (Sadamatsu *et al.*, 1999; Tomita *et al.*, 1999; Hattori *et al.*, 2000; Swoboda *et al.*, 2000; Thiriaux *et al.*, 2002).

PD look much more heterogeneous in and between the families. In the first ICCA families (Szepetowski et al. 1997), the patients had spontaneous or exercise-induced dystonic movements. In contrast, PD was clearly of the kinesigenic type in other families (Tomita *et al.*, 1999; Swoboda *et al.*, 2000). The attacks may also be exercise-induced (Sadamatsu *et al.* 1999). Interestingly, the type of PD may even change with time in the same patient (Caraballo *et al.*, 2001). Overall, this may signify that common pathophysiological pathways exist between at least a subset of the different types of PD. Indeed, most – if not all – the families with PD – whatever the type – and BIS associated together, show genetic linkage to the same genomic region *(Tables I & II)*.

It is worth mentioning that the association of epilepsy with paroxysmal abnormal movement disorder may also occur in the context of other epilepsy types. Idiopathic generalized epilepsy (Cuenca-Leon *et al.*, 2002), and especially absence epilepsy (Guerrini *et al.*, 2002; Bing *et al.*, 2005; Du *et al.*, 2005), as well as mixed epileptic phenotypes (Singh *et al.*, 1999) can be co-inherited with PD in some families. Even in ICCA families, epilepsy may recur later in life (Lee *et al.*, 1998). Another syndrome related to ICCA could be that of rolandic epilepsy with PED and writer's cramp, inherited as an autosomal recessive trait in three members of an Italian family (Guerrini *et al.*, 1999).

Aetiology and pathophysiology

Given the association of BIS with PD in patients and families, it obviously is necessary to consider the current knowledge on each disorder separately, as the same basic mechanisms may well lead to either type of clinical manifestations, or both associated.

Aetiology and pathophysiology of paroxysmal dyskinesia

Most PD are idiopathic and can be inherited as monogenic (usually autosomal dominant) traits (see below) or can be sporadic. In a few cases, PD look secondary (Blakeley & Jankovic, 2002). Causes for secondary PD include multiple sclerosis, hypoxic encephalopathy, diabetes mellitus, infarctions, and hypoparathyroidism (see also below) (Guerrini, 2001). Although little is known on the pathophysiology of the PD, it has been hypothesized that PD are ion channel disorders because channelopathies include some forms of inherited epilepsies (Szepetowski & Roll, 2002) as well as other types of paroxysmal movement disorders (Kullmann, 2002). Generally, mutations in ion channel genes represent a major cause of paroxysmal neurological disorders (Singh *et al.*, 1999; Berkovic, 2000). PD have also been viewed as subcortical epilepsy that involves the thalamus or the basal ganglia (Margari *et al.*, 2005), because of the paroxysmal character of the attacks, the detection of specific lesions of the basal ganglia in some secondary PKD, the possible existence of aura symptoms, and the neuroimaging abnormalities that have been reported. Abnormal cortical and spinal functioning has also been proposed. Recently, electrophysiological analyses detected abnormal patterns of cortical and spinal inhibition pathways in a series of 11 patients with idiopathic PKD (Mir *et al.*, 2005). The impaired patterns looked different from those described in primary dystonia and in epilepsy.

Table I. The genetic loci for BFIS, PD, ICCA, ICCA-like (BIS + PD), and related syndromes

Syndrome	Locus	Gene	Function	Special features	References
BFIS	16p12-q12			A homozygous patient had BIS with PD	Caraballo et al., 2001 Weber et al., 2004 Callenbach et al., 2005 Striano et al., 2006 Guipponi et al., 1997 Zara et al., 2001 Vanmolkot et al., 2003
	19q13				
	2q24				
	1q23	ATP1A2	Na/K pump subunit	BIS is associated with hemiplegic migraine	
PD					
PKD	1p34-p33			PKD is associated with episodic ataxia and spasticity	Auburger et al., 1996
	16p12-q12				Bennett et al., 2000 Cuenca-Leon et al., 2002 Valente et al., 2000
	16q12-q21				
PNKD	2q35	MR1	Unknown		Lee et al., 2004 Rainier et al., 2004
ICCA/ICCA-like	16p12-q12			Six out of eight PKD families had BIS Nine out of ten PKD families had BIS	Szepetowski et al., 1997 Lee et al., 1998 Tomita et al., 1999 Swoboda et al., 2000
Related syndromes					
RE-PED-WC	16p12			Consanguinity	Guerrini et al., 1999
Absence Epilepsy + PD	10q22	KCNMA1	Ca-activated K channel subunit	One single family	Du et al., 2005
BFIS/BFNS	2q24	SCN2A	Na channel subunit	Neonatal/Infantile intermediate phenotype	Heron et al., 2002 Berkovic et al., 2004

BFIS: benign familial infantile seizures. BFNS: benign familial neonatal seizures. PD: paroxysmal dyskinesia. PKD: paroxysmal kinesigenic dyskinesia. PNKD: paroxysmal non-kinesigenic dyskinesia. ICCA: infantile convulsions and paroxysmal choreoathetosis. RE-PED-WC: rolandic epilepsy, paroxysmal exercice-induced dystonia, and writer's cramp. Na: sodium. K: potassium. Ca: calcium.

Aetiology and pathophysiology of benign infantile seizures

Both familial and non-familial forms of BIS have been described (see Chapter 3). Familial BIS, or benign familial infantile convulsions (BFIC), are inherited as autosomal dominant traits and numerous genetic studies have proved successful (see below).

Table II. 16p12-q12 is a major genetic locus for autosomal dominant** BFIS, PKD, ICCA, and ICCA-like syndromes

Syndrome	Critical markers	Size (Mb)	Number of families	Position	References
BFIS					
	D16S401-D16S415	27,6	7	16p12-q12	Caraballo et al., 2001
	D16S690-D16S3136	21,4	14	16p11-q12	Weber et al., 2004
	D16S403-D16S685	7,6	2	16p12-p11	Callenbach et al., 2005
	D16S313-D16S415	25,2	16*	16p12-q12	Striano et al., 2006
PKD					
	D16S3100-D16S771	26,6	1	16p12-q12	Bennett et al., 2000
	D16S3145-D16S3398	35,6	1	16p12-q21	Cuenca-Leon et al., 2002
	D16S416-D16S503	12	1	16q12-q21	Valente et al., 2000
ICCA/ICCA-like					
	D16S401-D16S517	23,6	4	16p12-q12	Szepetowski et al., 1997
	D16S420-D16S416	26	1	16p12-q12	Lee et al., 1998
	D16S3093-D16S416	23,5	8 (2 with PKD only)	16p12-q12	Tomita et al., 1999
	D16S3131-D16S3396	23,8	10 (1 with PKD only)	16p12-q12	Swoboda et al., 2000
RE-PED-WC					
	D16S3133-D16S3131	1,3	1**	16p12	Guerrini et al., 1999

BFIS: benign familial infantile seizures. PKD: paroxysmal kinesigenic dyskinesia. ICCA: infantile convulsions and paroxysmal choreoathetosis. RE-PED-WC: rolandic epilepsy, paroxysmal exercice-induced dystonia, and writer's cramp. Mb: Megabases. *: One patient in a family had brief episodes of dystonia. **: RE-PED-WC syndrome has recessive mode of inheritance.

Non-familial forms could have genetic or non-genetic bases. Possible genetic causes may be *de novo* mutations, either in the genes that also underlie the familial forms, or in other types of genes. Somatic mutations and RNA editing cannot be excluded. Viral aetiology has also been proposed, as a subset of infantile seizures has been associated with mild gastroenteritis caused by rotavirus infection (Abe et al., 2000). The viral hypothesis remains speculative, but it is noteworthy that rotavirus has neuronal tropism and that non-cytolytic neuronal infection may cause alterations in the polarized sorting of neuronal proteins such as MAP2 (Microtubule-associated protein 2) (Weclewicz et al., 1993).

Aetiology and pathophysiology of ICCA/ICCA-like (BIS + PD) syndrome

Again, mutations in ion channel genes could provide a single explanation for the pathophysiology of the link between epilepsy and PD. As a matter of fact, a missense mutation in the potassium channel gene *KCNMA1* located onto human chromosome 10q22, has been found in a single family where absence epilepsy and PD co-segregated (Du et al., 2005). Association and inheritance as a single monogenic trait of BIS with PD has been observed in several families and one major gene has been mapped, albeit not identified yet, onto chromosome 16 (see below) *(Tables I & II)*.

Only very few sporadic cases have been reported (Koch *et al.*, 1999). A patient with idiopathic hypoparathyroidism and calcifications in the basal ganglia (Hattori & Yorifuji, 2000) had epileptic and dyskinetic manifestations indistinguishable from those of the familial ICCA syndrome (Szepetowski *et al.*, 1997). Paroxysmal dyskinesia with secondary generalization of tonic-clonic seizures has also been reported in a case of pseudohypoparathyroidism (Huang *et al.*, 2005). Hypoparathyroidism with hypocalcemia and calcifications in the basal ganglia have also been described as a secondary cause of PKD (Tabaee-Zadeh *et al.*, 1972; Christiansen & Hansen, 1972; Barabas & Tucker, 1988).

Genetics

Genetics of paroxysmal dyskinesia

Paroxysmal kinesigenic dyskinesia

Sporadic and familial cases of PKD have been described, and some genetic studies have been performed successfully *(Table I)*. An autosomal dominant and peculiar form of PKD associated with episodic ataxia and spasticity has been mapped at chromosome 1p (Auburger *et al.* 1996). More recently, one PKD locus (namely PKC1) has been mapped at the ICCA locus (see below) onto chromosome 16 in one large family of Afro-Caribean origin (Bennett *et al.*, 2000) *(Fig. 1)*. Other so-called PKD families have also been mapped to the same locus (Tomita *et al.*, 1999; Swoboda *et al.*, 2000) *(Fig. 1, Tables I & II)*. However, nearly all families in the two studies displayed patients with BIS too – so they should better be considered as ICCA or ICCA-like families rather than pure PKD families. One additional PKD family of Indian origin has also been mapped to human chromosome 16 (Valente *et al.*, 2000) but the locus (EKD2) apparently does not overlap that of the other ICCA and PKD families *(Fig. 1)*. This may well be due to the existence of two different PKD genes on chromosome 16. However, errors in the genetic and physical maps must also be considered. To date, no PKD gene is identified yet and the pathophysiology of those PKD that have genetic basis remains unknown.

Paroxysmal non-kinesigenic dyskinesia

Familial PNKD is classically inherited as an autosomal dominant disorder. It is characterized by spontaneous hyperkinetic attacks that can be triggered by a large variety of stimuli, including fatigue, stress, menstruation, coffee and alcohol. Genetic linkage had been obtained at chromosome 2q35 (Fouad *et al.*, 1996; Fink *et al.*, 1996; Hofele *et al.*, 1997) *(Table I)* and two recurrent missense mutations (*i.e.* gene mutations that change an aminoacid for a different one in the corresponding protein) in the non-ion channel gene *MR1* have been identified in the 14 families tested so far (Lee *et al.*, 2004; Rainier *et al.*, 2004). The two mutations, A7V and A9V, are located in the same N-terminal alpha helix of the protein. MR1 codes for a protein that may act as a myofibrillogenesis regulator but its actual function, in the brain particularly, remains unknown. The *MR1* gene is expressed in various areas of the brain, such as the spinal cord, the cerebellum,

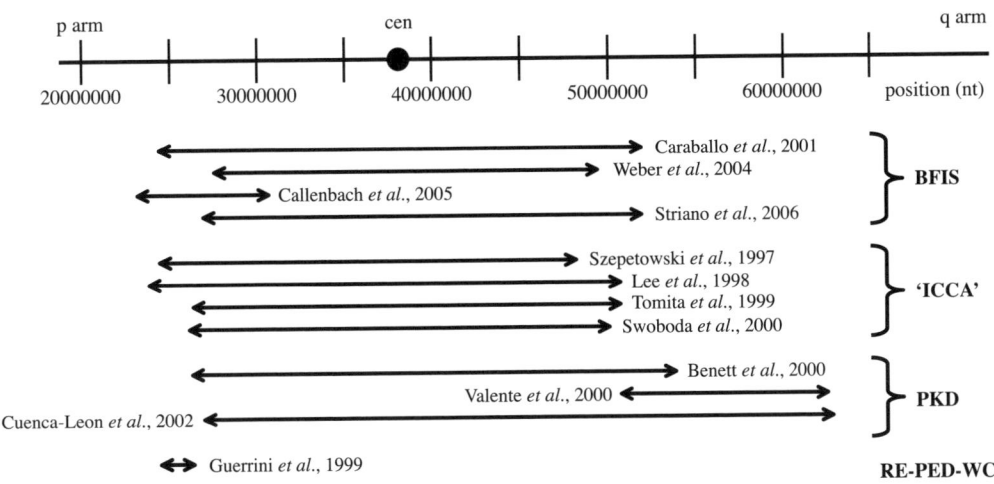

Figure 1. A map of the major ICCA/BFIS/PKD locus at the pericentromeric region of human chromosome 16. The boundaries of the critical areas are taken from the references as mentioned in the figure and their respective locations are taken from the March 2006 (NCBI Build 36.1) human genome sequence assembly at the UCSC (University of California Santa Cruz) website (http://genome.ucsc.edu). Positions are given in nucleotides (nt).

cen: centromere. BFIS: benign familial infantile seizures. "ICCA": infantile convulsions with paroxysmal choreoathetosis, and ICCA-like syndromes. PKD: paroxysmal kinesigenic dyskinesia. RE-PED-WC: rolandic epilepsy with paroxysmal exercise-induced dystonia and writer's cramp.

and the basal ganglia. These structures are known to play a crucial role in motor function. How *MR1* mutations may cause the disease remains elusive. Interestingly, the MR1 protein displays amino acid sequence homology to that of the HAGH (hydroxyacylglutathione hydrolase) protein. HAGH participates in the glyoxalase system – which detoxifies methylglyoxal. Coffee and alcohol are well known triggering factors for PNKD attacks and they indeed contain high levels of methylglyoxal. However, whether MR1 plays similar detoxifying role remains unknown.

Genetics of benign infantile seizures

Familial BIS, or benign familial infantile convulsions (BFIC), is an autosomal dominant disorder with incomplete penetrance. Several BFIC genes have been mapped to various genetic loci, thus demonstrating genetic heterogeneity *(Table I)*. One BFIC gene has been mapped to chromosome 19q in five families of Italian origin (Guipponi et al., 1997). At 16p12-q12, linkage has been demonstrated in several independent studies *(Table II)*, representing more than 30 families in total (Caraballo et al., 2001; Weber et al., 2004; Callenbach et al., 2005; Striano et al., 2006). A third locus at 2q24 has been proposed in four additional Italian families (Malacarne et al., 2001). The 16p12-q12 locus not only is the most frequently involved, but also is major in those familial BIS that are associated with PD *(Table II)*. A fourth BFIC locus associated with an atypical form of BIS has been postulated in a Chinese family as all three other BFIC loci were excluded (Xiao et al., 2005). In one Dutch-Canadian family where BIS and hemiplegic migraine co-segregated, a R689Q missense mutation in the *ATP1A2* gene that encodes a sodium/potassium pump subunit has been identified (Vanmolkot *et al.*, 2003). The *ATP1A2* gene maps at chromosome 1q23 and mutations in pure familial hemiplegic migraine had been previously reported (De Fusco *et al.*, 2003). Despite these promising findings, *ATP1A2* may not be involved in pure familial BIS (Martinelli Boneschi *et al.*, 2005). Further genetic heterogeneity is indicated by genetic exclusion of 1q23, 2q24, 16p12-q12 and 19q in at least one more BFIC family of Dutch origin (Callenbach *et al.*, 2005). Higher level of complexity might exist, as demonstrated by the recent definition of an intermediate phenotype of benign familial neonatal-infantile convulsions (BFNIC) with mutations in the sodium channel gene *SCN2A* (Heron *et al.*, 2002, Berkovic *et al.*, 2004).

Genetics of ICCA/ICCA-like (BIS + PD)

The ICCA syndrome is an autosomal dominant trait with incomplete penetrance and phenotypic variability. It had initially been characterized by the familial association of BIS with PNKD but familial BIS can be associated with PKD too. Pure BIS apparently are not distinguishable from those BIS that occur in the context of the ICCA syndrome. The first four ICCA families originated from Northwestern France (Szepetowski *et al.*, 1997). Earlier descriptions of sporadic or familial cases had been reported (Pryles *et al.*, 1952; Hudgins & Corbin, 1966). The ICCA syndrome has been linked genetically to the pericentromeric region of chromosome 16 (Szepetowski *et al.*, 1997) *(Tables I & II)*. This represented the first genetic evidence for shared mechanisms between these two paroxysmal disorders. The ICCA locus appears to be by far the most important in the BIS that are associated with various subtypes of PD, whether kinesigenic or not (Lee *et al.*, 1998; Tomita *et al.*, 1999; Swoboda *et al.*, 2000) *(Tables I & II)*. Moreover, pure BFIC have also been linked to the ICCA region in several independent studies (Caraballo *et al.*, 2001; Weber *et al.*, 2004; Callenbach *et al.*, 2005) *(Table II)*. One patient in a peculiar BIS family deserves more attention, as he inherited two copies of the disease haplotype because of consanguinity (Caraballo *et al.*, 2001). While all his relatives (who were heterozygous for the mutant allele) had typical BIS only, this patient had both BIS and early-onset PD. This raised the possibility that, at least in this case, whether BIS associates with PD or not may have genetic basis. A different and quite related syndrome, called autosomal recessive RE-PED-WC (rolandic epilepsy with paroxysmal dystonia and writer's cramp), has also been linked to the ICCA locus in one consanguine family (Guerrini *et al.*, 1999). The region of homozygosity entirely lies within the 10-cM ICCA area (Szepetowski *et al.*, 1997) *(Fig. 1)*.

The ICCA gene remains unidentified to date. A large number of genes still lie within the critical area(s). Numerous genes have been screened unsuccessfully (Roll *et al.*, 2002. Kato *et al.*, 2006). The disease gene might well be one with unknown function – and this type of gene usually is screened only after better candidates have been excluded. 16p12-q12 is a pericentromeric region. This genomic area shows very complex genomic structure with highly duplicated large DNA sequence (see the human genome sequence website at http://genome.ucsc.edu) and this makes it the mutation search more complicated, with the existence of nearly identical copies of a given gene lying close to each other at the same chromosomal locus. Although those BIS, PKD and ICCA syndromes that are linked to 16p12-q12 might well be allelic (*i.e.* caused by mutations within the same gene), the existence of several homologous disease genes in this particular chromosomal region cannot be ruled out. Moreover, the occurrence of large-scale genomic rearrangements such as deletions, duplications, and inversions cannot be excluded, as these events would be favoured in the context of a complicated genomic architecture. Whatever its function, the identification of the causative gene will shed new and important insights on the pathophysiology of BIS, PD, and of their close relationship in the context of ICCA and ICCA-like syndromes.

References

- Abe T, Kobayashi M, Araki K, *et al*. Infantile convulsions with mild gastroenteritis. *Brain Dev* 2000; 22: 301-6.

- Auburger G, Ratzlaff T, Lunkes A, *et al*. A gene for autosomal dominant paroxysmal choreoathetosis/spasticity (CSE) maps to the vicinity of a potassium channel gene cluster on chromosome 1p, probably within 2 cM between D1S443 and D1S197. *Genomics* 1996; 31: 90-4.

- Barabas G, Tucker SM. Idiopathic hypoparathyroidism and paroxysmal dystonic choreoathetosis. *Ann Neurol* 1988; 24: 585.

- Beaumanoir ML, Mira L, Van Lierde A. Epilepsy or paroxysmal kinesigenic choreoathetosis? *Brain Dev* 1996; 18: 139-41.

- Bennett LB, Roach ES, Bowcock AM. A locus for paroxysmal kinesigenic dyskinesia maps to human chromosome 16. *Neurology* 2000; 54: 125-30.

- Berkovic SF. Paroxysmal movement disorders and epilepsy: links across the channel. *Neurology* 2000; 55: 169-70.

- Berkovic SF, Heron SE, Giordano L, *et al*. Benign familial neonatal-infantile seizures: characterization of a new sodium channelopathy. *Ann Neurol* 2004; 55: 550-7.

- Bigal ME, Lipton RB, Cohen J, Silberstein SD. Epilepsy and migraine. *Epilepsy Behav* 2003; Suppl 2: S13-24.

- Bing F, Dananchet Y, Vercueil L. A family with exercise-induced paroxysmal dystonia and childhood absence epilepsy. *Rev Neurol* (Paris) 2005; 161: 817-22.

- Blakeley J, Jankovic J. Secondary causes of paroxysmal dyskinesia. *Adv Neurol* 2002; 89: 401-20.

- Boel M, Casaer P. Paroxysmal kinesigenic choreoathetosis. *Neuropediatrics* 1984; 15: 215-7.

- Bruno MK, Hallett M, Gwinn-Hardy K, *et al*. Clinical evaluation of idiopathic paroxysmal kinesigenic dyskinesia: new diagnostic criteria. *Neurology* 2004; 63: 2280-7.

- Callenbach PM, van den Boogerd EH, de Coo RF, *et al*. Refinement of the chromosome 16 locus for benign familial infantile convulsions. *Clin Genet* 2005; 67: 517-25.

- Caraballo R, Pavek S, Lemainque A, *et al*. Linkage of benign familial infantile convulsions to chromosome 16p12-q12 suggests allelism to the infantile convulsions and choreoathetosis syndrome. *Am J Hum Genet* 2001; 68: 788-94.

- Christiansen NJ, Hansen PF. Choreiform movements in hypoparathyroidism. *N Engl J Med* 1972; 287: 569-70.

- Cuenca-Leon E, Cormand B, Thomson T, Macaya A. Paroxysmal kinesigenic dyskinesia and generalized seizures: clinical and genetic analysis in a Spanish pedigree. *Neuropediatrics* 2002; 33: 288-93.

- De Fusco M, Marconi R, Silvestri L, *et al*. Haploinsufficiency of ATP1A2 encoding the Na+/K+ pump alpha2 subunit associated with familial hemiplegic migraine type 2. *Nat Genet* 2003; 33: 192-6.

- Demirkiran M, Jankovic J. Paroxysmal dyskinesias: clinical features and classification. *Ann Neurol* 1995; 38: 571-9.

- Du W, Bautista JF, Yang H, *et al*. Calcium-sensitive potassium channelopathy in human epilepsy and paroxysmal movement disorder. *Nat Genet* 2005; 37: 733-8.

• Fink JK, Rainer S, Wilkowski J, et al. Paroxysmal dystonic choreoathetosis: tight linkage to chromosome 2q. *Am J Hum Genet* 1996; 59: 140-5.

• Fouad GT, Servidei S, Durcan S, Bertini E, Ptacek LJ. A gene for familial paroxysmal dyskinesia (FPD1) maps to chromosome 2q. *Am J Hum Genet* 1996; 59: 135-9.

• Fukuyama Y, Okada R. Hereditary kinesigenic reflex epilepsy. Report of five families of peculiar seizures induced by sudden movements. *Adv Neurol Sci* 1967; 11: 168-97.

• Guerrini R, Bonanni P, Nardocci N, et al. Autosomal recessive rolandic epilepsy with paroxysmal exercise-induced dystonia and writer's cramp: delineation of the syndrome and gene mapping to chromosome 16p12-11.2. *Ann Neurol* 1999; 45: 344-52.

• Guerrini R. Idiopathic epilepsy and paroxysmal dyskinesia. *Epilepsia* 2001; 42 Suppl 3: 36-41.

• Guerrini R, Sanchez-Carpintero R, Deonna T, et al. Early-onset absence epilepsy and paroxysmal dyskinesia. *Epilepsia* 2002; 43: 1224-9.

• Guipponi M, Rivier F, Vigevano F, et al. Linkage mapping of benign familial infantile convulsions (BFIC) to chromosome 19q. *Hum Mol Genet* 1997; 6: 473-7.

• Hattori H, Fujii T, Nigami H, Higuchi Y, Tsuji M, Hamada Y. Co-segregation of benign infantile convulsions and paroxysmal kinesigenic choreoathetosis. *Brain Dev* 2000; 22: 432-5.

• Hattori H, Yorifuji T. Infantile convulsions and paroxysmal kinesigenic choreoathetosis in a patient with idiopathic hypoparathyroidism. *Brain Dev* 2000; 22: 449-50.

• Heron SE, Crossland KM, Andermann E, et al. Sodium-channel defects in benign familial neonatal-infantile seizures. *Lancet* 2002; 360: 851-2.

• Hirata K, Katayama S, Saito T, et al. Paroxysmal kinesigenic choreoathetosis with abnormal electroencephalogram during attacks. *Epilepsia* 1991; 32: 492-4.

• Hofele K, Benecke R, Auburger G. Gene locus FPD1 of the dystonic Mount-Reback type of autosomal-dominant paroxysmal choreoathetosis. *Neurology* 1997; 49: 1252-7.

• Huang CW, Chen YC, Tsai JJ. Paroxysmal dyskinesia with secondary generalization of tonic-clonic seizures in pseudohypoparathyroidism. *Epilepsia* 2005; 46: 164-5.

• Hudgins RL, Corbin KB. An uncommon seizure disorder: familial paroxysmal choreoathetosis. *Brain* 1966; 89: 199-204.

• Jankovic J, Demirkiran M. Classification of paroxysmal dyskinesias and ataxias. *Adv Neurol* 2002; 89: 387-400.

• Kato N, Sadamatsu M, Kikuchi T, Niikawa N, Fukuyama Y. Paroxysmal kinesigenic choreoathetosis: from first discovery in 1892 to genetic linkage with benign familial infantile convulsions. *Epilepsy Res* 2006; 70 Suppl 1: S174-84.

• Kinast M, Erenberg G, Rothner AD. Paroxysmal choreoathetosis: report of five cases and review of the literature. *Pediatrics* 1980; 65: 74-7.

• Koch C, Bednarek N, Motte J. Benign epileptic seizures in infancy followed by paroxysmal choreo-athetosis during adolescence. *Epileptic Disord* 1999; 1: 141-2.

• Lee WL, Tay A, Ong, HT, Goh LM, Monaco AP, Szepetowski P. Association of infantile convulsions with paroxysmal dyskinesias (ICCA syndrome): confirmation of linkage to human chromosome 16p12-q12 in a Chinese family. *Hum Genet* 1998; 103: 608-12.

• Lee HY, Xu Y, Huang Y, et al. The gene for paroxysmal non-kinesigenic dyskinesia encodes an enzyme in a stress response pathway. *Hum Mol Genet* 2004; 13: 3161-70.

• Lombroso C. Paroxysmal choreoathetosis: an epileptic or non-epileptic disorder? *Ital J Neurol Sci* 1995; 16: 271-7.

- Malacarne M, Gennaro E, Madia F, et al. Benign familial infantile convulsions: mapping of a novel locus on chromosome 2q24 and evidence for genetic heterogeneity. *Am J Hum Genet* 2001; 68: 1521-6.

- Margari L, Presicci A, Ventura P, Margari F, Perniola T. Channelopathy: hypothesis of a common pathophysiologic mechanism in different forms of paroxysmal dyskinesia. *Pediatr Neurol* 2005; 32: 229-35.

- Martinelli Boneschi F, Aridon P, Zara F, et al. No evidence of ATP1A2 involvement in 12 multiplex Italian families with benign familial infantile seizures. *Neurosci Lett* 2005; 388: 71-4.

- Mir P, Huang YZ, Gilio F, et al. Abnormal cortical and spinal inhibition in paroxysmal kinesigenic dyskinesia. *Brain* 2005; 128: 291-9.

- Mount LA, Reback S. Familial paroxysmal choreoathetosis; preliminary report on a hitherto undescribed clinical syndrome. *Arch Neurol Psychiatr* 1940; 44: 841-7.

- Pryles CV, Livingston S, Ford FR. Familial paroxysmal choreoathetosis of Mount and Reback: study of a second family in which this condition is found in association with epilepsy. *Pediatrics* 1952; 9: 44-7.

- Rainier S, Thomas D, Tokarz D, et al. Myofibrillogenesis regulator 1 gene mutations cause paroxysmal dystonic choreoathetosis. *Arch Neurol* 2004; 61: 1025-9.

- Richards RN, Barnett HJ. Paroxysmal dystonic choreoathetosis. A family study and review of the literature. *Neurology* 1968; 18: 461-9.

- Roll P, Szepetowski P. Epilepsy and ionic channels. *Epileptic Disord* 2002; 4: 165-72.

- Roll P, Massacrier A, Pereira S, Robaglia-Schlupp A, Cau P, Szepetowski P. New human sodium/glucose cotransporter gene (KST1): identification, characterization, and mutation analysis in ICCA (infantile convulsions and choreoathetosis) and BFIC (benign familial infantile convulsions) families. *Gene* 2002; 285: 141-8.

- Roll P, Rudolf G, Pereira S, et al. SRPX2 mutations in disorders of language cortex and cognition. *Hum Mol Genet* 2006; 15: 1195-207.

- Sadamatsu M, Masui A, Sakai T, Kunugi H, Nanko S, Kato N. Familial paroxysmal kinesigenic choreoathetosis: an electrophysiologic and genotypic analysis. *Epilepsia* 1999; 40: 942-9.

- Singh R, Macdonell RA, Scheffer IE, Crossland KM, Berkovic SF. Epilepsy and paroxysmal movement disorders in families: evidence for shared mechanisms. *Epileptic Disord* 1999; 1: 93-9.

- Stevens HF. Paroxysmal choreoathetosis: a form of reflex epilepsy. *Arch Neurol* 1966; 14: 415-20.

- Striano P, Lispi ML, Gennaro E, et al. Linkage analysis and disease models in benign familial infantile seizures: a study of 16 families. *Epilepsia* 2006; 47: 1029-34.

- Swoboda KJ, Soong B, McKenna C, et al. Paroxysmal kinesigenic dyskinesia and infantile convulsions: clinical and linkage studies. *Neurology* 2000; 55: 224-30.

- Szepetowski P, Rochette J, Berquin P, Piussan C, Lathrop GM, Monaco AP. Familial infantile convulsions and paroxysmal choreoathetosis: a new neurological syndrome linked to the pericentromeric region of human chromosome 16. *Am J Hum Genet* 1997; 61: 889-98.

- Tabaee-Zadeh MJ, Frame B, Kapphahn K. Kinesiogenic choreoathetosis and idiopathic hypoparathyroidism. *N Engl J Med* 1972; 286: 762-63.

- Thiriaux A, de St Martin A, Vercueil L, et al. Co-occurrence of infantile epileptic seizures and childhood paroxysmal choreoathetosis in one family: clinical, EEG, and SPECT characterization of episodic events. *Mov Disord* 2002; 17: 98-104.

- Tomita H, Nagamitsu S, Wakui K, et al. Paroxysmal kinesigenic choreoathetosis locus map to chromosome 16p11.2-q12.1. *Am J Hum Genet* 1999; 65: 1688-97.

- Tuchman R, Rapin I. Epilepsy in autism. *Lancet Neurol* 2002; 1: 352-8.

- Valente EM, Spacey SD, Wali GM, *et al*. A second paroxysmal kinesigenic choreoathetosis locus (EKD2) mapping on 16q13-q22.1 indicates a family of genes which give rise to paroxysmal disorders on human chromosome 16. *Brain* 2000; 123: 2040-5.

- Vanmolkot KR, Kors EE, Hottenga JJ, *et al*. Novel mutations in the Na+, K+-ATPase pump gene ATP1A2 associated with familial hemiplegic migraine and benign familial infantile convulsions. *Ann Neurol* 2003; 54: 360-6.

- Weber YG, Berger A, Bebek N, *et al*. Benign familial infantile convulsions: linkage to chromosome 16p12-q12 in 14 families. *Epilepsia* 2004; 45: 601-9.

- Weclewicz K, Svensson L, Billger M, Holmberg K, Wallin M, Kristensson K. Microtubule-associated protein 2 appears in axons of cultured dorsal root ganglia and spinal cord neurons after rotavirus infection. *J Neurosci Res* 1993; 36: 173-82.

- Xiao B, Deng FY, Xiong G, *et al*. Clinical and genetic study on a new Chinese family with benign familial infantile seizures. *Eur J Neurol* 2005; 12: 344-9.

Benign infantile focal epilepsy with midline spikes and waves during sleep

Giuseppe Capovilla, Francesca Beccaria
Mantova, Italy

The scenario of early onset focal epilepsies has been changed with years and, nowadays, the existence of idiopathic cases has been accepted worldwide. In fact, cases of focal idiopathic infantile epilepsies with benign outcome have been repeatedly described in many countries (Fukuyama, 1963; Watanabe *et al.*, 1987, 1990, 1996; Vigevano *et al.*, 1992, 1994; Lee *et al.*, 1993; Echenne *et al.*, 1994; Okumura *et al.*, 1996; Caraballo *et al.*, 1997, 2003; Capovilla *et al.*, 1998; Gautier *et al.*, 1999; Capovilla & Vigevano, 2002; Fejerman, 2002; Vigevano & Bureau, 2005; Franzoni *et al.*, 2005; Cahine & Mikati, 2006; Kaleyias *et al.*, 2006; Specchio & Vigevano, 2006) and their existence has been accepted by the international scientific community, and two specific syndromes of non-familial and familial benign infantile seizures were included in the ILAE's proposed diagnostic scheme for people with epileptic seizures and with epilepsy (Engel, 2001). Diagnosis of these two conditions, in particular for non-familial cases, is difficult and often retrospective (Okumura *et al.*, 2000), mostly due to the lack of a specific interictal pattern. Moreover, even if some authors recently described some cases with interictal epileptic discharges localized in the frontal or occipital lobes in different patients (Weber, 2004), one of the inclusion criteria to consider these forms as idiopathic continues to be the absence of interictal EEG abnormalities, both at the awake state and during sleep. (Watanabe *et al.*, 1987, 1990, 1996; Vigevano *et al.*, 1992, 1994; Lee *et al.*, 1993; Echenne *et al.*, 1994; Okumura *et al.*, 1996, 2000; Caraballo *et al.*, 1997, 2003; Franzoni *et al.*, 2005; Kaleyias *et al.*, 2006). In the clinical practice, the consequences are that the epileptologists themselves are cautios when they see interictal spikes, and an uncertain prognosis is often made.

In 2000, Capovilla and Beccaria described an electroclinical picture of focal benign infantile seizures characterized by the presence of peculiar sleep EEG abnormalities in the vertex regions and called it "benign partial epilepsy in infancy and early childhood with vertex spikes and waves during sleep (BVSE)". Clinical seizures are different from Watanabe's and Vigevano's cases. Without delineating a specific syndrome, the same EEG pattern was observed and described previously as an indicator of benignity in children of the same age (Bureau & Maton, 1998). Later on, this same group published a series of ten cases adding more data on the semciology of the seizures and reinforcing the value of the particular EEG marker (Bureau *et al.*, 2002). Regarding the presence of the interictal EEG abnormalities, there is some contradiction in not considering idiopathic the cases of babies with clinical features of benign seizures if they present EEG paroxysms, and on the side we use the findings of certain Rolandic or occipital spikes to reinforce our diagnosis of benign epilepsies of childhood.

Recently, we proposed to change the name and the acronym of BVSE and named this form "benign focal epilepsy in infancy with midline spikes and waves during sleep" (BIMSE), to avoid a confusing terminology with physiological sleep vertex spikes (Capovilla *et al.*, 2006). Interestingly, after the first described epileptic cases, we observed the peculiar EEG marker that characterizes this syndrome both in non-epileptic and febrile convulsion patients, similarly to functional focal spikes we observe at an older age. Some authors (Bureau *et al.*, 2002) think that midline spikes and waves, due to their difficult recognition, could have been overlooked by the authors that stressed the absence of interictal EEG paroxysms in their published series of benign focal infantile epilepsies. This possibility cannot be excluded, as midline spikes are difficult to recognize and, often, electrodes in the vertex regions are not placed at this age. We are sure that we didn't miss midline spikes in our first series of 12 sporadic non-Japanese patients with the clinical features described as benign complex partial epilepsy in infancy (Watanabe *et al.*, 1987, 1990), neither did we find those spikes in our personal non-familial or familial cases of benign infantile seizures (BIS) (Capovilla, 2002).

Epidemiology

The prevalence of BIMSE among our epileptic patients under two years of age was 11.5%, but no other data about the frequence of this particular condition have been reported. The prevalence of familial and non-familial BIS has already been described in Chapter 3. The wide variations, ranging from 6% to more than 30% in children under 2 years of age [Okumura *et al.*, 2000; Nelson *et al.*, 2002; Caraballo & Fejerman (Chapter 3)] may point two a possible recruiting bias. In our center we have a total prevalence (including BIMSE cases) of 30.5% of idiopathic cases among all the infant with focal epilepsies. These higher prevalence figures reflect a better awareness of the existence of these conditions.

General clinical features

Personal and familial history

Pre-, peri- and post-natal personal history was negative in all patients. Psychomotor development was normal, both before and after seizure onset. A positive family history of epilepsy was present in 48% of cases. An additional 15% had a positive family history for febrile seizures.

Neuroimaging studies

The first patients we observed were subjected to neuroradiological scans (CAT and/or MRI) and all of them had normal results. In the subsequent patients, the electroclinical picture and, in particular, the presence of interictal spikes permitted the diagnosis so that neuroradiological investigation had been exceptionally made.

Age at onset

In our first description (Capovilla & Beccaria, 2000), we wrote that age at onset was comprised between 13 and 30 months, with a peak between 16 and 20 months. But, subsequently, we observed cases with an earlier onset age. The younger personal observed case started with seizures at age 4 months and some colleagues from Italy referred to us about other typical cases whose seizure onset was in the second trimester of life. Our opinion is that, because the clinical symptomatology is often difficult to detect by parents, the first episodes can be unrecognized and the onset could be earlier than we reported for the first described patients, in particular for those patients with an onset after the second year of life. However, the majority of the patients (62%) presented their first seizure in the middle semester of the second year of life and our opinion is that the second year of life is the typical age onset period (80% of cases).

Seizure recurrence and age of seizure disappearance

About one third of our BIMSE patients presented a unique seizure. In the remaining patients, the attacks ceased mostly between the second and the third year of life. In all cases seizures were sporadic. In about one third of the cases, seizures clustered in 24-48 hours with up to 6-8. Some of the patients that clustered did not present any other attacks during evolution.

Seizure manifestations

Cyanosis (90%), in particular of the perioral region of the face, motion arrest (84%) and/or staring (90%) were the predominant ictal signs. Stiffening, in particular of the arms, was present in 47% of cases. Automatisms or lateralizing signs were rarely present (15%). Often, at the end of the attack, the infant felt asleep. Secondary generalization was never referred. Regarding loss of consciousness, we can say that it is often difficult, at this age, to distinguish between staring and loss of consciousness, also because that the parents are frightened by the seizure. Moreover, the attacks are rarely observed by epileptologists. In the case we video-recorded, loss of consciousness was not clear. Seizure length, as referred by parents, was comprised between 1 and 5 minutes. In all patients, the seizures occurred while awake but in about one quarter of the cases also during sleep. We had the opportunity to record on video-EEG a typical fit in an eighteen month old infant. The seizure was characterized by cyanosis and staring, without a complete loss of consciousness. The attack was stopped by the rectal administration of 10 mg Diazepam after 4 minutes from the onset.

EEG features

The peculiar EEG feature of this form is the presence of typical focal EEG paroxysms in the midline regions, spreading to the central and, more rarely, temporal regions *(Fig. 1)*. Such abnormalities appear only during sleep. They can be isolated or grouped in short sequences, in sleep

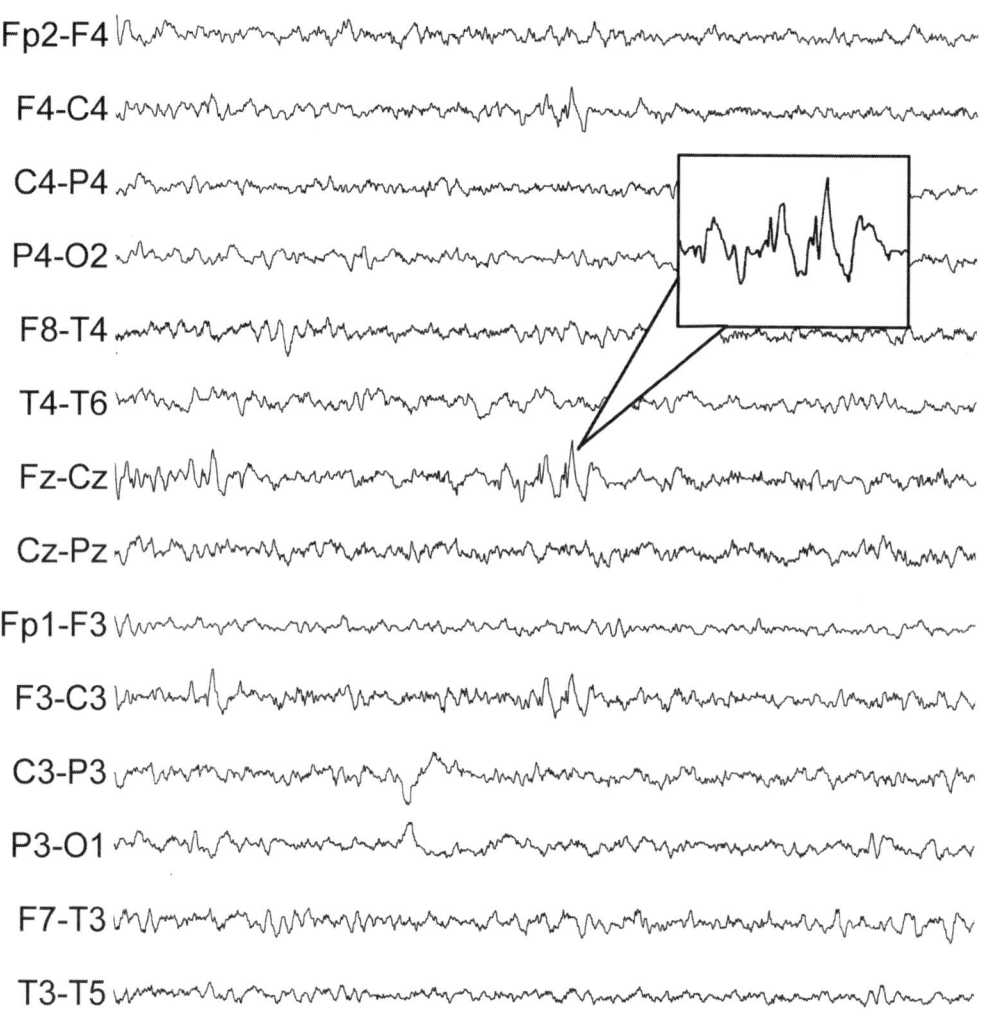

Figure 1. Two year 11 month old male infant. Typical spikes, followed by a bell shaped slow wave, are evident in the midline regions. They spread to both central areas.

stage I, but are more frequent during stage II. We described them as "a low voltage fast spike followed by a higher bell-shaped slow wave" (Capovilla & Beccaria, 2000; Capovilla & Vigevano, 2001; Capovilla *et al.*, 2006). This morphology is clearly different both from physiological sleep vertex spikes and from the EEG abnormalities observed in idiopathic focal epilepsies at an older age, like benign epilepsy with centrotemporal spikes and benign epilepsy with occipital spikes *(Fig. 2)*. The age of disappearance of midline spikes ranged from three years to 5 years and 6 months, even if, recently we observed their persistence in an eight years old healthy girl. We wrote, in previous papers, that this EEG trait was never found in normal infants (Capovilla

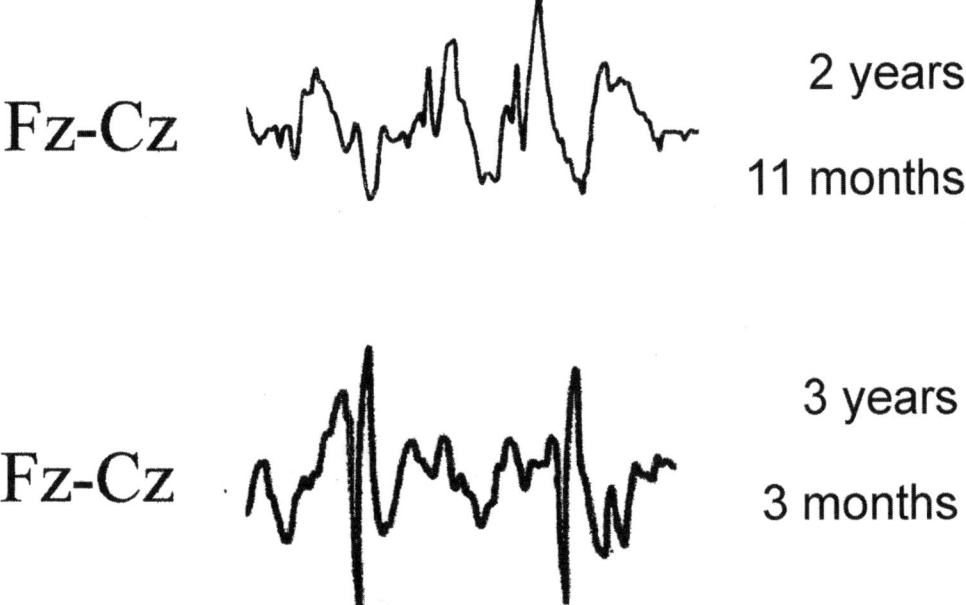

Figure 2. Top: Two typical BIMSE abnormalities. Clear morphological differences are evident with BCECTS abnormalities (bottom).

& Beccaria, 2000; Capovilla & Vigevano, 2001). But, recently, we found midline spikes in some patients presenting with a febrile convulsion and in three other patients with breath holding spells, who felt spontaneously asleep during their EEG records. In agreement with Bureau et al. (2002), we think that midline spikes can represent a EEG marker of benignity in infancy, similarly to functional spikes at an older age.

Aetiology and pathophysiology

On account of the low frequency of seizures and of the absence of epileptic status, as well as on its systematically favourable outcome and the neurological, neuroradiological and intellectual normality of the infants, we are convinced that BIMSE is an idiopathic epilepsy of infancy. This conviction is reinforced by the high rate of positive family history of epilepsy and by the recent observation of some familial cases. Moreover, we think that midline spikes are an EEG marker of benignity and their significance is similar to functional spikes in childhood.

The correlation between the topography of the EEG abnormalities and the clinical symptoms is unclear. In older papers, midline abnormalities have been often correlated to generalized mostly nocturnal seizures and were interpreted as fragments of generalized discharges (Ehle et al., 1981; Nelson et al.; 1983, Pourmand et al., 1984). It was reported that patients with midline spikes often present focal spikes arising from the mesial cerebral structures, both at pediatric and adult age (Mc Lachlan & Girvin, 1989, Kutluay *et al.*, 2001). Therefore, midline spikes should be interpreted as a pure focal EEG trait. Interestingly, in many papers published in the eighties, midline spikes were absent or scarce at awake state in many patients and they appeared or increased very much during sleep. (Ehle *et al.*, 1981; Nelson *et al.*, 1983; Pourmand *et al.*, 1984; Kutluay *et al.*, 2001). It is possible that, in BIMSE, the appearance of midline spikes only during sleep could be explained as an age-dependent over expression of this specific feature.

Diagnostic work up

Diagnostic steps in these infants comprise a neurological and developmental evaluation and an EEG captured both at awake state and, mainly, during sleep. We recommend to place always vertex electrodes since we know that, with the traditional EEG equipment, vertex electrodes are often excluded, in particular in infancy. Nowadays, the advent of the modern digital EEG technologies permits better to record from vertex electrodes, so that the typical EEG abnormalities could be easily detected. Neuroradiological investigations, in our opinion, could be avoided in the presence of a typical electroclinical context.

Differential diagnosis and relations with other epilepsy syndromes

Differential diagnosis includes both sporadic and familial benign focal seizures in infancy (BIS). As can be seen in *table I*, in these syndromes, which on average start at an earlier age, seizure frequency is much higher than in BIMSE. In addition, the clinical picture is characterized by a high presence of both lateralizing signs, automatisms and secondary generalized seizures in BIS, which are instead very rare in BIMSE. On the contrary, cyanosis is an almost constant symptom in BIMSE but much rarer in BIS. From the EEG point of view, the basic difference is the presence in BIMSE of paroxysmal abnormalities during sleep which are morphologically very typical. We know instead that in BIS the interictal picture is absolutely normal both while awake but above all during sleep.

Another possibility we have to consider in differential diagnosis, is that seizures in these infants may be early manifestations of benign partial epilepsies in childhood, namely of benign epilepsy with centrotemporal spikes (BCECTS) and Panayiotopoulos syndrome (PS). Cases of BIMSE with later onset and with EEG abnormalities spreading to the central, temporal or occipital regions may make diagnosis more difficult. The clinical semiology highlights clear differences between the benign focal epilepsies in infancy and the benign idiopathic syndromes in childhood, as shown in *table I*. As is well-known (Lerman, 1992; Dalla Bernardina *et al.*, 2005), BCECTS seizures occur characteristically mainly during sleep and they frequently appear with clonic activity of face or arms; focal signs are a rule, loss of consciousness is rare, and cyanosis absent. Moreover, even though rarely, seizures can present secondary generalization. In BIMSE, seizures occur

Table I. Distinctive features in BIMSE, BIS, BCECTS and PS

	BIMSE	BIS	BCECTS	PS
Familiarity	++	Familial: always Non familial: +	+	+
Age of onset	4-30 months	3-18 months	> 36 months	> 24 months
Seizure frequency	+	+++	+	+
Treatment	-	+++	+	+
Cyanosis	+++	+	-	+
Loss of consciousness	+	+++	-	++
Lateralizing Signs	+	++	+++	+++
Automatisms	+	++	+	+
Secondary Generalization	-	+++	+	++
Post-ictal sleep	+++	++	-	+
Awake EEG	Normal	Normal	C-T spikes	O-FT
Sleep EEG	Midline spikes	Normal	C-T spikes	O-FT

BIMSE, Benign focal epilepsy in infancy with vertex spikes and waves; BIS, benign infantile seizures (familial and non-familial); BCECTS, benign childhood epilepsy with centrotemporal spikes; PS, Panayiotopoulos syndrome; C-T, centro-temporal; O, Occipital; FT, Frontal/temporal.

preferentially at awake state and are usually accompanied by loss of consciousness, even if, in infancy, it is often difficult to understand if a true loss of consciousness is present. Focal signs and clonic activity are rarely present, while cyanosis is one of the most common symptoms and secondary generalization is never clearly evident. Moreover, the EEG picture appears completely different. The morphology of BCECTS abnormalities, usually present at awake state too, is characteristic, with high-voltage diphasic spikes followed by a slow wave, that recur at short interval, often in clusters (Nayrac & Beaussart, 1958; Lerman, 1992; Dalla Bernardina et al., 2005). In BIMSE spikes are present only during sleep and their voltage is much lower. They recur at long interval and they frequently appear isolated. Clusters are very rare. Abnormalities are localized primitively in the midline regions even though they tend to spread to the central areas and very little to the temporal regions. The morphological differences are clearly shown in *figure 3*. During evolution none of our cases ever showed EEG abnormalities evoking those of BCECTS, neither while awake nor during sleep.

Partial symptomatic or cryptogenic epilepsy is a differential diagnosis to consider. Neurological, neuroradiological and intellectual normality in BIMSE, both before and after seizures, is in contrast with this possibility. Moreover, after the disappearance of seizures, no relapses occur at follow-up, even in the children not undergoing therapy or who have discontinued it.

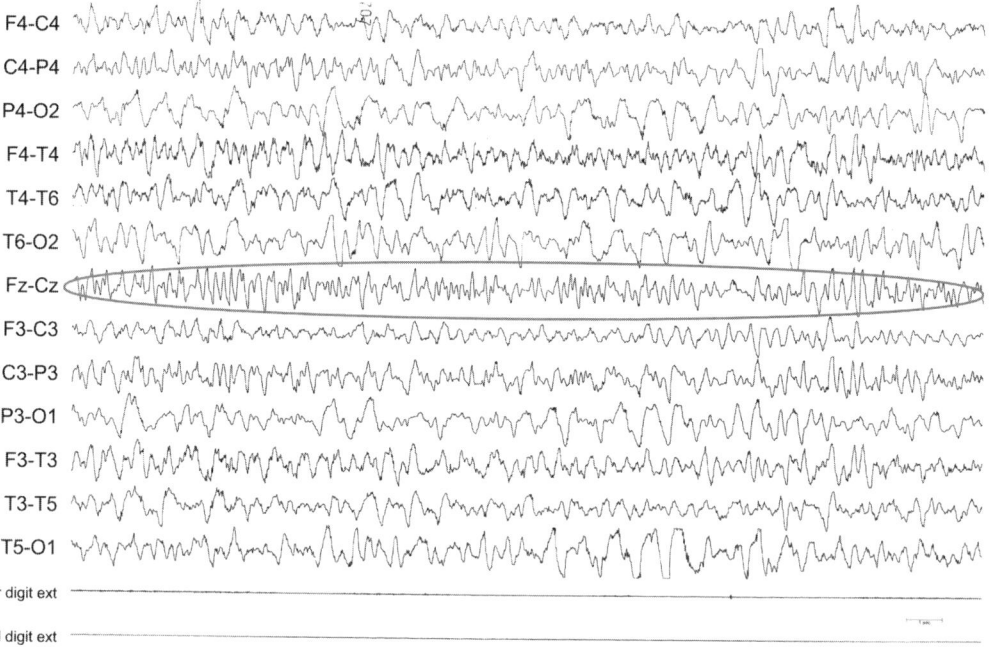

Figure 3. Eighteen month old normal infant. A focal rhythmic discharge of theta activity is evident in the vertex areas (ellipsis). The seizure was characterized by cyanosis and unresponsiveness, without clonic movements or automatisms.

Treatment

We understand that in infants having clusters of BIS and in cases with clinical-EEG features of BIMSE the first intention may be to use some antiepileptic drugs. However, we think that the latter group of patients should not be treated, because seizures are rare and show a spontaneous benign course. In the case of seizures in clusters, rectal or intravenous diazepam should be used, without a subsequent antiepileptic treatment.

Prognosis and long-term evolution

Prognosis is excellent, both for the spontaneous remission of the seizures and the absolute neurological and intellectual normality of the patients. Long-term follow-up of our patients (many of them have a follow-up period more than 5 years, some more than ten years) confirms the absolute benignity of BIMSE.

Data about our series of patients

Up to now, we collected more than 30 cases of BIMSE, even if some of these cases were not included in the papers we wrote because they were lost at follow-up. Here we report the descriptions of two of our patients.

Case 1

This neurologically and mentally normal boy presented, when he was 18-month-old, an awake afebrile seizure characterized by perioral cyanosis and staring, without automatisms or lateralizing signs, lasting about 5 minutes. An awake EEG was normal. While the infant was being prepared for a sleep-EEG recording, he presented a similar seizure captured by video-EEG after one minute from the onset *(Fig. 3)*. After that this attack was stopped with rectal diazepam, the infant fell asleep and his EEG was normal, but pharmacological fast rhythms altered the record. No therapy was started. One month later, typical midline spikes were recorded during a sleep EEG. At follow-up, when the child was 6.9 year old, he continued to have a normal psychomotor development. Midline spikes disappeared at age 3.

Case 2

This is a 8.5 year old neurologically and mentally normal child who presented, at age 17 months, a one-minute seizure characterized by stiffening of the arms, cyanosis, staring and motion arrest. After a few ours the infant repeated three similar attacks and the fourth seizure was stopped with rectal diazepam. He repeated similar seizures at age 2.2 and 3 years. His 11-year-old brother presented with two simple febrile convulsions in the same day at age 2 years. The EEG was not done at that moment but was normal at age 7 years. Based on the patient's positive familial history, we recorded the EEG of his younger sister when she was 9 month old which was normal. Later, when she was 14 month old, she had a brief afebrile seizure characterized by staring and motion arrest. Her sleep EEG evidenced the presence of typical midline spikes. Two episodes of simple clonic febrile seizures occurred at age 15 months and 2 years. One first cousin, now 8 year old, had two simple febrile seizures, while his younger brother, now 4 year old, had breath holding spells at age 8 months. Both had typical sleep midline spikes in the EEGs.

References

- Bureau M, Maton B. Valeur de l'EEG dans le pronostic précoce des épilepsies partielles non idiopathiques de l'enfant. In: Bureau M, Kahane P, Munari C (eds). *Épilepsies partielles graves pharmaco-résistantes de l'enfant : stratégies diagnostiques et traitements chirurgicaux*. London: John Libbey, 1998: 67-78.

- Bureau M, Cokar O, Maton B, Genton P, Dravet C. Sleep-related, low voltage Rolandic and vertex spikes: an EEG marker of benignity in infancy-onset focal epilepsies. *Epileptic Disord* 2002; 4: 15-22.

- Capovilla G, Beccaria F. Benign partial epilepsy in infancy and early childhood with vertex spikes and waves during sleep: a new epileptic form. *Brain Dev* 2000; 22: 93-9.

- Capovilla G, Giordano L, Tiberti S, Valseriati D, Menegati E. Benign partial epilepsy in infancy with complex partial seizures (Watanabe's syndrome): 12 non-Japanese new cases. *Brain Dev* 1998; 20: 105-11.

- Capovilla G. About benign idiopathic partial epilepsies in infancy. *Epileptic Disord* 2002; 4: 227.

- Capovilla G, Vigevano F. Benign idiopathic partial epilepsies in infancy. *Review J Child Neurol* 2001; 16: 874-81.

- Capovilla G, Beccaria F, Montagnini A. Benign focal epilepsy in infancy with vertex spikes and waves during sleep. Delineation of the syndrome and recalling as 'benign infantile focal epilepsy with midline spikes and waves during sleep' (BIMSE). *Brain Dev* 2006; 28: 85-91.

- Caraballo R, Cersosimo RO, Galicchio S, Fejerman N. Epilepsies during the first year of life. *Rev Neurol* 1997; 25: 1521-4.

- Caraballo RH, Cersosimo RO, Espeche A, Fejerman N. Benign familial and non-familial infantile seizures: a study of 64 patients. *Epileptic Disord* 2003; 5: 45-9.

- Chahine LM, Mikati MA. Benign pediatric localization-related epilepsies. Part I. Syndromes in infancy. *Epileptic Disord* 2006; 8: 169-83.

- Dalla Bernardina B, Sgrò V, Fejerman N. Epilepsy with centrotemporal spikes and related syndromes. In: Roger J, Bureau M, Dravet C, Genton P, Tassinari CA & Wolf P. *Epileptic syndromes in infancy, childhood and adolescence* (4th ed). London: John Libbey, 2005: 203-25.

- Echenne B, Humbertclaude V, Rivier F, Malafosse A, Cheminal R. Benign infantile epilepsy with autosomal dominant inheritance. *Brain Dev* 1994; 16: 108-11.

- Ehle A, Co S, Jones MG. Clinical correlates of midline spikes. An analysis of 21 patients. *Arch Neurol* 1981; 38: 355-7.

- Engel J Jr; International League Against Epilepsy (ILAE). A proposed diagnostic scheme for people with epileptic seizures and with epilepsy: report of the ILAE Task Force on Classification and Terminology. *Epilepsia* 2001; 42: 796-803.

- Fejerman N. Benign focal epilepsies in infancy, childhood and adolescence. *Rev Neurol* 2002; 34: 7-18.

- Franzoni E, Bracceschi R, Colonnelli MC, *et al*. Clinical features of benign infantile convulsions: familial and sporadic cases. *Neurology* 2005; 11; 65: 1098-100.

- Fukuyama Y. Borderland of epilepsy with special reference to febrile convulsions and so-called infantile convulsions. *Seishing-Igaku* (Clin Psychiatry) 1963; 5: 211-23.

- Gautier A, Pouplard F, Bednarek N, *et al*. Benign infantile convulsions. French collaborative study. *Arch Pediatr* 1999; 6: 32-9.

- Kaleyias J, Khurana DS, Valencia I, Legido A, Kothare SV. Benign partial epilepsy in infancy: myth or reality? *Epilepsia* 2006; 47: 1043-9.

- Kutluay E, Passaro EA, Gomez-Hassan D, Beydoun A. Seizure semiology and neuroimaging findings in patients with midline spikes. *Epilepsia* 2001 Dec; 42: 1563-68.

- Lee WL, Low PS, Rajan U. Benign familial infantile epilepsy. *J Pediatr* 1993; 123: 588-90.

- Lerman P. Benign partial epilepsy with centrotemporal spikes. In: Roger J, Bureau M, Dravet C, Dreifuss FE, Perret A, Wolf P, eds. *Epileptic syndromes in infancy, childhood and adolescence*. London: John Libbey, 1992: 189-200.

- Mc Lachlan RS, Girvin JP. Electroencephalographic features of midline spikes in the cat penicillin focus and in human epilepsy. *Electroencephalogr Clin Neurophysiol* 1989; 72: 140-6.

- Nayrac P, Beaussart M. Les pointes-ondes prérolandiques : expression EEG très particulière. *Rev neurol* 1958 ; 99: 201-6.

- Nelson KR, Brenner RP, de la Paz D. Midline spikes. EEG and clinical features. *Arch Neurol* 1983; 40: 473-6.

- Nelson GB, Olson DM, Hahn JS. Short duration of benign partial epilepsy in infancy. *J Child Neurol* 2002; 17: 440-5.

- Okumura A, Hayakawa F, Kuno K, Watanabe K. Benign partial epilepsy in infancy. *Arch Dis Child* 1996; 74: 19-21.

- Okumura A, Hayakawa F, Kato T, Kuno K, Negoro T, Watanabe K. Early recognition of benign partial epilepsy in infancy. *Epilepsia* 2000; 41: 714-7.

- Pourmand RA, Markand ON, Thomas C. Midline spike discharges: clinical and EEG correlates. *Clin Electroencephalogr* 1984; 15: 232-6.

- Specchio N, Vigevano F. The spectrum of benign infantile seizures. *Epilepsy Res* 2006; 70 suppl 1: 156-67.

- Vigevano F, Fusco L, Di Capua M, Ricci S, Sebastianelli R, Lucchini P. Benign infantile familial convulsions. *Eur J Pediatr* 1992; 151: 608-12.

- Vigevano F, Sebastianelli R, Fusco L, *et al*. Benign infantile familial convulsions. In: Malafosse A, Genton P, Hirsch E, Marescaux C, Broglin D, Bernasconi R (eds). *Idiopathic Generalized Epilepsies: Clinical, Experimental and Genetic Aspects*. London: John Libbey, 1994: 45-9.

- Vigevano F, Bureau M. Idiopathic and/or benign localization-related epilepsies in infants and young children. In: Roger J, Bureau M, Dravet C, Genton P, Tassinari CA & Wolf P. *Epileptic syndromes in infancy, childhood and adolescence* (4th ed). London: John Libbey, 2005: 171-9.

- Watanabe K, Yamamoto N, Negoro T, *et al*. Benign complex partial epilepsies in infancy. *Pediatr Neurol* 1987; 3: 208-11.

- Watanabe K, Yamamoto N, Negoro T, Takahashi I, Aso K, Maehara M. Benign infantile epilepsy with complex partial seizures. *J Clin Neurophysiol* 1990; 7: 409-16.

- Watanabe K. Recent advances and some problems in the delineation of epileptic syndromes in children. *Brain Dev* 1996; 18: 423-37.

- Weber YG, Berger A, Bebek N, *et al*. Benign familial infantile convulsions: linkage to chromosome 16p12-q12 in 14 families. *Epilepsia* 2004; 45: 601-9.

Part III
Idiopathic focal epilepsies in childhood

Benign childhood epilepsy with centrotemporal spikes

Natalio Fejerman*, Roberto H. Caraballo*,
Bernardo Dalla Bernardina**
*Buenos Aires, Argentina
**Verona, Italy

The recognition of epilepsies in children associating focal clinical manifestations and unilateral EEG discharges, with the features of functional epilepsies and with benign evolution, was one of the most interesting contributions to pediatric epileptology in the last 50 years.

The concept of idiopathic and benign focal epilepsies in childhood is relevant not only from the theoretic point of view, but also as a practical tool because the term implies absence of structural brain lesions and genetic predisposition to present age-dependent seizures. Benign childhood epilepsy with centrotemporal spikes (BCECTS) is the most frequent of the benign focal epilepsies in childhood and represents 15% to 25% of epilepsy syndromes in children below 15 years of age. Besides it is the most frequent epilepsy syndrome in school age (Watanabe, 2004; Panayiotopoulos, 2005, Dalla Bernardina *et al.*, 2005).

Yvette Gastaut was the first to state in 1952 that "pre-rolandic spikes" could be "functional" instead of indicators of a cortical lesion. In 1958, Bancaud *et al.* and Nayrac and Beaussart reported the first series of patients emphasizing that Rolandic or pre-rolandic spikes or spike-waves constituted EEG features typical of childhood which should not induce "neurosurgical behaviors", although they didn't describe a clear electroclinical correlation. In 1960, Gibbs and Gibbs stated that prognosis was much better in children with centrotemporal spikes than in those with spikes in anterior temporal regions. In the same year, Faure and Loiseau (1960) spoke about "Rolandic spike-waves without focal significance", referring to age of onset and sleep as trigger of seizures, and to a spontaneous trend to electroclinical normalization in puberty. However clinical features of seizures were not defined because they found generalized seizures in 13 of their 15 cases. In 1966, Trojaborg published a longitudinal study in a cohort of 519 children with focal spike discharges. Two hundred and eighty of these patients had cerebral palsy. The main purpose of this work was a detailed analysis of the significance of acute waves in the EEG and their correlation with brain lesions. The author recognized a good prognosis in cases with centrotemporal spikes, but did not determine their clinical correlation. In the same year 1966 the most important series of children with temporal lobe epilepsy was published (Ounsted *et al.*,

1966). Among the 100 children followed-up, 33 constituted the subgroup without pathological history and with mean age of onset of seizures between 7 and 8 years. It is now easy to imagine that a significant proportion of these 33 children might have had the diagnosis of BCECTS.

One year later, two independent groups reported their series of patients with a peculiar form of epilepsy to be differentiated from other focal epilepsies, mainly from temporal lobe epilepsy. Loiseau et al. (1967) presented 122 cases with onset of seizures in school age and rolandic paroxysms in the EEG. In 80% of their patients, seizures occurred during sleep and were frequently motor with predominance in face. Lombrosso (1967) did a clear description of the seizures emphasizing about somatosensitive symptoms in tongue, oral mucose and gums, along with speech arrest and proposed the term of "Sylvian seizures" recognizing also the particular focal EEG features. Both Loisseau et al. and Lombrosso stressed the benign character of the condition regarding evolution of seizures and normalization of EEG. In 1969, Sorel and Rucquoy-Ponsar proposed the name of "functional epilepsy of maturation", and at the same time Aicardi and Chevrie (1969) published the report on 61 cases of "partial epilepsy with Rolandic foci in second infancy". In 1972 Blom et al. presented a prevalence and follow-up study proposing to name the condition "Benign epilepsy of children with centrotemporal EEG foci". In the same year, Beaussart selected 221 cases with epilepsy, Rolandic sharp-waves and absence of neuropsychologic abnormalities to emphasize the characterization of BCECTS. One year later Loiseau and Beaussart (1973) published a new paper describing the various types of "signs" present in seizures, pointing their origin in the activation of the lower portion of Rolandic area. Several long term follow-up studies confirmed the good prognosis (Beaussart, 1972; Lerman & Kivity, 1975; Beaussart & Faou, 1978; Loisseau et al., 1988). Atypical and not-so-benign evolutions have been reported in some patients with this form of epilepsy (Aicardi & Chevrie, 1982; Fejerman & Di Blasi, 1987; Fejerman, 1996; Fejerman et al., 2000, Hahn et al., 2001; Fejerman, 2002). Literature in Spanish language on BCECTS was scarce. Early papers were published at the end of the seventies (Nieto-Barrera et al., 1978, Fejerman & Medina, 1980; Prats Viñas, 1980). Interestingly, in the first edition of our book "Convulsiones en la infancia" we had included a description of BCECTS in the chapter of temporal lobe epilepsies, even knowing that it was not a temporo-limbic epilepsy (Fejerman & Medina, 1977). This form of epilepsy is now called benign childhood epilepsy with centrotemporal spikes and is placed in the group of idiopathic localization-related (focal, local, partial) epilepsies in the International Classification of Epilepsies and Epileptic Syndromes (Commission on classification, 1989). In *Table I* of Chapter 1 it can be seen that in the 2001 proposal of the Task Force on Classification of ILAE, BCECTS was included in the group of Idiopathic focal epilepsies of infancy and childhood (Engel, 2001) and in the last report of the Core Group on Classification of ILAE, BCECTS was again clearly identified as a recognized syndrome (Engel, 2006). We are aware of at least two thesis devoted to this syndrome (Prats Viñas, 1980; Lundberg, 2004). A book dealing with Benign childhood partial seizures and related epileptic syndromes included BCECTS as the first item (Panayiotopoulos, 1999).

The most common name besides BCECTS appearing in the literature referring to this condition is "Benign rolandic epilepsy". The term "benign" has been questioned for other epilepsy syndromes, because some epileptologists believe that benign implies a natural evolution to remission of seizures and EEG abnormalities even without treatment. In this sense BCECTS complies with the mentioned concept even when we must accept that there are exceptions confirming the rule.

Onset during childhood with motor hemifacial seizures, speech arrest and syalorrhea, recurring mostly during sleep, along with peculiar centrotemporal spikes in the EEG, are well defined features and lead to a prompt diagnosis and a good prognosis, although subsets of atypical cases with slight compromise of neuropsychological functions are increasingly reported (Weglage et al., 1997; Verrotti et al., 2002; Papavasiliou et al., 2005). Clear evidence exists of cases of BCECTS evolving into status of BCECTS and even into epileptic encephalopathies such as Landau-Kleffner syndrome and Continuous spike-and-waves during slow sleep syndrome (CSWSS) (Fejerman et al., 2000) (see Chapter 10).

Epidemiology

Benign childhood epilepsy with centrotemporal spikes accounts for about 15 to 25% of all epileptic syndromes in children between ages 4 and 12 (Cavazzuti, 1980; Panayiotopoulos 1999, 2005; Watanabe, 2004; Dalla Bernardina et al., 2005). Its annual incidence has been reported to be between 7.1 and 21 per 100,000 in children under age 15 (Heijbel et al., 1975a). Because nocturnal seizures can be easily missed in diagnosis, this disorder may be even more common than generally suspected. There is a slight male predominance (Lüders et al., 1987; Lerman, 1998; Panayiotopoulos, 1999). BCECTS has been recognized all over the world. In a recent retrospective study in China, 276 patients were enrolled and electroclinical features showed to be quite characteristic (Zhao et al., 2007).

The prevalence of epilepsy is much higher among close relatives of children with benign childhood epilepsy with centrotemporal spikes than in a matched control group (Bray & Wiser, 1964). In one study, 15% of siblings had seizures and rolandic spikes, 19% of siblings had rolandic spikes without attacks, and 11% of the parents had childhood seizures that had disappeared by adulthood (Heijbel et al., 1975b).

A series of epidemiological studies performed since 1988 were based on the ILAE's 1985 proposal and 1989 accepted classification of epileptic syndromes (Commission on Classification, 1989). In a 20 years cohort of 440 pediatric neurology outpatients with epilepsy, 8% had benign rolandic epilepsy of childhood (Kramer et al., 1998). Examining the clinical records of 645 consecutive patients between 1 month and 15 years followed at a Children's epilepsy center in Milan from 1977 through 1985, the authors were quite successful in recognizing epileptic syndromes. When considering the less biased example of children with newly diagnosed epilepsies, BCECTS was identified in 8.3% of the children (Viani et al., 1988). In a population study in Sweden, 155 children between 0-16 years with epilepsy were identified and BCECTS was diagnosed in 17.4% of them (Sidenvall et al., 1996). In a cohort of 407 children with a first unprovoked seizure prospectively recruited and followed up for a mean of 9.4 years, the 182 children who have had two or more seizures were studied for distribution of epilepsy syndromes: 27 (14%) of them were diagnosed as Rolandic localization-related idiopathic epilepsy (Shinnar et al., 1999). In a survey made by 14 epilepsy centers in Italy, a sample of 3,469 patients with ages 40-80 years was collected. Adults (age > 15 years) were 75% of the sample. Nevertheless, idiopathic localization related syndromes were recognized in 183 (5.3%) cases [Osservatorio Regionale per L'Epilessia (OREp), Lombardi, 1997]. If we consider that at the time the only other recognized idiopathic localization-related epilepsy syndrome was Childhood epilepsy with occipital paroxysms, and that 75% of the patients were adults, the mentioned 5.3% of diagnosed cases become much more significant. The most comprehensive epidemiologic study of newly diagnosed unprovoked epileptic seizures covering 1942 patients from 1 month to 95 years was done with data provided by 243 child and adult neurologists in France (Jallon et al., 2001). The whole sample was divided in two groups, one with a single seizure at diagnosis and the other with more than one seizure at diagnosis. All patients with idiopathic (localization-related or generalized epilepsies) had at least one EEG. Among 80 patients with idiopathic localization-related epilepsy within the 926 cases of the single seizure group, 66 (7.1%) had BCECTS, and among the 48 cases within the 1,016 of the more than one seizure group, 39 (3.8%) had BCECTS. As can be seen, these figures point to a much higher prevalence of BCECTS than previously reported if we consider that this epilepsy syndrome appears after 3-4 years of age and disappears around puberty. Quite recently a population-based study using hospital data register selected 205 children 1 month to 16 years old with epilepsy. A majority of the patients (54%) had focal seizures and the most common syndrome recognized was Rolandic epilepsy occurring in 17% (Larsson & Eeg-Olofson, 2006).

Clinical Features

A high incidence of familial antecedents of epilepsy (18-36%) has been confirmed by all investigators, and we'll see later that there are different genetic interpretations of these findings. About 7-10% of children with BCECTS have a personal history of febrile seizures. Absence of neurological and intellectual deficits are part of the definition. Obviously in subjects with a fixed neurological or intellectual deficit, the diagnosis of BCECTS must not be excluded "a priori", but considered with reserve and only in presence of all other diagnostic parameters (Herranz, 2002). Some cases have been reported in the literature on BCECTS in subjects with cerebral lesions documented neuroradiologically (Santanelli et al., 1989; Deggen et al., 1999). Thus we must point out how difficult it can be, in some of these cases, to distinguish between a symptomatic epilepsy with favorable evolution and a casual association of cerebral lesions and BCECTS (Lerman, 1985; Fejerman et al., 1998). Coincidental associations with rare metabolic encephalopathies might also occur due to the frequency of BCECTS (Polychronopoulos, 2006).

We are going to see the main clinical features of BCECTS assuming that this is an idiopathic focal epilepsy, which appears in children with normal neuropsychological development:

1. The age of onset is between 4 and 10 years in 90% of the patients and the median age of onset is around 7 years. There are no references about BCECTS occurring during the first year of life or after age 15, and cases with seizure onset before the age of 2 years are extremely rare (Fejerman et al., 1998; Dalla Bernardina et al., 2005).

2. BCECTS is seen more frequently in males with a relation to females of 3:2.

3. Seizures are clearly related to sleep, whether during the night or the day. This is seen in 80% to 90% of the patients. Seizures during waking hours are more likely to occur shortly after awakening (Luders et al., 1987), although in many occasions, in the episodes occurring during early morning the child wakes up with the seizure which really started during sleep. In about 15% of the cases seizures occur both during sleep and while awake, and in near 10% only in waking states. Seizure frequency is usually low and around 10% of cases present only one seizure. However, in about 20% of the children, seizures are frequent and may even occur several times per day (Dalla Bernardina et al., 2005). Each individual patient has a single type of seizure, but 20-25% of children experience more than one type (Loiseau & Duche, 1989). Typical seizures last from 30-60 seconds to no more than 2-3 minutes. Loiseau and Beaussart (1972) described 35 signs or components of 275 seizures analyzed in 190 children with BCECTS. Nevertheless, we can reduce this number to a small group of characteristic manifestations of seizures (Fejerman, 2007):

A. *Orofacial motor signs*, specially tonic or clonic contractions of one side of the face with predilection of the labial commissure (contralateral to centrotemporal spikes). Involvement of the ipsilateral eyelids is not unusual. More rarely, clonic convulsions may appear simultaneously in the ipsilateral upper extremity, while involvement of the leg is even rarer. There are also contractions of the tongue or jaw, guttural sounds, and drooling from hypersalivation and swallowing disturbance.

B. *Speech arrest*, most probably due to tonic contractions of pharyngeal and bucal muscles, constituting anarthric seizures. Laryngeal sounds may be uttered, particularly at the beginning. There is no impairment of the cortical language mechanism, and this may explain why ictal arrest of speech is equally common in left or right sided seizures (Panayiotopoulos, 1999). In fact, what happens is that the patient can not speak during the seizure, either because he wakes up with hemifacial contractions, or because having a fit while awake, he opens the mouth with the intention to speak and stays blocked in that position. In exceptional cases post-ictal disarthria may persist for a few minutes after the seizure.

C. *Somatosensory symptoms*. Unilateral numbness or paresthesia of the tongue, lips, gums, and inner cheek are frequent, but sometimes have to be looked for in the anamnesis.

D. *Sialorrhea*. It is not clear whether it corresponds to increased salivation, a swallowing disturbance, or both. Sialorrhea is a characteristic ictal symptom of BCECTS and may be associated with oro-facial motor signs, with speech arrest, or with both.

E. *Less frequent ictal manifestations*. Although partial seizures are characteristic of this disorder, generalized seizures are not infrequently observed, particularly in younger children (Luders et al., 1987; Lerman, 1998; Chahine & Mikati, 2006). The initial event is often a nocturnal hemifacial convulsion, which may spread to the arm and the leg or may become secondarily generalized. It is highly probable that in these cases the child starts with a focal seizure during sleep with a rapid generalization with loss of consciousness which impairs the child to remember what happened. This idea is in line with the fact that almost all seizures starting while awake are focal. In children aged 2-5 years, hemiclonic seizures last sometimes more than 30 minutes and may be followed by a transient homolateral deficits, generally not including the face (Dalla Bernardina *et al.*, 1992, 2002). In a review of 70 patients with BCECTS searching for the presence of post-ictal paresis, this finding was reported in 8 of the cases, and in all of them the hemiparesis resolved within 60 minutes. The authors concluded that the presence of post-ictal paresis should not exclude the diagnosis of BCECTS (Dai and Weinstock, 2005). In anecdotal cases, the combination of sialorrhea and contraction of pharyngeal muscles, specially when laying on the bed, produced a "choking" sensation. Paroxysmal tooth ache was also reported (Stephani, 2000). Transient oromotor deficits with intermittent dysarthria and drooling not in the context of typical clinical seizures were reported (Roulet *et al.*, 1989, Kramer *et al.*, 2001), but we'll deal with this phenomenae in the chapter on atypical evolutions.

4. Behavioral and learning problems are less frequent than in other forms of childhood epilepsy. It was frequently mentioned that children with BCECTS were free of neuropsychological impairments (Heijbel & Bohman, 1975; Fejerman & Medina, 1986; Fejerman *et al.*, 1997; Lerman, 1998). Not only the IQ, the neuropsychologic functions, or the eventual risks of neuropsychological impairment have to be looked for, but also the emotional impact of seizures in the child's behavior should be considered. We studied long ago a small number of children with BCECTS with the Bender, WISC and Rorschach tests. IQs ranged between 81 and 126 with a mean of 99, but certain impairment in the non verbal items of the WISC were detected. Regarding the Rorschach test no abnormalities were found (Fejerman & Medina, 1980). We also emphasized at the time the presence in the child of anxiety both during the anarthric seizures while awake and when waking up with hemiclonic facial seizures and sialorrhea, and this was clearly found every time we asked about it. In the last years several reports based on meta-analysis of published series, retrospective analysis of patients, or prospective cohort studies reported a higher incidence of learning and/or language difficulties in these children. In a study of 40 children with centrotemporal spikes with and without seizures compared with 40 healthy controls, patients were significantly impaired in IQ, visual perception, short-term memory, and psychiatric status. The deficits in IQ were more correlated with frequency of spikes in the EEG than with the frequency of seizures (Weglage *et al.*, 1997). Similar findings were reported in 19 children with this syndrome (Deonna *et al.*, 2000). In a study of 17 children 7-14 years old with BCECTS matched with controls, the patients had significantly lower scores than their controls on the neuropsychological items. However, intellectual abilities did not differ and neither did school functioning or behavior according to teachers (Croona *et al.*, 1999). Another interesting finding is that in children with "attention deficit hyperactivity disorder," an increased frequency of Rolandic spikes was found (Holtmann *et al.*, 2003). In one study, a consistent pattern of language dysfunction was found in 13 of 20 children with BCECTS suggesting an interictal dysfunction of the perisylvian language areas (Staden *et al.*, 1998). A longitudinal study of 1 boy with acquired epileptic dysgraphia was reported. Most probably, in this case, the acquired regression of graphomotor skills was associated with an increase in spike frequency as happens in the cases with atypical evolutions of this syndrome (Dubois *et al.*, 2003). In a more recent report, 32 children with typical BCECTS were compared with 36 controls regarding written language skills. As a group, the

patients with BCECTS performed significantly worst than controls in spelling, reading aloud and reading comprehension; presented dyslexic-type errors and frequently had below-average school performance (Papavasiliou et al., 2005). The language assessment in 16 children with BCECTS also showed that the domains of expressive grammar and literacy skills were affected in a significant proportion of the cases (Monjauze et al., 2005). A comprehensive study of neuropsychological and language profiles of 42 children with BCECTS selected with strict clinical and EEG criteria showed that the patients have normal intelligence and language ability although a specific pattern of difficulties in memory and phonologic awareness was found. No correlation between EEG features and the mentioned impairments was demonstrated (Northcott et al., 2005).

Atypical features in benign childhood epilepsy with centrotemporal spikes can be seen on clinical grounds (daytime-only seizures, post-ictal Todd paresis, prolonged seizures, or even status epilepticus), or in EEG features (atypical spike morphology, unusual location, or abnormal background) (Aicardi, 2000). In a retrospective case series, atypical clinical features were seen in 50% of patients and atypical electrographic features in 31% (Wirrell et al., 1995). A follow-up study of 74 children with typical rolandic epilepsy and 14 with atypical features was reported and a significant higher percentage of learning and behavioral disabilities was found in the second group (Verrotti et al., 2002).

Transient cognitive disorders can occur in typical BCECTS in the active phase of the disease (Deonna, 2000; Deonna et al., 2000). They seem to correlate with an increase in epileptic activities during this period. In a prospective study of 9 children with marked evidence of activation of epileptic discharges compared with 9 unaffected controls, the BCECTS patients showed normal IQ scores, but presented disorders in visuospatial short-term memory, attention, picture naming, visuospatial skills. After the time of interictal epileptic discharges remission, their performance did not differ from the controls (Baglietto et al., 2001). Several recent reports emphasized again that BCECTS can be accompanied by specific cognitive disorders and low academic achievement. Eighteen children were studied in terms of neuropsychological and learning abilities. IQ and verbal functions were normal, but reading, numeracy and/or spelling abilities were significantly delayed by one academic year or more in ten of the children (Pinton et al., 2006). Neuropsychological functioning and mathematics achievement were investigated in 30 children with idiopathic partial epilepsies and 30 healthy controls. Results suggested cautiousness regarding academic prognosis in children with benign partial epilepsies at childhood (Hande Sart et al., 2006). In 22 children with BCECTS compared with 22 controls, a comprehensive neuropsychological tests battery demonstrated significant deficits in higher functions of spatial perception, including spatial orientation in the patients (Volkl-Kernstock et al., 2006).

Excluding the patients with atypical evolutions with continuous spike-and-waves activities and severe language or behavior impairments, which account for around 5% of BCECTS patients in our tertiary epilepsy center for children, we have to be cautious with conclusions. Even when a significant number of children with BCECTS show some learning difficulties, the vast majority of them are able to attend normal schools. Besides, in most of the mentioned studies, the types of antiepileptic drugs and their blood levels are not reported, neither are they considered as eventual cause of the neuropsychological findings.

EEG and other neurophysiological studies

Electroencephalographic findings

After recognition of typical seizures, the cornerstone of the diagnosis of BCECTS lies in the characteristic interictal EEG pattern and its following features:

1. <u>Background EEG activity</u>: is symmetrical, well organized and normally reactive during wakefulness, and the physiological patterns of sleep are also normal (Dalla Bernardina *et al.*, 1991, 2005).

2. <u>Interictal epileptic discharges and location of spikes</u>:
   a. *Characteristics of spikes*: the typical spikes (CTS) are located in centrotemporal or Rolandic areas *(Fig. 1)*. They are broad, diphasic, high-voltage (100-microvolts to 300-microvolts) spikes, with a transverse dipole, and they are often followed by a slow wave. The spikes may occur isolated or in clusters *(Fig. 2)*. (Loiseau & Duche, 1989). Focal rhythmic slow activity is occasionally observed in the region where the spikes are seen (Mitsudome *et al.*, 1997a). The spikes may be seen in only one hemisphere or as bilateral synchronic discharges in both hemispheres. These bilateral, synchronic or independents CTS appear in wakefulness or sleep in about one third of cases. (Loiseau *et al.*, 1967; Dalla Bernardina *et al.*, 1992, 2002; Holmes, 1992; Lerman, 1998; Pan & Luders, 2000; Engel & Fejerman, 1999-2006) *(Fig. 3)*. The CTS tend to diffuse to adjacent regions. *(Fig. 4)* Several authors emphasized the characteristic dipolar pattern in the EEG (Gregory & Wong, 1984; Lischka & Graf, 1992; Tsai & Hung, 1998). Two groups of patients have been disclosed according to EEG findings (maximal negativity was registered in high– and low-central regions, but never in midtemporal regions), a high-central region group with more frequent hand involvement and the low-central group with common orofacial symptoms (Legarda *et al.*, 1994). The source distribution of benign rolandic spikes of childhood along and across the central sulcus in 15 patients aged between 7 and 15 years, were evaluated. The equivalent current dipoles of the spikes measured by whole-head magnetoencephalography were compared to the spike distributions detected by simultaneous scalp EEG. Rolandic spikes can be explained by a pre-central origin, assuming that the surface negative potential is continuous from the gyral to fissural cortices (Ishitobi *et al.*, 2004).
   b. *Enhancement of discharges*: the centrotemporal spikes are not enhanced by eye opening or closure, by hyperventilation, or by photic stimulation. Even more, it has been reported that hyperventilation reduces the frequency of Rolandic spikes (Fejerman & Medina, 1986; Watanabe, 2004). The discharge rate is increased in drowsiness and in all stages of sleep *(Fig. 5)*, and in about one third of children, the spikes appear only in sleep (Lombroso, 1967). The sleep EEG organization is preserved *(Fig. 6)* (Dalla Bernardina & Beghini, 1976). In spite of their increasing frequency during sleep, the CTS show the same morphology as during wakefulness. A change in morphology, particularly the appearance of fast spikes or polyspikes, or a marked increase in the slow component, or a brief depression of voltage, evoke an organic etiology even when the ictal features are suggestive of BCECTS (Dalla Bernardina *et al.*, 2005). There is no correlation between intensity of spike discharges in the EEG and frequency, length, or duration of clinical seizures (Lerman &

Kivity, 1975). In fact, extreme discrepancies between the rarity of seizures and the activity of the EEG foci are not uncommon and clinical experience indicates that the EEG is often relatively unchanged, even with effective treatment (Arzimanoglou et al., 2004).

c. *Spikes in other areas, multifocal paroxysms, and spike-wave discharges*: from the first EEG recording or during evolution spikes may appear in other areas. *(Fig. 7)* (Dalla Bernardina et al., 1991; Herranz Tanarro et al., 1984; Panayiotopoulos, 1999). In some cases, multifocal paroxysms are specially evident during sleep *(Fig. 8)*. The possible presence of multifocal paroxysms with the same morphology and behavior both during wakefulness and sleep, does not seem correlated with the frequency of seizure recurrence (Massa et al., 2001). Generalized spike-wave discharges are rarely seen in the waking state, but are not infrequent during drowsiness and sleep (Fejerman & Medina, 1986; Beydoun et al., 1992) *(Fig. 9)*. The real incidence of spike-wave discharges in children with BCECTS is not well known, since numbers vary between 7 and 65% (Degen & Degen, 1990; Dalla Bernardina et al., 2005). However, we must be cautious in its interpretation because bursts of slow waves with spikes in drowsiness are seen in up to 20% of children between 3 and 6 years, especially with history of febrile seizures (Alvarez et al., 1983).

3. Frequency of discharges and its correlation with cognitive deficits: the association of more frequent discharges or multifocal paroxysms with complicated evolutions in BCECTS is a debated subject (Massa et al., 2001; Dalla Bernardina et al., 2005). However, it is clear that the appearance of bilateral synchronies leading to continuous spikes and wave during sleep are frequently associated with severe cognitive and language impairment (Fejerman et al., 2000). In a study of

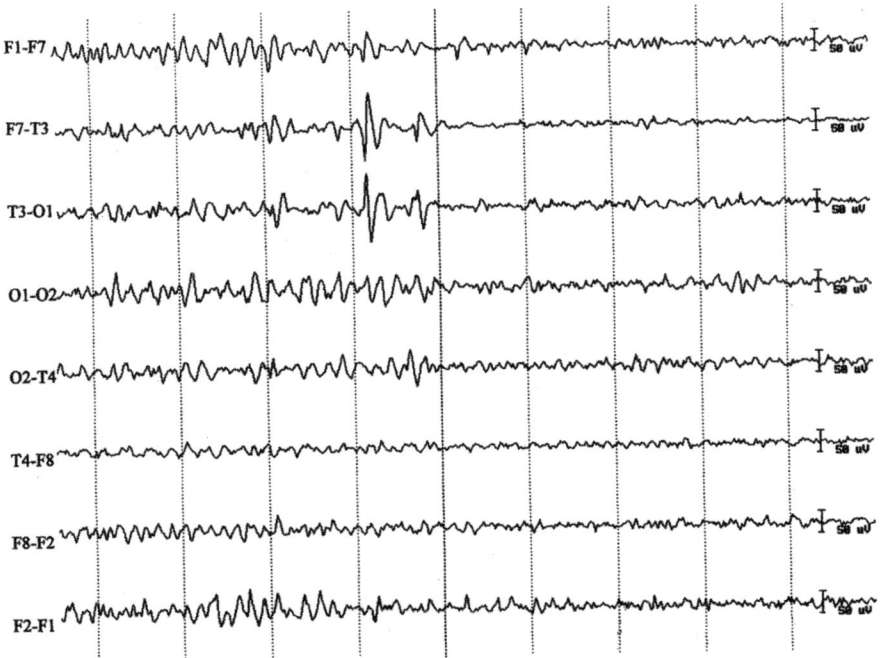

Figure 1. Seven years old boy. EEG while awake shows left centrotemporal spikes.

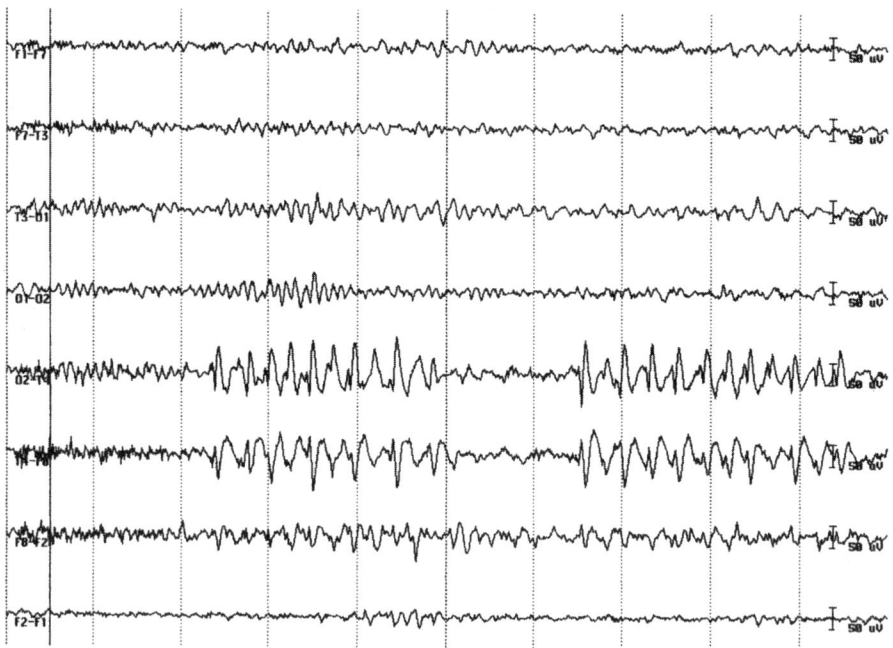

Figure 2. Eight years old girl. EEG while awake with clusters of right centrotemporal spikes.

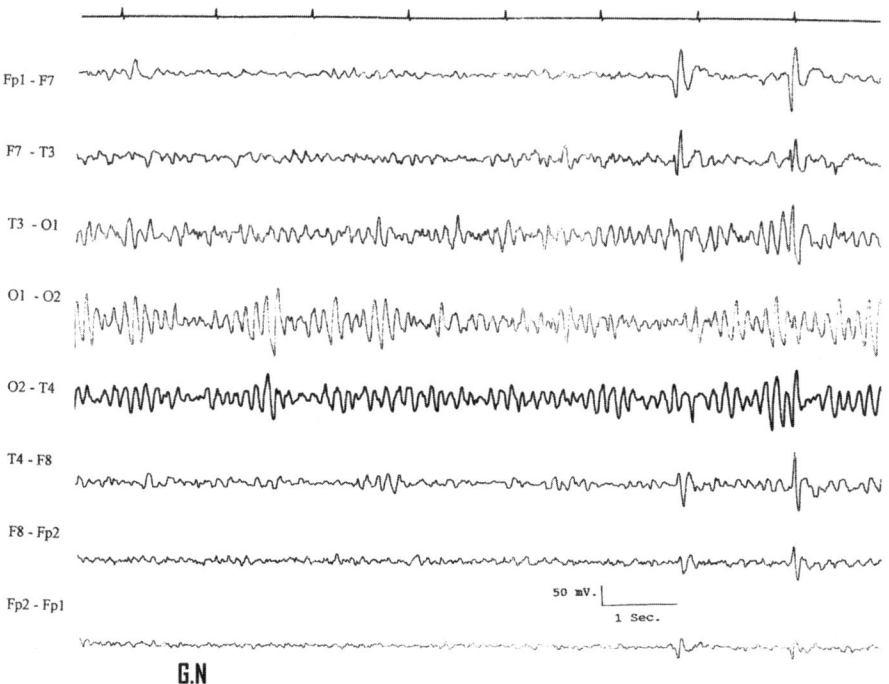

Figure 3. Eight years old girl. EEG while awake shows synchronic bilateral centrotemporal spikes.

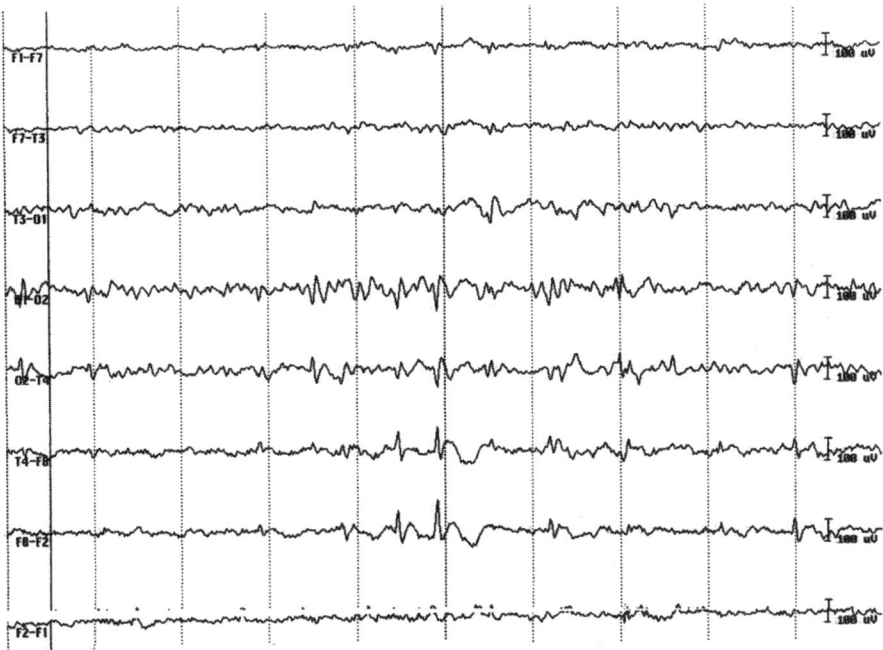

Figure 4. Seven years old boy. EEG while awake shows centrotemporal spikes diffusing to adjacent regions.

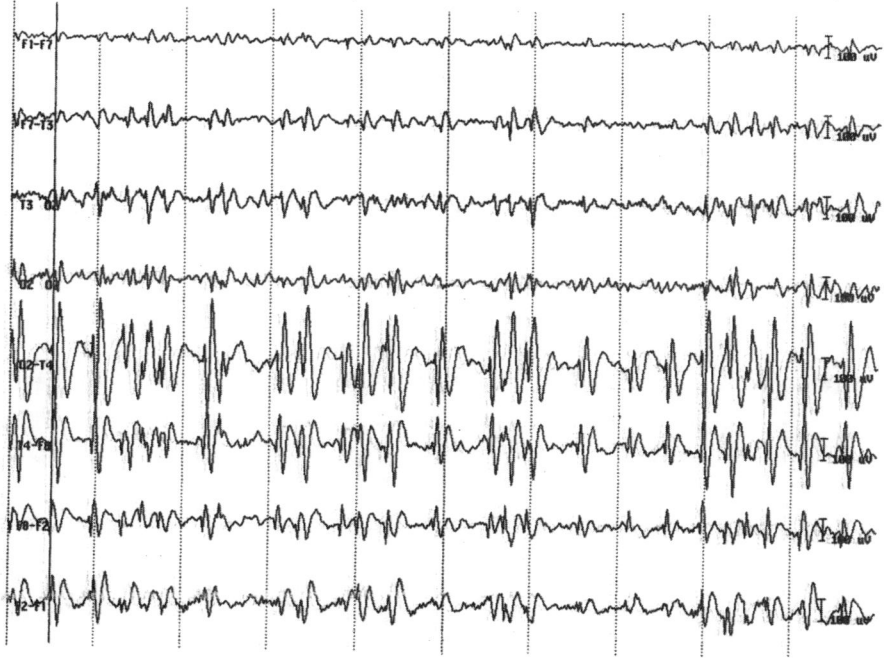

Figure 5. Sleep EEG of the patient presented in *Fig. 2* shows high frequency bilateral spikes dominant on right centrotemporal region.

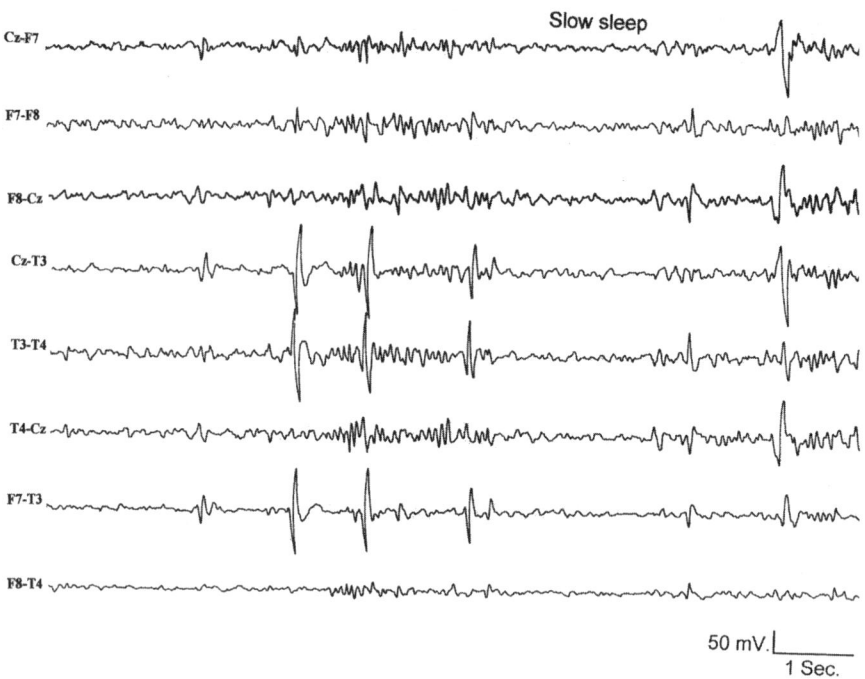

Figure 6. Eight years old boy. Sleep EEG shows left centrotemporal spikes and clear preservation of the background rhythm.

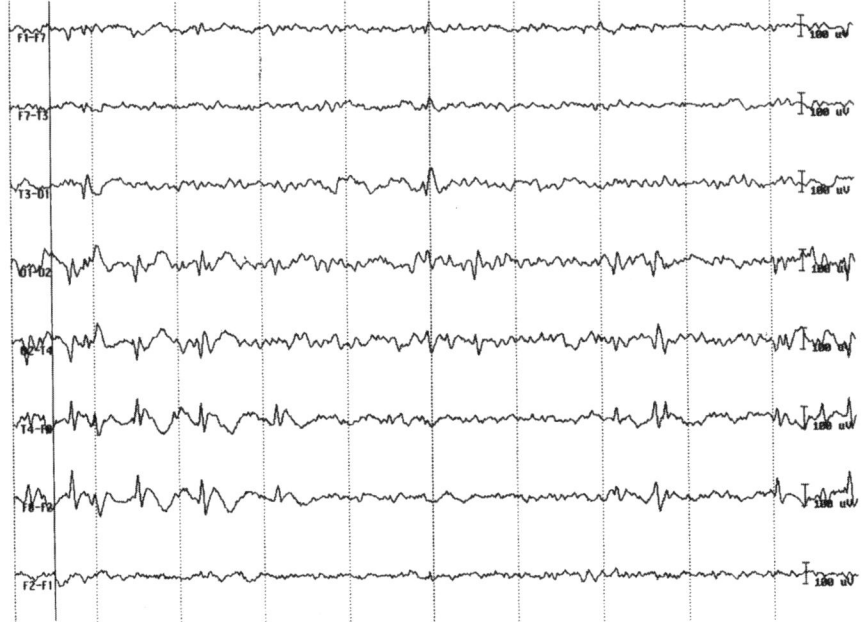

Figure 7. Eight years old boy. EEG while awake shows frequent right centrotemporal spikes and occasional independent spikes in occipital areas.

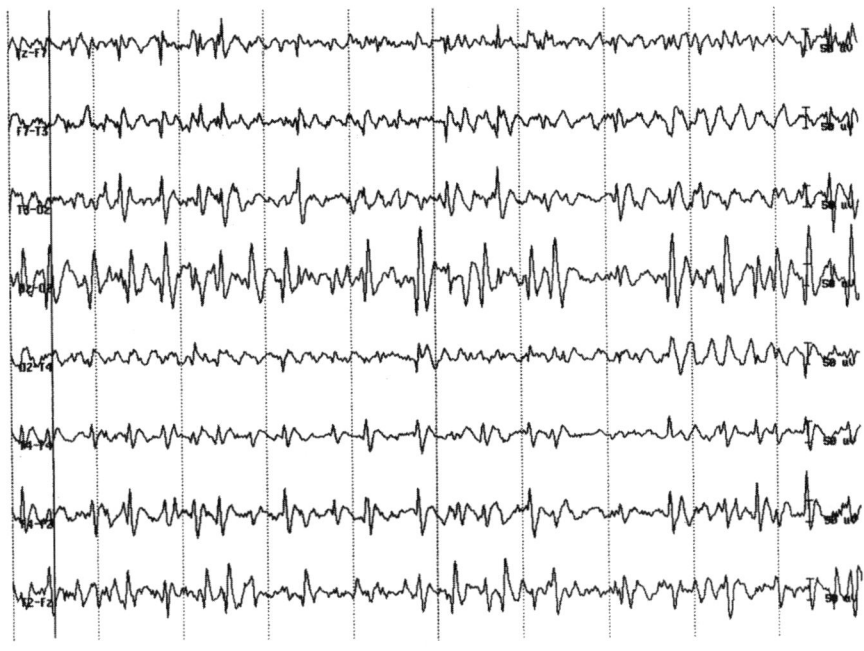

Figure 8. Nine years old girl. Sleep EEG shows multifocal spikes.

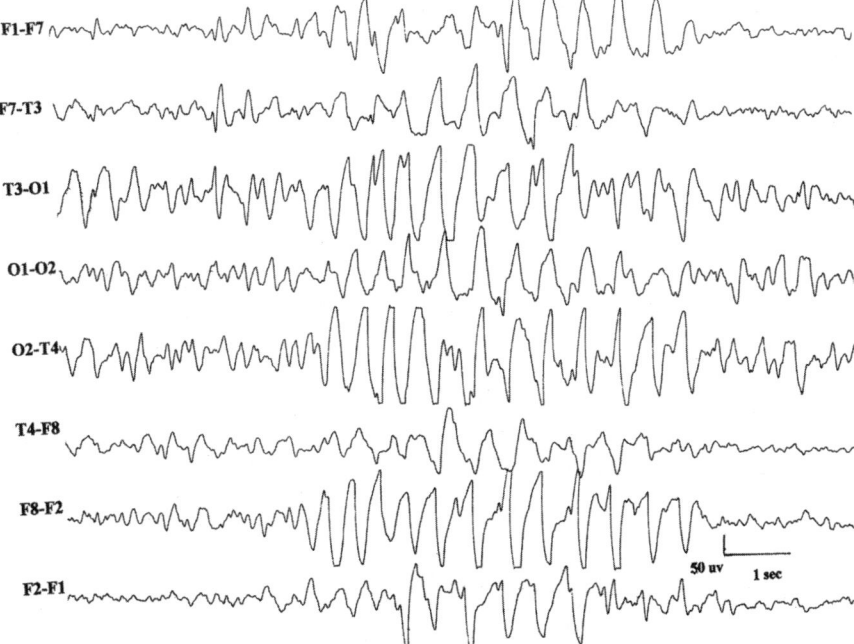

Figure 9. Seven years old boy. Sleep EEG shows a left centrotemporal spike followed by a generalized spike-wave discharge.

20 children with diagnosis of benign partial epilepsies examined by combined EEG, magnetoencephalography and MRI, location of spikes was determined by dipole source estimates. A correlation was shown between location of spikes and selective cognitive deficits, with left perisylvian spikes associated with lower language test in 11 cases, while 6 children with right perisylvian location performed within normal ranges in all parts of the tests (Wolff et al., 2005). Hemispheric lateralization of cognitive functions in children with centrotemporal spikes was recently studied in 6 children with BCECTS and left sided focus, 6 with BCECTS and right sided focus, and 12 controls. The typical left hemisphere advantage in the verbal tasks was not reported in children with left foci, while the children with right foci showed lack of the classic global superiority effect due to impaired performance of the specialized global level processing (Bedoin et al., 2006). In a small group of patients with status epilepticus in benign childhood epilepsy with centrotemporal spikes the finding of independent right and left seizures was considered a risk factor (Gregory et al., 2002). A study of 21 children with BCECTS compared to controls showed that the patient have mild language defects, revealed by tests measuring phonemic fluency, verbal re-elaboration of semantic knowledge, and lexical comprehension. Interictal EEG discharges demonstrated that a high rate of occurrence while awake, multifocal location, and temporal prominence seem to impair the efficiency of some of the neuropsychological functions investigated (Riva et al., 2007). In a recent prospective study of 44 children with BCECTS they were divided into two groups. The first group (n = 28) was referred as typical BCECTS. The second group (n = 16) referred as "atypical" showed in the early EEGs atypical features as slow spike wave focus, as synchronous foci, or generalized 3 Hz spike wave discharges. The results showed that the atypical group had significant lower full scale IQ and verbal IQ and differences in certain tasks of the performance scale were also observed (Metz-Lutz & Filippini, 2006). This group showed, after recovery of epilepsy, a significant improvement in all the cognitive domains investigated, except the verbal short-term memory. Even when there is consensus that several atypical EEG characteristics are related to cognitive or behavioral problems, it remains to be shown whether antiepileptic drug treatment of nocturnal discharge in children with BCECTS is indicated to improve cognitive and behavioral problems (Nicolai et al., 2006).

4. Centrotemporal spikes in normal children: several EEG studies in large numbers of healthy children were performed. Centrotemporal spikes were found in 2.1% of 533 children between 6 and 15 years (Eeg Olofsson et al., 1971), in 2.4% of 3,726 children between 6 and 13 years (Cavazzutti, 1980) and in 3.5% of 1,057 children between 6 and 12 years (Okubo et al., 1994). Considering that in many of the cases the EEGs were performed in waking state, we may assume that real figures should be higher. The fact is that in a vast majority of children with CTS, a genetically determined cortical excitability produces the EEG abnormalities, which in a few patients are associated with clinical seizures. It has been estimated that less than 25% of children with CTS have seizures (Luders et al., 1987). The presence of CTS was also reported in children with Rett syndrome, fragile X syndrome and even in children with brain tumors (Niedermeyer & Naidu, 1990; Musumeci et al., 1988; Kraschnitz et al., 1988). Centrotemporal spikes apparently increase impulsivity in ADHD patients. This was the conclusion of a neuropsychological assessment of 16 ADHD children with Rolandic spikes, 16 ADHD children with epileptiform abnormalities in the EEG, and 16 healthy controls (Holtman et al., 2006).

5. Ictal EEGs: reports in the literature about the ictal EEGs in children with BCECTS are scarce and only with isolated cases (Dalla Bernardina & Tassinari, 1975; Ambrosetto & Gobbi, 1975). The ictal pattern is generally characterized by a sequence of rhythmic spikes remaining quite monomorphous throughout the discharge. Lerman described a diurnal seizure with local decremental activity followed by dense spikes confined to the centrotemporal area during the tonic phase and with spike-waves during the clonic phase (Lerman, 1998).

Evoked potentials

Evoked potentials have been studied in children with idiopathic focal epilepsies.

Peripheral stimulation can both inhibit centrotemporal spikes (CTS) or trigger them. In fact CTS may be attenuated by contralateral hand-movements, tongue movements (Niedermeyer & Naidu, 1990; Veggiotti et al., 1999) or electrical stimulation on fingers (Manganotti et al., 1998a). In the case report by Vegiotti et al. (1999), tongue protrusion was also able to stop the seizure. On the contrary, tapping of hands and/or feet or electrical stimulation of the fingers at 1 Hz elicited, in some cases, extreme somatosensory evoked potentials (ESEPs) on the contralateral hemisphere (De Marco & Tassinari, 1981; Dalla Bernardina et al., 1991; Manganotti et al., 1998b). As confirmed by Langill and Wong (2003), these ESEPs are not correlated to a specific type of epilepsy. Similar ESEPs had been seen in subjects without epilepsy as well.

Mismatch negativity (MMN) is a cognitive event-related potential component, a brain automatic response to change in auditory stimulation. MMN was recorded 23 children with BCECTS (16 typical and 7 atypical cases), and 10 controls. Even when no significant results were found, in individual patients with atypical BCECTS and learning difficulties the smallest MMN, compared to the other groups, were recorded (Metz-Lutz & Filippini, 2006).

Magnetoencephalography (MEG)

We are going to comment later on MEG as a tool to improve our understanding of patophysiology of epileptic discharges and dipole analysis. Whether MEG or EEG is superior remains controversial and they often provide complementary information. An interesting review of selected studies relevant to epilepsy, including BCECTS, has recently been published (Cappell et al., 2006).

Etiology

There is enough evidence regarding the high incidence of a positive family history for epilepsy and focal EEG abnormalities suggesting the importance of genetic factors in the etiology of BCECTS (Blom et al., 1972; Bray & Wiser, 1964; Luders et al., 1987; Degen & Degen, 1990). Most of the authors speak about an autosomal dominant trait with variable penetrance

(Heijbel *et al.*, 1975b; Bray & Wiser, 1964). This type of inheritance was also suggested by studies of monozygotic twins with rolandic discharges (Kajitani *et al.*, 1980), and HLA antigens and their haplotypes (Egg-Olofson, 1992). However, in another study of clinical and genetic aspects in children with benign focal sharp waves, including 134 probands with seizures (24% of which had typical rolandic seizures), the findings were in agreement with a multifactorial pathogenesis of epilepsies with "benign" focal epileptiform sharp waves (Doose *et al.*, 1997). Expression of the gene may be influenced by other genetic and environmental factors (Loiseau & Duche, 1989; Berkovic & Scheffer, 1999). The mentioned series of papers were thoroughly analyzed on account of patients selection and interpretation of the EEGs, and doubts were casted regarding their methodology (Panayiotopoulos, 1999). The same criticism is valid for the findings in siblings of patients with BCECTS, specially when they are compared to the known 2-3% of EEG abnormalities in general childhood population. Near 10% of patients have a history of previous febrile seizures and this suggests also a genetic predisposition for febrile seizures expressed at earlier ages in children with BCECTS (Kajitani *et al.*, 1992; Lerman, 1998). However, previous interpretations or speculations regarding genetic influence on BCECTS have recently been questioned. In a study using population-based twin registries of epilepsy from Denmark, USA, Norway and Australia, 18 twin pairs were identified (10 monozygous; 8 dizygous) of whom at least one twin was diagnosed with classic BCECTS on the basis of electroclinical criteria with normal neurologic development. Patients with a compatible electroclinical picture but abnormal development were termed non-classic BCECTS. The twin data didn't show any concordant twin pair with classic BCECTS, suggesting that non-inherited factors are of major importance in BCECTS. The authors found that genetic factors are probably more important in non-classic BCECTS. The conclusion at present is that the etiology and mode of inheritance are much more complicated than initially thought (Vadlamudi *et al.*, 2006). Linkage to chromosome 15q14 was found in 54 patients of 22 families with benign childhood epilepsy with centrotemporal spikes (Neubauer *et al.*, 1998). However, in a study of 70 families with the same syndrome in Italy, the mentioned linkage could not be found (Pruna *et al.*, 2000). A similar seizures and EEG phenotype of BCECTS was found in 3 children with "de novo" terminal deletions of the long arm of chromosome 1q and the authors suggested that it could be a potential site for a candidate gene (Vaughn *et al.*, 1996).

The potassium chloride cotransporter KCC3 was looked for as a candidate gene in 16 families with rolandic epilepsy, but the results did not support a role of KCC3 in the etiology of BCECTS (Steinlein *et al.*, 2001).

The association of an Autosomal recessive rolandic epilepsy with paroxysmal dystonia induced by exercise and writer's cramp and its gene mapping to chromosome 16p12-11.2 was described (Guerrini *et al.*, 1999).

A family with nine affected individuals in three generations was reported showing the features of rolandic epilepsy associated with oral and speech dyspraxia and cognitive impairment (Scheffer *et al.*, 1995; Scheffer, 1999). (See Chapter 13).

Pathophysiology

Although the pathophysiology of BCECTS is unknown, and there is no associated structural lesion, the typical focal ictal clinical behavior and EEG discharge indicate a disturbance in the sylvian and rolandic areas (Engel & Fejerman, 1999-2006). Electrophysiologic studies, however, fail to demonstrate a discrete generator, and a large, shifting area of dysfunction may be present. In some patients with BCECTS, the occurrence of generalized spike-wave EEG discharges, as well as focal spikes in other areas, suggests a relationship between this disorder and the idiopathic generalized epilepsies, as well as with other idiopathic localization-related partial epilepsies (Luders et al., 1987; Lerman & Kivity, 1991). Ten percent to 20% of patients with centrotemporal spikes may also have sharp slow wave complexes in other cortical locations (Panayiotopoulos, 1999).

Combined recording of interictal spikes and somatosensory-evoked potentials concluded that in some patients multiple simultaneous neuronal populations are active within the central region (Baumgartner et al., 1996).

Magnetoencephalographic analysis of generator and propagation of rolandic discharges in BCECTS with neuromagnetic three-dimensional dipole localization suggested that rolandic discharges are generated through a mechanism similar to that of somatosensory-evoked responses (Minami et al., 1996). A localization analysis of spontaneous magnetic brain activities also suggested the value of magnetoencephalography for pathophysiological elucidation (Kamada et al., 1998). Six children with bilateral centrotemporal synchronous discharges were studied using magnetoencephalography and EEG with equivalent current dipole modeling. Results implied cortical epileptogeneicity in bilateral perirolandic areas (Lin et al., 2003). Interictal spikes were recorded during fMRI acquisition in a MR-compatible digital EEG system in 7 children, and the spike-related activation in the perisylvian central region was found in 3 of them (Boor et al., 2003). Using high resolution EEG and MEG and a realistic volume conductor model, spacio-temporal aspect of the sources of spikes in children with BCECTS were investigated. Results for the EEG and MEG were different. Both high resolution EEG and MEG revealed that in some cases sources well separated in space and time exist, whereas in other cases only single source activity can be resolved (Huiskamp et al., 2004). In a more recent study of 10 children combining MEG and EEG to elucidate the oscillatory dynamics with respect to interictal spike occurrence in BCECTS, bilateral increase of 0.5-25 Hz oscillations during unilateral spike formation was found, suggesting that by using wavelet transform analysis, one could be able to detect irritative features not detected in visual analysis (Lin et al., 2006).

In a recent paper on BCECTS, Landau Kleffner syndrome and Electrical status epilepticus in sleep were considered as a spectrum of disorders with a common transient, age dependent, non-lesional, genetically based epileptogenic abnormality implying the role of a perisylvian epileptic network. The authors speak about "mild to severe epileptic encephalopathy limited to the perisylvian network, were the cognitive impairment is caused by epileptic discharges interfering with cognitive development" (Halasz et al., 2005).

Diagnostic work-up

EEG and other neurophysiologic studies have been considered in detail. Abnormal processing of auditory information in children with BCECTS was detected through a study with event related auditory potentials (Liasis *et al.*, 2006). In a previous study of dichotic listening in 13 children with BCECTS, auditory discrimination problems were found in patients compared to controls (Lundberg *et al.*, 2004).

Structural and functional neuroimaging

When the clinical and EEG features are typical, the diagnosis is certain, and therefore neuroimaging in BCECTS has been regarded as superfluous by many authors (Lerman, 1998; Arzimanoglou *et al.*, 2004). However, several reports called attention to a higher percentage of brain abnormalities in children with typical BCECTS. Gelisse *et al.* (1999) presented a 10-year-old-boy disclosing a very marked right hippocampal atrophy, although they concluded that the seizure disorder could not be ascribed to this abnormality. The same group reported CT or MRI abnormalities in 10 of 71 consecutive patients with BCECTS, but the sample was most probably biased because 2 of the 5 children showing enlargement of the lateral ventricle had shunted hydrocephalus (Gelisse *et al.*, 2003). Hippocampal asymmetries and white matter abnormalities in MRI have been reported in 33% of 18 children with BCECTS, but their etiology was considered unclear (Lundberg *et al.*, 1999). In a further study of 13 electroclinically typical cases of BCECTS compared with 13 healthy controls, metabolic changes were analyzed in the hippocampal region with proton magnetic resonance spectroscopy (^{1}H-MRS). Lateralization of the interictal epileptiform activity corresponded with the lower tNAA/tCr ratio in 10 of 13 patients. Hippocampal asymmetry was again found in 4 of 13 patients (Lundberg *et al.*, 2003). However, the finding of subtle MRI asymmetries in the control group casts doubt about the interpretation of these imaging findings.

A few cases were reported with electroclinical phenotypes of BCECTS associated with cortical dysplasia (Ambrosetto, 1992; Sheth *et al.*, 1997). One of us (NF) had the chance to follow a boy with a clear heterotopic mass on the same region were the spikes arised from. Medication stopped the Rolandic seizures and after puberty the patient remained with clinical and EEG normalization (Fejerman, 1996, 2002). A "pseudo-BCECTS" syndrome was reported in 5 children with brain tumors (Shevell *et al.*, 1996), but 2 of the cases had deep thalamic tumors making not clear the cause-effect relation between the pathology and the centrotemporal spikes with Rolandic seizures of these patients. On the other hand, the group of Marseille had presented before the coincidental finding of non-evolutive brain lesions and electroclinical features of BCECTS in 3 patients (Santanelli *et al.*, 1989).

On account of these findings, and the evaluation of what happens in everyday practice, we believe that it is licit to obtain an MRI study to avoid the phantoms of ignoring existing abnormalities.

EEG-assisted functional MRI (fMRI) was used in 7 children with BCECTS and the authors were able to demonstrate a spike-related fMRI activation in the perisylvian central region, although they accept that further improvements in the techniques are needed to evaluate the clinical application of this method (Boor *et al.*, 2003).

Very few functional neuroimaging studies utilizing PET have been performed in children with BCECTS. De Saint-Martin *et al.* (1999) reported a longitudinal study of a child with BCECTS using F-fluorodeoxyclucose (FDG) PET. They found a bilateral increase of glucose metabolism in the temporal opercular regions interictally during the "active" phase of the epilepsy. In 11 children with BCECTS studied with FDG-PET no interictal side differences in glucose metabolism were demonstrated (Van Bogaert *et al.*, 1998). These studies seem to confirm the hypothesis of a transient cortical modification with a bilateral increase in glucose metabolism in the central regions, in concordance with clinical oromotor symptoms and interictal EEG focus. These results are similar to those observed in Landau Kleffner syndrome or Continuous spike and wave during slow sleep syndrome (CSWSS) (Maquet *et al.*, 1995, 2000; da Silva *et al.* 1997; Guerreiro *et al.*, 1996).

Differential Diagnosis and relation with other epilepsy syndromes

In *Tables I and II* we summarize the alternatives of finding BCECTS phenotypes in children with cerebral pathology and the differential diagnosis between BCECTS and symptomatic, probably symptomatic, and other idiopathic epilepsy syndromes. Because of their prevalence, fortuitous associations may be found between benign childhood epilepsy with centrotemporal spikes and non-evolutive brain lesions (Santanelli *et al.*, 1989). Under diagnostic evaluation we already commented on these reported 3 patients. One of them had, for instance, a corpus callosum agenesis. One might speculate that this patient, studied at the time with TAC, probably had also some non-detected heterotopy and it would belong to the group with BCECTS phenotype and migrating disorders as described by several authors (Ambrosetto, 1992; Fejerman, 1996; Sheth *et al.*, 1997). We also mentioned and questioned if the 5 cases of "pseudo-BCECTS" associated with brain tumors really had a typical electroclinical phenotype (Shevell *et al.*, 1996), although we have to keep in mind the possibility of a mistake in the differential diagnosis. The last category in *Table I* refers to two possibilities: one, that children with cerebral palsy may also have a fortuitous association with CTS and Rolandic seizures; the second is constituted by a large series of patients that we are presenting in Chapter 11 who had congenital hemiparesis associated with

Table I. Diagnosis of BCECTS in children with cerebral pathology

- Occasional associations of BCECTS with non-evolutive cerebral lesions
- BCECTS "phenotype" and unilateral focal heterotopia
- BCECTS in children with cerebral palsy
  - As a fortuitous association
  - As a peculiar syndrome (not so benign) in children with unilateral polymicrogyria

Table II. Differential diagnosis between BCECTS and other epilepsy syndromes

- ■ With symptomatic or probably symptomatic epilepsies
  - Mesial temporal lobe epilepsy
  - Symptomatic lateral temporal lobe epilepsy
  - Other focal epilepsies with seizures arising from neocortical areas
  - Symptomatic epilepsies arising from Rolandic – Sylvian areas
- ■ With other idiopathic epilepsy syndromes
  - Benign infantile focal epilepsy with midline spikes and waves during sleep
  - Panayiotopoulos syndrome
  - Late-onset occipital lobe epilepsy (Gastaut type)
  - Other proposed benign focal epilepsy syndromes
  - Autosomal dominant partial epilepsy with auditory features
  - Autosomal dominant rolandic epilepsy with speech dyspraxia

unilateral polymicrogyria and behave electroclinically in a quite similar way to our cases of BCECTS who present an atypical evolution with bilateral secondary synchronies in the EEG and transient neuropsychologic deterioration.

Distinction between BCECTS and more serious non-idiopathic epileptic conditions, such as mesial temporal lobe epilepsy, can usually be made easily on the basis of history and the unique dipole pattern of the centrotemporal spike. However, benign focal epileptiform discharges were found in two of 17 preadolescent children who eventually underwent anteromesial temporal resection for refractory temporal lobe epilepsy due to hippocampal sclerosis and the authors suggested that it might not have been an incidental finding (Pan *et al.*, 2004).

Of course, frontal or parietal epilepsy syndromes may present motor or sensory seizures mimicking in some way the rolandic seizures, but the most difficult differential diagnosis are posed when the signs or symptoms arise from rolandic-sylvian areas. Five children with a so-called "malignant rolandic-sylvian epilepsy" secondary to neuronal migration disorders and gliosis were reported as presenting similar clinical and EEG features of benign childhood epilepsy with centrotemporal spikes. The authors emphasized the role of magnetoencephalography in the differential diagnosis (Otsubo *et al.*, 2001).

Differential diagnosis with other idiopathic epilepsy syndromes is not such a burden in the sense that if we miss it there will be not much harm to the patient, but nevertheless it is our responsibility. Besides, it opens an intriguing field to speculate about variable phenotypes. Onset of benign partial epilepsy with vertex spikes is before the age of BCECTS and details are given in chapter 5. Panayiotopoulos syndrome is the special case to discuss, since we and others have described patients presenting clinical and EEG features of both syndromes in the same episodes, in the same night, or in a time sequence (Caraballo *et al.*, 1998; Covanis *et al.*, 2003). The Gastaut type of childhood occipital epilepsy presents quite different clinical and EEG features. As for the other proposed benign focal epilepsies, specially the one with affective symptomatology described by Dalla Bernardina *et al.* (1980), the author is now thinking that it is a variant of BCECTS, and he is covering extensively the subject in Chapter 9.

Relations with other idiopathic epileptic syndromes

It is not so difficult to envisage that the not exceptional findings of two idiopathic benign focal epilepsy syndromes occurring in the same patients might suggest that they constitute phenotypic variants of a single condition. In 1998 we reported 10 neurologically normal children who presented the following features: ictal vomiting in 10 cases, ictal anarthria in 10 cases, oculocephalic deviation in 9 cases, clonic partial seizures in 7 cases, 2 of them with secondary generalization. Seizures were prevalent during sleep. The EEGs showed occipital spikes during sleep in all cases and on wakefulness in 7 patients. The same EEGs showed independent centrotemporal spikes in 9 cases. We disclosed three well-defined groups: five children started with Panayiotopoulos syndrome (PS) and after certain time presented seizures typical of BCECTS. The second group comprised three patients who featured in the same attack typical seizures of PS and BCECTS. Other two cases presented in different occasions independent seizures of BCECTS and PS (Caraballo et al., 1998). The association of BCECTS and Childhood absence epilepsy has also been reported. Three children had typical BCECTS and 1-4 years after recovering from the electroclinical picture, presented typical absences with generalized spike-wave discharges. Their long term course was excellent (Gambardella et al., 1996). Generalized synchronous 3Hz spike and wave complexes, as well as CTS, in the same EEG or in different recordings were also reported in five children. Two of them showed clinically both absences and focal motor seizures. Other two had only absences, and the other patient presented only focal motor seizures (Ramelli et al., 1998). Among our 398 cases of BCECTS we registered two patients who later presented typical absences. We have also presented clinico-EEG evidence of cases showing the association of other Benign focal epilepsies with absence epilepsy, namely, patients with Panayiotopoulos syndrome and late-onset occipital epilepsy of the Gastaut type evolving into typical childhood absence epilepsies (Caraballo et al., 2004, 2005). It is also very interesting to quote the report of two siblings with Benign familial neonatal convulsions who presented a few years later typical features of BCECTS (Maihara et al., 1999). In Chapter 3 we already mentioned that three of our patients with familial and non familial Benign infantile seizures prented during childhood typical electroclinical features of BCECTS, while other two only showed CTS.

Finally, we also have a chapter devoted to familial (autosomal dominant) focal epilepsies, including the autosomal dominant partial epilepsies with auditory features (Ottman et al., 1995, 1995) and autosomal dominant rolandic epilepsy with speech dyspraxia (Scheffer et al., 1995; Scheffer, 1999).

Another interesting association to consider is between idiopathic benign focal epilepsies and migraine. Relationship between epilepsies and migraine have been visualized since long-time ago (Andermann & Lugaresi, 1987). We know that the prevalence of migraine in children is around 5% (Di Blasi et al., 2007), while the prevalence of epilepsy is 1%. Therefore chances exist of coincidental coexistence of both conditions in the same persons. However, epidemiological data were collected showing that the prevalence of migraine in populations with epilepsy is around 10%, and the prevalence of epilepsy in migraineous populations is also significantly higher than in the general population (Andermann & Andermann, 1987). The concept of migraine epilepsy syndrome or migralepsy is intermittently activated in the literature making things even more difficult (Panayiotopoulos, 1987; Andermann, 2000; Milligan & Bromfield, 2005). We know that migraine symptoms are part of the Gastaut type of childhood occipital epilepsy, and we'll comment on all the details in Chapter 8. In a chapter of the book "Migraine and epilepsy" (Andermann & Lugaresi, 1987), Bladin presented evidence of association between BCECTS and migraine through the 5 to 8 years follow-up of 30 patients with BCECTS. In a more recent report, prevalence of migraine was compared in 3 cohorts of 53 childrens each: a) children with BCECTS; b) patients with cryptogenic/symptomatic partial epilepsy; c) children with no history of seizures (Wirrell & Hamiwka, 2006). The conclusion was that partial epilepsy, regardless of etiology, is associated with higher rates of migraine in children. In our series of 398 patients with BCECTS we also found an increased history of migraine in first degree relatives and in the patients. This intriguing association of two conditions which have different pathophysiology clearly requires further investigations.

Treatment

When we consider outcome in children with BCECTS, we have to talk about control of seizures on one side, and incidence of neuropsychological impairments, either transitory or persistent, on the other side. Regarding control of seizures, treatment is usually effective although many colleagues think that drug treatment is not necessary in the benign focal epilepsies of childhood (Panayiotopoulos, 1999; Galanopoulou et al., 2000; Dalla Bernardina et al., 2005). Therefore, continuous treatment should be considered only in subjects with frequent seizures and when the ictal events are disruptive to the patient or family. However, it is difficult to evaluate the degree of distress in the family after a seizure, specially in cases in which the first seizure occurred at night and motivated a hospital admission.

Carbamazepine was always the drug of choice (Fejerman & Medina, 1986; Watanabe, 2004; Lundberg, 2004; Chahine & Mikati, 2006). However, it has been demonstrated that Carbamazepine can induce an increase in spike-wave activity and negative myoclonus (Shields & Saslow, 1983; Caraballo et al., 1989; Prats et al., 1998; Kochen et al., 2002), and therefore should not be used in BCECTS cases showing spike-wave discharges, either during sleep or while awake. In a retrospective study of 98 consecutive cases of BCECTS, 40 of them were exposed to Carbamazepine and only 1 case of electroclinical aggravation was found (Corda et al., 2001). Phenobarbital, Phenytoin and Valproic acid had been reported as equally effective but are less used. Besides, all three drugs have also induced atypical evolutions in children with BCECTS (Fejerman et al., 2000; Prats et al., 1998). Benzodiazepines were also repeatedly recommended, in one report only for several weeks (De Negri et al., 1997). In comparison with Valproate and Carbamazepine, Clonazepam showed to be more efficient in making rolandic discharges disappear after four weeks of treatment (Mitsudome et al., 1997b). However, clinicians shouldn't look only to EEG abnormalities and their fast disappearance under treatment, but should also evaluate the control of seizures and the adverse effects of medicaments. At present, the use of Benzodiazepines at night is one of the first choices in those children who only have seizures during sleep. We are using now 10 mg of Clobazam given at night in the children with seizures during night sleep. It doesn't seem to interfere with day time activities. Besides, it is well known that Benzodiazepines do not worsen the EEG discharges and do not induce the mentioned complications of BCECTS. We'll see later in chapter10 how Clobazam or Diazepam become the drugs of choice in cases showing an atypical clinico-EEG evolution. As always, a recent report constitutes the exception: the case of a 10-year old girl who presented severe somnolence and daily enuresis one month after receiving 0.6 mg/kg/day of Clobazam. After finding very high plasma levels of Clobazam, mutations in the CYP2C19 were demonstrated and symptoms disappeared after withdrawal of Clobazam (Parmeggiani et al., 2004).

Sulthiame was recommended in several reports (Doose et al., 1988; Lerman & Lerman-Sagie, 1995; Lerman, 1998; Ben-Zeev et al., 2004). In a double blind, placebo controlled study of 66 children with benign childhood epilepsy with centrotemporal spikes, Sulthiame was found to be remarkably effective in preventing seizures and well tolerated (Rating et al., 2000). Another report also shows the benefits of Sulthiame (Engler et al., 2003). Therapeutic efficacy of Carbamazepine *versus* Sulthiame was compared in 38 patients who received Carbamazepine and 18 patients who received Sulthiame. Cessation of seizures was observed in 73.6% of the former and in 76.7% of the latter. Normalization of interictal epileptiform activity was seen in 71% of the patients with Sulthiame and in 42% of those with Carbamazepine. The authors concluded that no significant differences between these two medications were found in the treatment of BCECTS (Kramer et al., 2002a). Tachypnea, hyperpnea, paraesthesia and headache are well known side-effects of high doses of Sulthiame (Gross-Selbeck, 1995), but again, one case was reported showing depressed mode, fatigue and lack of drive with only 5 mg/kg/day of this drug. Symptoms disappeared after withdrawal of Sulthiame, although no data on EEG during the worsening period was given in this letter to the Editor (Weglage et al., 1999).

Almost all of the new drugs had been used, at least anecdotally, to treat children with BCECTS. Oxcarbazepine monotherapy in 70 newly diagnosed patients with BCECTS followed up during 18 months was considered effective in preventing seizures, normalizing EEGs, and even in preserving cognitive functions and behavioral abilities (Tzitiridou et al., 2005). Oxcarbazepine induced epileptic negative myoclonus in a child with symptomatic focal epilepsy (Hahn et al., 2004). More recently, Oxcarbazepine was considered responsible of atypical evolutions in 3 patients with BCECTS who already had some atypical features (Grosso et al., 2006). We also saw 2 patients who evolved into Atypical benign focal epilepsy of childhood while on treatment with Oxcarbazepine.

In 1998 a double blind, randomized, placebo-controlled study of gabapentin (GBP) in BCECTS was reported. A total of 225 patients was enrolled and received either GBP, 30 mg/kg/day or placebo. The study lasted 36 weeks and authors concluded that GBP monotherapy was effective in controlling seizures in children with BCECTS (Bourgeois et al., 1998; Bourgeois, 2000).

Lamotrigine also induced seizure aggravation and negative myoclonus in 2 children with BCECTS (Catania et al., 1999, Cerminara et al., 2004) and we are not aware of any large series of patients with BCECTS treated with this drug. The same is true for Topiramate, although there is an anecdotal report of CSWSS induced by Topiramate (Montenegro & Guerreiro, 2002). We also saw one patient with bilateral secondary synchronies and atonic seizures induced by this drug. However, it must be kept in mind, that probably both drugs are added in cases which already had showed resistance to other drugs and are more prone to present atypical evolutions.

Levetiracetam showed to be efficacious and well tolerated as add-on therapy in children with resistant partial seizures (Glauser *et al.*, 2006). Levetiracetam has been used in a few children with BCECTS with good results (Bello-Espinosa & Roberts, 2003). In a recent comparative study between Levetiracetam and Oxcarbazepine, 39 children with BCECTS were randomly allocated to one of these drugs. Preliminary findings suggested that both drugs where effective (Coppola *et al.*, 2006). A recent monotherapy non-controlled study with Levetiracetam in 21 children with BCECTS showed that it is effective and well tolerated in children using dosis ranging from 1,000 to 2,500 mg per day (Verrotti *et al.*, 2007). However, more Levetiracetam monotherapy trials in children with BCECTS are still needed.

Curiously enough, through an ictal clinical and EEG study in 1 child, it was suggested that voluntary protrusion of the tongue could stop seizures and EEG discharges (Veggiotti *et al.*, 1999).

In a prospective study of treatment in childhood epilepsy, it was concluded that 1 year of treatment can be recommended in children with benign childhood epilepsy with centrotemporal spikes (Braathen *et al.*, 1996). In fact, once the decision to treat is taken, we cannot speak of a given term of time, but there is no need to wait for the normalization of the EEG to stop medication (Shorvon, 2005). Relapse of seizures, however, may occur after premature withdrawal (Loiseau & Duche, 1989).

If we consider that there is risk for an atypical evolution due to the finding of worsening of the EEG, or increase of number of seizures, or presence of inhibitory seizures, or evidence of neuropsychological impairments, the steps should be: first stop the previous medications, be they Carbamazepine, Oxcarbazepine, Phenytoin or Valproic acid and then switch to benzodiazepine, Ethosuximide or Sulthiame. We'll enter more in detail about this subject in Chapter 10.

Prognosis and long-term evolution

In general, BCECTS is associated with excellent prognosis. Seizures eventually disappear and EEGs normalize irrespective of treatment. Over 90% of the cases are in remission by 12 years of age (Watanabe, 2004). Seizures are difficult to control in only a small number of cases (Beaussart & Faou, 1978; Blom & Heijbel, 1982). The prognosis is favorable even for those whose seizures are difficult to control, and seizures almost always remit spontaneously in adolescence. In their investigation of 168 patients 7 to 30 years after cessation of epilepsy with centrotemporal spikes, Loiseau and colleagues reported that seizures occurred in only three cases after adulthood (Loiseau *et al.*, 1988). The seizure types were all generalized tonic-clonic seizures. Two of the three had obviously isolated incidences. This incidence of generalized seizures in adults with a history of epilepsy with centrotemporal spikes in childhood is nevertheless higher than that of seizures in the general population (Loiseau *et al.*, 1988). We had the same experience as is shown in *Table III*. Cognitive functions were evaluated in 23 adolescents and young adults in complete

Table III. Long-term follow-up of 58 patients with BCECTS*

1. Population: 58 patients aged now between 21 and 41 years
2. Gender: 33 (57% males), 25 (43% females)
3. Age at onset: mean 6.9 years (range 3-12)
4. Seizures: last seizure before the age of 16 years in all cases (range 5-16 years)
5. Treatment: 21 subjects have never been treated
6. Evolution during long-term follow-up:
   - 2 patients died (1 car accident, 1 leukemia)
   - 3 patients suffered from other seizures after the age of 18 years
   - 36 have a satisfactory working career according to education degree achieved
   - 16 are still attending school with normal results
   - 6 have severe learning and working difficulties but only one with IQ lower than 70

* *Unit of child neuropsychiatry, University of Verona.*

remission from benign childhood epilepsy with centrotemporal spikes showing no significant differences with controls. However, qualitative analysis suggested a different organizational pattern for cerebral language in adolescents and young adults in remission from this syndrome (Hommet et al., 2001).

A meta-analysis of the course of patients with BCECTS, based on 794 patients in 13 cohorts, concluded that the early prediction of seizure outcome in the new patient cannot be given with certainty (Bouma et al., 1997).

Prognosis was evaluated on account of clinical and EEG parameters in children with BCECTS. The presence of atypical interictal epileptiform EEG patterns did not appear to alter prognosis in one study (Beydoun et al., 1992). Clinical and EEG markers for risk of behavioral problems and cognitive dysfunctions were looked-for in a prospective study of 35 unselected children with BCECTS, followed until complete remission of seizures and normalization of the EEGs. The authors were able to disclose two groups at the end of follow-up. Group 1 did not display any relevant behavior or cognitive problem, while group 2 developed serious difficulties that impaired the quality of life, both at home and at school. Different combinations of six distinct interictal EEG patterns seemed to be the hallmarks of patients at risk of neuropsychological impairments (Massa et al., 2001) *(Figs. 10, 11)*. In another report, clinical characteristics were used to identify patients at risk for multiple seizures, and the only predictor for a disease course with multiple seizures was an onset prior to 3 years of life (Kramer et al., 2002b). An eight years follow-up study of 85 children with BCECTS separated patients into two groups. Group A (74 patients) with typical BCECTS and group B (11 children) with atypical features. No patient of either group developed status epilepticus, Landau Kleffner syndrome, or CSWSS syndrome. The responses to treatment were similar in the two groups of children, but a significant higher percentage of learning and behavioral disabilities were found in children of group B (Verrotti et al., 2002). Poor response to treatment in association with early onset of seizures was again recently reported in a retrospective study of 144 patients (You et al., 2006).

Atypical features and atypical evolutions of BCECTS have been considered in a recent comprehensive review of the subject (Chahine & Mikati, 2006).

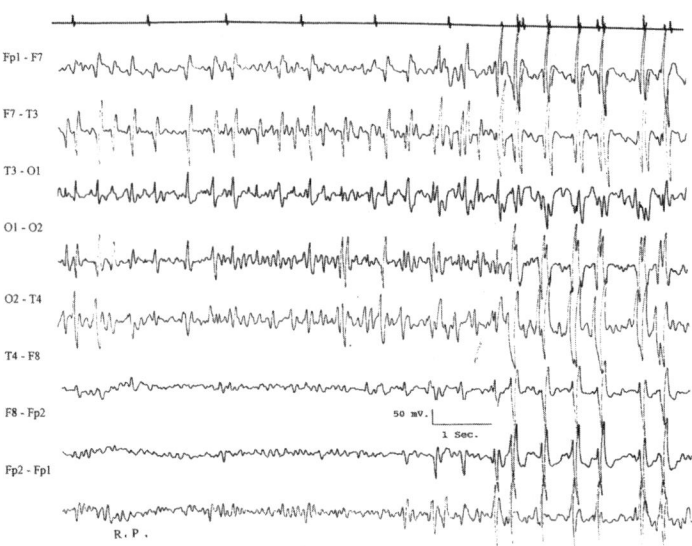

Figure 10. Six years old boy. Sleep EEG during the period of typical BCECTS seizures. Shows very frequent centrotemporal spikes with marked diffusion within the same hemisphere and synchronic discharges in the other hemisphere. This child did present several months later frequent inhibitory seizures with falls and ESES in the EEG.

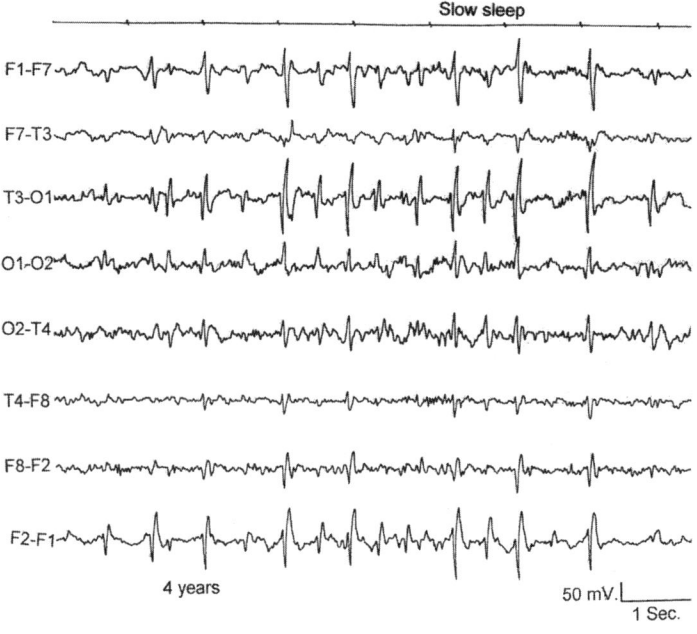

Figure 11. Four years old boy. EEG shows propagation of centrotemporal spikes to anterior areas. Several months later the patient presented the clinico-EEG features of an atypical evolution of BCECTS.

Of course, prognosis will be quite different in the cases evolving into Atypical benign partial epilepsy of childhood, Status of BCECTS, Landau-Kleffner syndrome or CSWSS syndrome. As we'll see in Chapter 10, early recognition of these atypical evolutions is crucial to the decision of switching antiepileptic drugs and treating adequately these cases.

Coming back to what we said earlier, the great majority of children with BCECTS are able to attend normal schools. Interestingly, in a recent study investigating the influence of cognition on the quality of life of 30 children with BCECTS, parental emotional impact was considered the major independent predictor of quality of life (Connolly et al., 2006).

Table III includes data about long-term follow-up of 58 patients in Verona (Bernardo Dalla Bernardina).

References

- Aicardi J, Chevrie JJ. Épilepsie partielle avec foyer rolandique de la secoónde enfance. *J Paris Pediatr* 1969; 4: 125-42.

- Aicardi J, Chevrie JJ. Atypical benign partial epilepsy of childhood. *Dev Med Child Neurol* 1982; 24: 281-92.

- Aicardi J. Atypical semiology of Rolandic epilepsy in some related syndromes. *Epileptic Disorders* 2000; 2 (Suppl 1): S5-S10.

- Alvarez N, Lombroso CT, Medina C, Cantlon B. Paroxysmal spike and wave activity in drowsiness in young children: its relationship to febrile convulsions. *Electroenceph and Clin Neurophysiol* 1983; 56: 406-13.

- Ambrosetto G, Gobbi G. Benign epilepsy of childhood with Rolandic spikes or a lesion? EEG during a seizure. *Epilepsia* 1975; 16: 793-6.

- Ambrosetto G. Unilateral opercular macrogyria and benign childhood epilepsy with centrotemporal (rolandic) spikes. *Epilepsia* 1992; 33: 499-503.

- Andermann E, Andermann F. Migraine epilepsy relationship: Epidemiological and genetic aspects. In: Andermann F, Lugaresi E (Eds). *Migraine and Epilepsy*. Boston: Butterworths, 1987: 281-92.

- Andermann F, Lugaresi E (Eds). *Migraine and Epilepsy*. Boston: Butterworths, 1987.

- Andermann F. Migraine and the benign partial epilepsies of childhood: evidence for an association. *Epileptic Disorders* 2000; 2 (Suppl 1), S37-S40.

- Arzimanoglou A, Guerrini R, Aicardi J. Epilepsies characterized by partial seizures. In: Arzimanoglou A, Guerrini R, Aicardi J. (Eds). *Aicardi's epilepsy in children*. 3rd Edition. Philadelphia: Lippincott Williams & Wilkins, 2004: 114-75.

- Baglietto MG, Battaglia FM, Nobili L, et al. Neuropsychological disorders related to interictal epileptic discharges during sleep in benign epilepsy of childhood with centrotemporal or Rolandic spikes. *Dev Med Child Neurol* 2001; 43: 407-12.

- Bancaud J, Colomb D, Dell MB. Les pointes rolandiques : un symtôme EEG propre à l'enfant. *Rev Neurol* (Paris) 1958 ; 99: 206-9.

- Baumgartner C, Graf M, Doppelbauer A, et al. The functional organization of the interictal spike complex in benign rolandic epilepsy. *Epilepsia* 1996; 37 (12): 1164-74.

- Beaussart M. Benign epilepsy of children with rolandic (centrotemporal) paroxysmal foci. *Epilepsia* 1972; 13: 795-811.

- Beaussart M, Faou. Evolution of epilepsy with rolandic paroxysmal foci: a study of 324 cases. *Epilepsia* 1978; 19: 337-42.

- Bedoin N, Herbillon V, Lamoury I, et al. Hemispheric lateralization of cognitive functions in children with centrotemporal spikes. *Epilepsy Behav* 2006; 9 (2): 268-74.

- Bello-Espinosa LE, Roberts SL. Levetiracetam for benign epilepsy of childhood with centrotemporal spikes – three cases. *Seizure* 2003; 12: 157-9.

- Ben-Zeev B, Watemberg N, Lerman P, et al. Sulthiame in childhood epilepsy. *Pediatr Int* 2004; 46 (5): 521-4.

- Berkovic SF, Scheffer IE. Genetics of partial epilepsies: new frontiers. In: Berkovic SF, Genton P, Hirsch E, Picard F (Eds). *Genetic of focal epilepsies*. London: John Libbey, 1999: 7-14.

- Beydoun A, Garofalo EA, Drury I. Generalized spike-waves, multiple loci, and clinical course in children with EEG features of benign epilepsy of childhood with centrotemporal spikes. *Epilepsia* 1992; 33: 1091-6.

- Bladin PF. The association of Benign rolandic epilepsy with migraine. In: Andermann F, Lugaresi E (Eds). *Migraine and Epilepsy*. Boston: Butterworths, 1987: 145-52.

- Blom S, Heijbel J, Bergfors PG. Benign epilepsy of children with centrotemporal foci: prevalence and follow-up study of 40 patients. *Epilepsia* 1972; 13: 609-19.

- Blom S, Heijbel J. Benign epilepsy of children with centrotemporal EEG foci: a follow-up study in adulthood of patients initially studied as children. *Epilepsia* 1982; 23: 629-31.

- Boor S, Vucurevic G, Pfleiderer C, et al. EEG-related functional MRI in benign childhood epilepsy with centrotemporal spikes. *Epilepsia* 2003; 44 (5): 688-92.

- Bouma PA, Bovenkerk AC, Westendorp RG, Brouwer OF. The course of benign partial epilepsy of childhood with centrotemporal spikes: a meta-analysis. *Neurology* 1997; 48 (2): 430-7.

- Bourgeois B, Brown W, Pellock JM, et al. Gabapentin (Neurontin) monotherapy in children with Benign childhood epilepsy with centrotemporal spikes (BECTS): A 36-week, double blind, placebo-controlled study. *Epilepsia* 1998; 39 (6): 163 (Abstract).

- Bourgeois B. Drug treatment of benign focal epilepsies of childhood. *Epilepsia* 2000; 41 (8): 1057-8.

- Braathen G, Andersson T, Gylje H, et al. Comparison between one and three years of treatment in uncomplicated childhood epilepsy: a prospective study. I. Outcome in different seizure types. *Epilepsia* 1996; 37 (9): 822-32.

- Bray PF, Wiser WC. Evidence for a genetic etiology of temporal central abnormalities in focal epilepsy. *N Engl J Med* 1964; 271: 926-33.

- Cappell J, Schevon C, Emerson RG. Magnetoencephalography in epilepsy: tailoring interpretation and making inferences. *Curr Neurol Neurosci Rep* 2006; 6 (4): 327-31.

- Caraballo R, Fontana E, Michelizza B, et al. CBZ inducing atypical absences, drop-spells and continuous spike and waves during slow sleep (CSWS). *Boll Lega It Epil* 1989; 66/67: 379-81.

- Caraballo R, Cersosimo R, Fejerman N. Idiopathic partial epilepsies with rolandic and occipital spikes appearing in the same children. *J Epilepsy* 1998; 11: 261-4.

- Caraballo RH, Sologuestua A, Granana N, et al. Idiopathic occipital and absence epilepsies appearing in the same children. *Pediatr Neurol* 2004; 30 (1): 24-8.

- Caraballo RH, Cersosimo RO, Fejerman N. Late-onset, "Gastaut type", childhood occipital epilepsy: an unusual evolution. *Epileptic Disord* 2005; 7 (4): 341-6.

- Catania S, Cross H, de Sousa C, Boyd S. Paradoxic reaction to lamotrigine in a child with benign focal epilepsy of childhood with centrotemporal spikes. *Epilepsia* 1999; 40 (11): 1657-60.

- Cavazzuti GB. Epidemiology of different types of epilepsy in school age children of Modena, Italy. *Epilepsia* 1980; 21: 57-62.

- Cerminara C, Montanaro ML, Curatolo P, Seri S. Lamotrigine-induced seizure aggravation and negative myoclonus in idiopathic rolandic epilepsy. *Neurology* 2004; 63 (2): 373-5.

- Chahine LM, Mikati MA. Benign pediatric localization-related epilepsies. Syndromes in childhood. *Epileptic Disord* 2006; 8: 243-58.

- Colamaria V, Sgro V, Caraballo R, et al. Status epileptics in benign rolandic epilepsy manifesting as anterior operculum syndrome. *Epilepsia* 1991; 32: 329-34.

- Commission on Classification and Terminology of the International League Against Epilepsy. Proposal for revised classification of epilepsies and epileptic syndromes. *Epilepsia* 1989; 30: 389-99.

- Connolly AM, Northcott E, Cairns DR, et al. Quality of life of children with benign rolandic epilepsy. *Pediatr Neurol* 2006; 35 (4): 240-5.

- Coppola G, Franzoni E, Verrotti A, et al. Levetiracetam or oxcarbazepine as monotherapy in newly diagnosed benign epilepsy of childhood with centrotemporal spikes (BECTS): An open-label, parallel group trial. *Brain Dev* 2007; 29 (5): 281-4.

- Corda D, Gelisse P, Genton P, et al. Incidence of drug-induced aggravation in benign epilepsy with centrotemporal spikes. *Epilepsia* 2001; 42 (6): 754-9.

- Covanis A, Lada C, Skiadas K. Children with Rolandic spikes and ictal vomiting: Rolandic epilepsy or Panayiotopoulos syndrome? *Epileptic Disorders* 2003; 5 (3): 139-43.

- Croona C, Kihlgren M, Lundberg S, et al. Neuropsychological findings in children with benign childhood epilepsy with centrotemporal spikes. *Dev Med Child Neurol* 1999; 41: 813-8.

- Dai AI, Weinstock A. Post-ictal paresis in children with benign rolandic epilepsy. *J Child Neurol* 2005; 20 (10): 834-6.

- Dalla Bernardina B, Tassinari CA. EEG of a nocturnal seizure in a patient with benign epilepsy of childhood with rolandic spikes. *Epilepsia* 1975; 16: 497-501.

- Dalla Bernardina B, Beghini G. Rolandic spikes in children with and without epilepsy. *Epilepsia* 1976; 17: 161-7.

- Dalla Bernardina B, Bureau M, Dravet C, et al. Épilepsie bénigne de l'enfant avec crises à séméiologie affective. *Rev EEG Neurophysiol* 1980; 10: 8-18.

- Dalla Bernardina B, Sgro V, Caraballo R, et al. Sleep and benign partial epilepsies of childhood: EEG and evoked potential study. In: Degen R, Rodin EA (Eds). *Epilepsy, sleep and sleep deprivation*. Amsterdam: Elsevier, 1991: 83-96.

- Dalla Bernardina B, Sgro V, Fonatana E, et al. Idiopathic epilepsies in children. In: Roger J, Bureau M, Dravet C, et al. (Eds). *Epileptic syndromes in infancy, childhood and adolescence* (2nd Ed.). London: John-Libbey, 1992: 173-88.

- Dalla Bernardina B, Sgro V, Fejerman N. Epilepsy with centrotemporal spikes and related syndromes. In: Roger J, Bureau M, Dravet C, et al. (Eds). *Epileptic syndromes in infancy, childhood and adolescence* (3rd Ed.). London: John Libbey, 2002: 181-202.

- Dalla Bernardina B, Sgro V, Fejerman N. Epilepsy with centrotemporal spikes and related syndromes. In: Roger J, Bureau M, Dravet Ch, Genton P, Tassinari CA, Wolf P (Eds). *Epileptic syndromes in infancy, childhood and adolescence* (4rd Ed.). Montrouge: John Libbey, 2005: 203-25.

- Da Silva EA, Chugani DC, Muzik O, Chugani HT. Landau-Kleffner syndrome: metabolic abnormalities in temporal lobe are a common feature. *J Child Neurol* 1997; 12: 489-95.

- De Marco P, Tassinari CA. Extreme somatosensory evoked potentials (ESEP): a EEG sign forecasting the possible occurrence of seizures in children. *Epilepsia* 1981; 22: 569-85.

- De Negri M, Baglietto MG, Gaggero R. Benzodiazepine (BDZ) treatment of benign childhood epilepsy with centrotemporal spikes. *Brain Dev* 1997; 19 (7): 506.

- De Saint-Martin A, Petiau C, Massa R, et al. Idiopathic Rolandic epilepsy with "interictal" facial myoclonia and oromotor deficit: a longitudinal EEG and PET study. *Epilepsia* 1999; 40: 614-20.

- Degen R, Degen HE. Some genetic aspects of Rolandic epilepsy: waking and sleep EEGs in siblings. *Epilepsia* 1990; 31: 795-801.

- Degen R, Holthausen H, Pieper T, et al. Benign discharges in patients with lesional partial epilepsies. *Pediatr Neurol* 1999; 20: 354-9.

- Deonna T, Zesiger P, Davidoff V, Maeder M, Mayor C, Roulet E. Benign partial epilepsy of childhood: a longitudinal neuropsychological and EEG study of cognitive function. *Dev Med Child Neurol* 2000; 42 (9): 595-603.

- Deonna T. Rolandic epilepsy: neuropsychology of the active epilepsy phase. *Epileptic Disorders* 2000; 2 (Suppl 1): S59-S62.

- Di Blasi AM, Arroyo H, Fejerman N. Cefaleas y migrañas. In: Fejerman N, Fernadez-Alvarez E (Eds). *Neurologia Pediatrica* (3rd Ed.). Buenos Aires: Editorial Panamericana, 2007: 675-90.

- Doose H, Baier WK, Ernst JP, Tuxhorn I, Volzke E. Benign partial epilepsy: treatment with sulthiame. *Dev Med Child Neurol* 1988; 30: 683-4.

- Doose H, Brigger-Heuer B, Neubauer B. Children with focal sharp waves: clinical and genetic aspects. *Epilepsia* 1997; 38 (7): 788-96.

- Dubois CM, Zesiger P, Perez ER, Ingvar MM, Deonna T. Acquired epileptic dysgraphia: a longitudinal study. *Dev Med Child Neurol* 2003; 45 (12): 807-12.

- Eeg-Olofsson O, Petersen I, Selden U. The development of the electroencephalogram in normal children from the age of 1 through 15 years. *Neuropediatrie* 1971; 2: 375-404.

- Eeg-Olofsson O. Further genetic aspects in benign localized epilepsies in early childhood. In: Degen R, Dreifuss FE (Eds). *Benign localized and generalized epilepsies of early childhood. Epilepsy Research*. Suppl 6. Amsterdam: Elsevier, 1992: 117-9.

- Engel J Jr. A proposed diagnostic scheme for people with epileptic seizures and with epilepsy: Report of the ILAE Task Force on Classification and Terminology. *Epilepsia* 2001; 42 (6): 796-803.

- Engel J, Fejerman N. Benign childhood epilepsy with centrotemporal spikes. In: Engel J, Fejerman N (Eds). *MedLink Neurology* (Section of Epilepsy). San Diego: MedLink Corporation, 1999-2006. Available at www.medlink.com.

- Engel J. Report of the ILAE Classification Core Group. *Epilepsia* 2006; 47 (9): 1558-68.

- Engler F, Maeder-Ingvar M, Roulet E, Deonna T. Treatment with sulthiame (Ospolot) in benign partial epilepsy of childhood and related syndromes: an open clinical and EEG study. *Neuropediatrics* 2003; 34 (2): 105-9.

- Faure J, Loiseau P. Une corrélation clinique particulière des pointes-ondes sans signification focale. *Rev Neurol* 1960; 102: 399-406.

- Fejerman N, Medina CS (Eds). *Convulsiones en la infancia*. Buenos Aires: Editorial Ergon, 1977.

- Fejerman N, Medina CS. Epilepsia benigna de la infancia con espiga temporal media. In: Fernández Alvarez E, Fejerman N, Campos-Castelló J (Eds). *Actualidades en Neuropediatria*. Volumen 1. Barcelona: Editorial Médica y Técnica, 1980: 41-66.

- Fejerman N, Medina CS. *Convulsiones en la infancia* (2nd Ed.). Buenos Aires: Editorial El Ateneo, 1986: 166-78.

- Fejerman N, Di Blasi AM. Status epilepticus of benign partial epilepsies in children: report of two cases. *Epilepsia* 1987; 28: 351-5.

- Fejerman N. Atypical evolutions of benign partial epilepsies in children. *Int Pediatr* 1996; 11 (6): 351-6.

- Fejerman N, Medina CS, Caraballo R. Síndromes epilepticos en la infancia y adolescencia. In: Fejerman N, Fernadez-Alvarez E (Eds). *Neurologia Pediátrica* (2nd Ed.). Buenos Aires: Panamericana, 1997: 536-8.

- Fejerman N, Caraballo R, Tenembaum S. Epilepsias parciais idiopaticas. In: Costa da Costa J, Palmini A, Yacubian EMT, Cavalheiro EA (Eds). *Fundamentos Neurobiologicos das Epilepsias*. Sao Paulo: Lemos, 1998.

- Fejerman N, Caraballo R, Tenembaum SN. Atypical evolutions of benign localization-related epilepsies in children: are they predictable? *Epilepsia* 2000; 41 (4): 380-90.

- Fejerman N. Benign focal epilepsies in infancy, childhood and adolescence. *Rev Neurol* 2002; 34 (1): 7-18.

- Fejerman N. Benign childhood epilepsy with centrotemporal spikes. In: Engel J, Pedley TA (Eds). *Epilepsy: a comprehensive textbook*. Philadelphia: Lippincott Williams & Wilkins, 2007, In Press.

- Galanopoulou A, Bojko A, Lado F, Moshe SL. The spectrum of neuropsychiatric abnormalities associated with electrical status epilepticus in sleep. *Brain Dev* 2000; 22: 279-95.

- Gambardella A, Aguglia U, Guerrini R, *et al*. Sequential occurrence of benign partial epilepsy and childhood absence epilepsy in three patients. *Brain & Dev* 1996; 18: 212-5.

- Gastaut Y. Un élément déroutant de la séméiologie électroencéphalographique : les pointes prérolandiques sans signification focale. *Rev Neurol* (Paris) 1952 ; 87: 488-90.

- Gélisse P, Genton P, Raybaud C, *et al*. Benign childhood epilepsy with centrotemporal spikes and hippocampal atrophy. *Epilepsia* 1999; 40: 1312-5.

- Gélisse P, Corda D, Raybaud C, *et al*. Abnormal neuroimaging in patients with benign epilepsy with centrotemporal spikes. *Epilepsia* 2003; 44 (3): 372-8.

- Gibbs EL, Gibbs FA. Good prognosis of mid-temporal epilepsy. *Epilepsia* 1960; 1: 448-53.

- Glauser TA, Ayala R, Elterman RD, *et al*. Double-blind placebo-controlled trial of adjunctive levetiracetam in pediatric partial seizures. *Neurology* 2006; 66 (11): 1654-60.

- Gregory DL, Wong PK. Topographical analysis of the centrotemporal discharges in benign Rolandic epilepsy of childhood. *Epilepsia* 1984; 25: 705-11.

- Gregory DL, Farrell K, Wong PK. Partial status epilepticus in benign childhood epilepsy with centrotemporal spikes: are independent right and left seizures a risk factor? *Epilepsia* 2002; 43 (8): 936-40.

- Grosso S, Balestri M, Di Bartolo RM, *et al*. Oxcarbazepine and atypical evolution of benign idiopathic focal epilepsy of childhood. *Eur J Neurol* 2003; 13 (10): 1142-5.

- Gross-Selbeck G. Treatment of "benign" partial epilepsies of childhood, including atypical forms. *Neuropediatrics* 1995; 26: 45-50.

- Guerreiro MM, Camargo EE, Kato M, *et al*. Brain single photon emission computed tomography imaging in Landau-Kleffner syndrome. *Epilepsia* 1996; 37: 60-7.

- Guerrini R, Bonanni P, Nardocci N, *et al*. Autosomal recessive rolandic epilepsy with paroxysmal exercise-induced dystonia and writer's cramp: delineation of the syndrome and gene mapping to chromosome 16p 12-11.2. *Ann Neurol* 1999; 45: 344-52.

- Hahn H. Atypical benign partial epilepsy/pseudo-Lennox syndrome. *Epileptic Disorders* 2000; 2 (Suppl 1); S11-S18.

- Hahn A, Pistohl J, Neubauer BA, Stephani U. Atypical "benign" partial epilepsy or pseudo-Lennox syndrome. Part I: symptomatology and long-term prognosis. *Neuropediatrics* 2001; 32 (1): 1-8.

- Hahn A, Fischenbeck A, Stephani U. Induction of epileptic negative myoclonus by oxcarbazepine in symptomatic epilepsy. *Epileptic Disord* 2004; 6 (4): 271-4.

- Halasz P, Kelemen A, Clemens B, *et al*. The perisylvian epileptic network. A unifying concept. *Ideggyogy Sz* 2005; 58 (3-4): 104.

- Hande Sart ZH, Demirbilek V, Korkmaz B, *et al*. The consequences of idiopathic partial epilepsies in relation to neuropsychological functioning: a closer look at the associated mathematical disability. *Epileptic Disord* 2006; 8 (1): 24-31.

- Heijbel J, Blom S, Bergfors PG. (1975a) Benign epilepsy of children with centrotemporal EEG foci. Study of incidence rate in outpatient care. *Epilepsia* 1975; 16: 657-64.

- Heijbel J, Blom S, Rasmuson M. (1975b) Benign epilepsy of childhood with centrotemporal EEG foci: a genetic study. *Epilepsia* 1975; 16: 285-93.

- Heijbel J, Bohman M. Benign epilepsy of children with centrotemporal EEG foci: intelligence, behavior and school adjustment. *Epilepsia* 1975; 16: 679-87.

- Herranz Tanarro FJ, Saenz Lope E, Sassot CS. La pointe-onde occipitale avec et sans épilepsie bénigne chez l'enfant. *Rev EEG Neurophysiol* 1984; 14: 1-7.

- Herranz JL. Broad clinical prognostic spectrum of Rolandic epilepsy: agreement, disagreement and open questions. *Rev Neurol* 2002; 35 (1): 79-81.

- Holmes GL. Rolandic epilepsy: clinical and electroencephalographic features. *Epilepsy Research* 1992; 6 (Suppl): 29-43.

- Holtmann M, Becker K, Kentner-Figura B, Schmidt MH. Increased frequency of Rolandic spikes in ADHD children. *Epilepsia* 2003; 44 (9): 1241-4.

- Holtmann M, Matei A, Hellmann U, *et al*. Rolandic spikes increase impulsivity in ADHD – A neuropsychological pilot study. *Brain Dev* 2006; 28 (10): 633-40.

- Hommet C, Billard C, Motte J, *et al*. Cognitive function in adolescents and young adults in complete remission from benign childhood epilepsy with centrotemporal spikes. *Epileptic Disord* 2001; 3 (4): 207-16.

- Huiskamp G, van Der Meij W, van Huffelen A, van Nieuwenhuizen O. High resolution spatio-temporal EEG-MEG analysis of rolandic spikes. *J Clin Neurophysiol* 2004; 21 (2): 84-95.

- Ishitobi M, Nakasato N, Yamamoto K, Iinuma K. Opercular to interhemispheric source distribution of benign rolandic spikes of childhood. *Neuroimage* 2004; 25 (2): 417-23.

- Jallon P, Loiseau P, Loiseau J. Newly diagnosed unprovoked epileptic seizures: presentation at diagnosis in CAROLE study. *Epilepsia* 2001; 42: 464-75.

- Kajitani T, Nakamura M, Ueoka K, Koduchi S. Three pairs of monozygotic twins with rolandic discharges. In: Wada J, Penny J (Eds). *Advances in Epileptology, the Xth International Symposium*. New York: Raven Press, 1980: 171-5.

- Kajitani T, Kimura T, Sumita M, Kaneko M. Relationship between benign epilepsy of children with centrotemporal EEG foci and febrile convulsions. *Brain Dev* 1992; 14: 230-4.

- Kamada K, Moller M, Saguer M, *et al*. Localization analysis of neuronal activities in benign rolandic epilepsy using magnetoencephalography. *J Neurol Sci* 1998; 154 (2): 164-72.

- Kochen S, Gigante B, Oddo S. Spike-and-wave complexes and seizure exacerbation caused by carbamazepine. *Eur J Neurol* 2002; 9: 41-7.

- Kramer U, Nevo Y, Neufeld MY, *et al*. Epidemiology of epilepsy in childhood: a cohort of 440 consecutive patients. *Pediatr Neurol* 1998; 18 (1): 46-50.

- Kramer U, Ben-Zeev B, Harel S, Kivity S. Transient oromotor deficits in children with benign childhood epilepsy with central temporal spikes. *Epilepsia* 2001; 42 (5): 616-20.

- Kramer U, Shahar E, Zelnik N, *et al*. (2002a) Carbamazepine versus sulthiame in treating benign childhood epilepsy with centrotemporal spikes. *J Child Neurol* 2002; 17 (12): 914-6.

- Kramer U, Zelnik N, Lerman-Sagie T, Shahar E. (2002b) Benign childhood epilepsy with centrotemporal spikes: clinical characteristics and identification of patients at risk of multiple seizures. *J Child Neurol* 2002; 17 (1): 17-9.

- Kraschnitz W, Scheer P, Korner K, *et al*. Rolandic spikes as an EEG manifestation of an oligodendro-glioma. *Pediatr Pathol* 1988; 23: 313-9.

- Langill L, Wong PK. Tactile-evoked rolandic discharges: a benign finding? *Epilepsia* 2003; 44 (2): 221-7.

- Larsson K, Eeg-Olofsson O. A population based study of epilepsy in children from a Swedish county. *Eur J Paediatr Neurol* 2006; 10 (3): 107-13.

- Legarda S, Jayakar P, Duchowny M, *et al*. Benign rolandic epilepsy: high central and low central subgroups. *Epilepsia* 1994; 35: 1125-9.

- Lerman P, Kivity S. Benign focal epilepsy of childhood. A follow-up study of 100 recovered patients. *Arch Neurol* 1975; 32: 261-4.

- Lerman P. Benign partial epilepsy with centrotemporal spikes. In: Roger J, Dravet C, Bureau M, Dreifuss FE, Wolf P (Eds). *Epileptic syndromes in infancy, childhood and adolescence* (1st ed.). London: John Libbey, 1985: 150-8.

- Lerman P, Kivity S. The benign partial nonrolandic epilepsies. *J Clin Neurophysiol* 1991; 8: 275-87.

- Lerman P, Lerman-Sagie T. Sulthiame revisited. *J Child Neurol* 1995; 10: 241-2.

- Lerman P. Benign childhood epilepsy with centrotemporal spikes. In: Engel J, Pedly TA (Eds). *Epilepsy: a comprehensive textbook*. Philadelphia: Lippincott-Raven, 1998: 2307-14.

- Liasis A, Bamiou DE, Boyd S, Towell A. Evidence for a neurophysiologic auditory deficit in children with benign epilepsy with centrotemporal spikes. *J Neural Transm* 2006; 113 (7): 939-49.

- Lin YY, Chang KP, Hsieh JC, *et al*. Magnetoencephalographic analysis of bilaterally synchronous discharges in benign rolandic epilepsy of childhood. *Seizure* 2003; 12 (7): 448-55.

- Lin YY, Hsiao FJ, Chang KP, *et al*. Bilateral oscillations for lateralized spikes in benign rolandic epilepsy. *Epilepsy Res* 2006; 69 (1): 45-52.

- Lischka A, Graf M. Benign rolandic epilepsy of childhood: topographic EEG analysis. *Epilepsy Res* 1992; Suppl 6: 53-8.

- Loiseau P, Cohadon F, Mortureux Y. À propos d'une forme singulière d'épilepsie de l'enfant. *Rev Neurol* (Paris) 1967 ; 116: 244-8.

- Loiseau P, Beaussart M. The seizures of benign childhood epilepsy with rolandic paroxysmal discharges. *Epilepsia* 1973; 14: 381-9.

- Loiseau P, Duche B, Cordova S, Dartigues JF, Cohadon S. Prognosis of benign childhood epilepsy with centrotemporal spikes. A follow-up study of 168 patients. *Epilepsia* 1988; 29: 229-35.

- Loiseau P, Duche B. Benign childhood epilepsy with centrotemporal spikes. *Cleve Clin J Med* 1989; 56: S17-S22.

- Lombroso CT. Sylvian seizures and midtemporal spike foci in children. *Arch Neurol* 1967; 17: 52-9.

- Luders H, Lesser RP, Dinner DS, Morris HH III. Benign focal epilepsy of childhood. In: Luders H, Lesser RP (Eds). *Epilepsy: electroclinical syndrome*. Berlin: Springer-Verlag, 1987: 303-46.

- Lundberg S, Eeg-Olofsson O, Raininko R, Eeg-Olofsson KE. Hippocampal assimetries and white matter abnormalities on MRI in benign childhood epilepsy with centrotemporal spikes. *Epilepsia* 1999; 40 (12): 1808-15.

- Lundberg S, Weis J, Eeg-Olofsson O, Raininko R. Hippocampal region asymmetry assessed by H-MRS in Rolandic epilepsy. *Epilepsia* 2003; 44 (2): 205-10.

- Lundberg S. *Rolandic epilepsy*. Thesis, Acta Universitatis Upsaliensis (Upsala), 2004.

- Lundberg S, Friylmark A, Eeg-Olofsson O. Children with rolandic epilepsy have abnormalities of oromotor and dichotic listening performance. In: Lundberg S (Ed). *Rolandic epilepsy*. Thesis, Acta Universitatis Upsaliensis (Upsala), 2004.

- Maihara T, Tsuji M, Higuchi Y, Hattori H. Benign familial neonatal convulsions followed by benign epilepsy with centrotemporal spikes in two siblings. *Epilepsia* 1999; 40 (1): 110-3.

- Manganotti P, Miniussi C, Santorum E. (1998a) Influence of somatosensory input on paroxysmal activity in Benign rolandic epilepsy with "extreme somatosensory evoked potentials". *Brain* 1998; 121: 647-58.

- Manganotti P, Miniussi C, Santorum E. (1998b) Scalp topography and source analysis of interictal spontaneous spikes and evoked spikes by digital stimulation in benign rolandic epilepsy. *Electroencephalogr Clin Neurophysiol* 1998 ; 107: 18-26.

- Maquet P, Hirsch E, Metz-Lutz MN, *et al*. Regional cerebral glucose metabolism in children with deterioration of one or more cognitive functions and continuous spike-and-wave discharges during sleep. *Brain* 1995; 188: 1497-520.

- Maquet P, Metz-Lutz MN, de Saint-Martin A, *et al*. Isotope tracer-techniques in rolandic epilepsy and its variants. *Epileptic Disord* 2000; 2 (Suppl 1): S55-S57.

- Massa R, de Saint-Martin A, Carcangiu R, *et al*. EEG criteria predictive of complicated evolution in idiopathic Rolandic epilepsy. *Neurology* 2001; 57: 1071-9.

- Metz-Lutz MN, Filippini M. Neuropsychological findings in rolandic epilepsy and Landau-Kleffner syndrome. *Epilepsia* 2006; 47 (Suppl 2): 71-5.

- Milligan T, Bromfield E. A case of "Migralepsy". *Epilepsia* 2005; 46 (Suppl 10): 2-6.

- Minami T, Gondo K, Yamamoto T, *et al*. Magnetoencephalographic analysis of rolandic discharges in benign childhood epilepsy. *Ann Neurol* 1996; 39 (3): 326-34.

- Mitsudome A, Ohu M, Yasumoto S, Ogawa A. (1997a) Rhythmic slow activity in benign childhood epilepsy with centrotemporal spikes. *Clin Electroencephalogr* 1997; 28 (1): 44-8.

- Mitsudome A, Ohfu M, Yasumoto S, *et al*. (1997b) The effectiveness of clonazepam on the rolandic discharges. *Brain Dev* 1997; 19 (4): 274-8.

- Monjauze C, Tuller L, Hommet C, *et al*. Language in benign childhood epilepsy with centrotemporal spikes abbreviated form: Rolandic epilepsy and language. *Brain Lang* 2005; 92 (3): 300-8.

- Montenegro MA, Guerreiro MM. Electrical status epilepticus of sleep in association with Topiramate. *Epilepsia* 2002; 43 (11): 1436-40.

- Musumeci SA, Colognola RM, Ferri R, *et al*. Fragile-X syndrome: a particular epileptogenic EEG pattern. *Epilepsia* 1988; 29: 41-7.

- Nayrac P, Beaussart M. Les pointes-ondes prérolandiques : expression EEG très particulière. Étude électroclinique de 21 cas. *Rev Neurol* (Paris) 1958; 99: 201-6.

- Neubauer BA, Fiedler B, Himmelein B, *et al*. Centrotemporal spikes in families with rolandic epilepsy: linkage to chromosome 15q14. *Neurology* 1998; 51 (6): 1608-12.

- Nicolai J, Aldenkamp AP, Arends J, *et al*. Cognitive and behavioural effects of nocturnal epileptiform discharges in children with benign childhood epilepsy with centrotemporal spikes. *Epilepsy Behav* 2006; 8 (1): 56-70.

- Niedermeyer E, Naidu S. Further EEG observations in children with the Rett syndrome. *Brain Dev* 1990; 12: 53-4.

- Nieto Barrera M, Jimenez Ayllon M, Lopez Guerrero D. Epilepsia com paroxismos rolándicos. *Anales Espan Pediatr* 1978; 11 (3): 195-204.

- Northcott E, Connolly AM, Berroya A, *et al*. The neuropsychological and language profile of children with benign rolandic epilepsy. *Epilepsia* 2005; 46 (6): 924-30.

- Okubo Y, Matsuura M, Asai T, *et al*. Epileptiform EEG discharges in healthy children: prevalence, emotional and behavioural correlates, and genetic influences. *Epilepsia* 1994; 35: 832-41.

- Osservatorio Regionale per l'Epilessia (OREp), Lombardy. The contribution of tertiary centers to the quality of the diagnosis and treatment of epilepsy. *Epilepsia* 1997; 38 (12): 1338-43.

- Otsubo H, Chitoku S, Ochi A, *et al*. Malignant rolandic-sylvian epilepsy in children: diagnosis, treatment, and outcomes. *Neurology* 2001; 57 (4): 590-6.

- Ottman R, Risch N, Hauser WA, *et al*. Localization of a gene for partial epilepsy to chromosome 10q. *Nat Genet* 1995; 10: 56-60.

- Ottman R, Barker-Cummings C, Lee JH, Ranta S. Genetics of autosomal dominant partial epilepsy with auditory features. In: Berkovic SF, Genton P, Hirsch E, Picard F (Eds). *Genetic of focal epilepsies*. London: John Libbey, 1999: 95-102.

- Ounsted C, Lindsay J, Norman R. *Biological factors in temporal lobe epilepsy. Clinics in developmental medicine #22*. London: W. Heinemann Medical Books, 1966.

- Pan A, Luders HO. Epileptiform discharges in benign focal epilepsy of childhood. *Epileptic Disorders* 2000; 2 (Suppl 1): S29-S36.

- Pan A, Gupta A, Wyllie, E, Luders H, Bingaman W. Benign focal epileptiform discharges of childhood and hippocampal sclerosis. *Epilepsia* 2004; 45 (3): 284-8.

- Panayiotopoulos CP. Difficulties in differentiating migraine and epilepsy based on clinical and EEG findings. In: Andermann F, Lugaresi E (Eds). *Migraine and epilepsy*. Boston: Butterworths, 1987: 31-46.

- Panayiotopoulos CP. *Benign childhood partial seizures and related epileptic syndromes*. London: John Libbey, 1999.

- Panayiotopoulos CP. *The Epilepsies*. Oxfordshire: Bladon publishing, 2005.

- Papavasiliou A, Mattheou D, Bazigou H, Kotsalis C, Paraskevoulakos E. Written language skills in children with benign childhood epilepsy with centrotemporal spikes. *Epilepsy Behav* 2005; 6 (1): 50-8.

- Parmeggiani A, Posar A, Sangioggi P, Giovanardi-Rossi P. Unusual side-effects due to Clobazam: a case with genetic study of CYP2C19. *Brain & Development* 2004; 26 (1): 63-6.

- Pinton F, Ducot B, Motte J, *et al*. Cognitive functions in children with benign childhood epilepsy with centrotemporal spikes (BECTS). *Epileptic Disord* 2006; 8 (1): 11-23.

- Polychronopoulos P, Argyriou AA, Papapetropoulos S, *et al*. Wilson's disease and benign epilepsy of childhood with centrotemporal (rolandic) spikes. *Epilepsy Behav* 2006; 8 (2): 438-41.

- Prats Viñas JM. *Epilepsia infantil y paroxismos rolándicos EEG*. Tesis doctoral, Bilbao, 1980: 234.

- Prats JM, Garaizar C, Garcia-Nieto ML, Madoz P. Antiepileptic drugs and atypical evolution of idiopathic partial epilepsy. *Pediatr Neurol* 1998; 18 (5): 402-6.

- Pruna D, Persico I, Serra D, *et al*. Lack of association with the 15q14 candidate region for benign epilepsy of childhood with centrotemporal spikes in a Sardinian population. *Epilepsia* 2000; 41: 164.

- Ramelli GP, Donati F, Moser H, Vassella F. Concomitance of childhood absence and Rolandic epilepsy. *Clin Electroencephalogr* 1998; 29 (4): 177-80.

- Rating D, Wolf C, Bast T. Sulthiame as monotherapy in children with benign childhood epilepsy with centrotemporal spikes: a 6-month randomized, double-blind, placebo-controlled study. Sulthiame Study Group. *Epilepsia* 2000; 41 (10): 1284-8.

- Riva D, Vago C, Franceschetti S, *et al*. Intellectual and language findings and their relationship to EEG characteristics in benign childhood epilepsy with centrotemporal spikes. *Epilepsy Behav* 2007; 10 (2): 278-85.

- Roulet E, Deonna T, Despland PA. Prolonged intermittent drooling and oromotor dyspraxia in benign childhood epilepsy with centrotemporal spikes. *Epilepsia* 1989; 30: 564-8.

- Santanelli P, Bureau M, Magaudda A, *et al*. Benign partial epilepsy with centrotemporal (or rolandic) spikes and brain lesion. *Epilepsia* 1989; 30 (2): 182-8.

- Scheffer IE, Jones L, Pozzebon M, *et al*. Autosomal dominant rolandic epilepsy and speech dyspraxia: a new syndrome with anticipation. *Ann Neurol* 1995; 38 (4): 633-42.

- Scheffer IE. Autosomal dominant rolandic epilepsy with speech dyspraxia. In: Berkovic SF, Genton P, Hirsch E, Picard F (Eds). *Genetic of focal epilepsies*. London: John Libbey, 1999: 109-14.

- Sheth RD, Gutierrez AR, Riggs JE. Rolandic epilepsy and cortical dysplasia: MRI correlation of epileptiform discharges. *Pediatr Neurol* 1997; 17 (2): 177-9.

- Shevell MI, Rosenblatt B, Watters GV, *et al*. "Pseudo-BECRS": intracranial focal lesions suggestive of a primary partial epilepsy syndrome. *Pediatr Neurol* 1996; 14 (1): 31-5.

- Shields WD, Saslow E. Myoclonic, atonic, and absence seizures following institution of carbamazepine therapy in children. *Neurology* 1983; 33 (11): 1487-9.

- Shinnar S, O'Dell C, Berg AT. Distribution of epilepsy syndromes in a cohort of children prospectively monitored from the time of their first unprovoked seizure. *Epilepsia* 1999; 40 (10): 1378-83.

- Shorvon S. *Handbook of epilepsy treatment* (2nd Ed.). Malden: Blackwell, 2005: 84.

- Sidenvall R, Forsgren L, Heijbel J. Prevalence and characteristics of epilepsy in children in northern Sweden. *Seizure* 1996; 5 (2): 139-46.

- Sorel L, Rucquoy-Ponsar M. L'épilepsie fonctionnelle de maturation. *Rev Neurol* (Paris) 1969 ; 121: 288-97.

- Staden U, Isaacs E, Boyd SG, *et al*. Language dysfunction in children with Rolandic epilepsy. *Neuropediatrics* 1998; 29: 242-8.

- Steinlein OK, Neubauer BA, Sander T, *et al*. Mutation analysis of the potassium chloride cotransporter KCC3 (SLC12A6) in rolandic and idiopathic generalized epilepsy. *Epilepsy Res* 2001; 44 (2-3): 191-5.

- Stephani U. Typical semiology of benign childhood epilepsy with centrotemporal spikes (BCECTS). *Epileptic Disorders* 2000; 2 (Suppl 1): S3-S4.

- Trojaborg W. Focal spike discharges in children: a longitudinal study. *Acta Paediatr Scand* 1966; Suppl: 168.

- Tsai ML, Hung KL. Topographic mapping and clinical analysis of BCECS. *Brain Dev* 1998; 20 (1): 27-32.

- Tzitiridou M, Panou T, Ramantani G, *et al*. Oxcarbazepine monotherapy in benign childhood epilepsy with centrotemporal spikes: A clinical and cognitive evaluation. *Epilepsy Behav* 2005; 7 (3): 458-67.

- Vadlamudi L, Kjeldsen MJ, Corey LA, *et al*. Analyzing the etiology of benign rolandic epilepsy: a multicenter twin collaboration. *Epilepsia* 2006; 47 (3): 550-5.

- Van Bogaert P, Wikler D, Damhaut P, *et al*. Cerebral glucose metabolism and centrotemporal spikes. *Epilepsy Res* 1998; 29 (2): 123-7.

- Vaughn BV, Greenwood RS, Aylsworth AS, Tennison MB. Similarities of EEG and seizures in del (1q) and benign rolandic epilepsy. *Pediatr Neurol* 1996; 15 (3): 261-4.

- Veggiotti P, Beccaria F, Gatti A, *et al*. Can protrusion of the tongue stop seizures in Rolandic epilepsy? *Epileptic Disord* 1999; 1 (4): 217-20.

- Verrotti A, Latini G, Trotta D, *et al.* Typical and atypical rolandic epilepsy in childhood: a follow-up study. *Pediatr Neurol* 2002; 26 (1): 26-9.

- Verrotti A, Coppola G, Manco R, *et al.* Levetiracetam monotherapy for children and adolescents with benign rolandic seizures. *Seizure* 2007; 16 (3): 271-5.

- Viani F, Beghi E, Atza MG, Gulotta MP. Classifications of epileptic syndromes: advantages and limitations for evaluation of childhood epileptic syndromes in clinical practice. *Epilepsia* 1988; 29: 440-5.

- Volkl-Kernstock S, Willinger U, Feucht M. Spacial perception and spatial memory in children with benign childhood epilepsy with centrotemporal spikes (BCECTS). *Epilepsy Res* 2006; 72 (1): 39-48.

- Watanabe K. Benign partial epilepsies. In: Wallace SJ, Farrell K (Eds). *Epilepsy in children* (2nd Ed.). London: Arnold, 2004: 199-220.

- Weglage J, Demsky A, Pietsch M, Kurlemann G. Neuropsychological, intellectual, and behavioral findings in patients with centrotemporal spikes with and without seizures. *Dev Med Child Neurol* 1997; 39 (10): 646-51.

- Weglage J, Pietsch M, Sprinz A, *et al.* A previously unpublished side effect of sulthiame in a patient with Rolandic epilepsy. *Neuropediatrics* 1999; 30 (1): 50.

- Wirrell EC, Camfield PR, Gordon KE, *et al.* Benign rolandic epilepsy: atypical features are very common. *J Child Neurol* 1995; 10 (6): 455-8.

- Wirrell EC, Hamiwka LD. Do children with benign rolandic epilepsy have a higher prevalence of migraine than those with other partial epilepsies or nonepilepsy controls? *Epilepsia* 2006; 47 (10): 1674-81.

- Wolff M, Weiskopf N, Serra E, *et al.* Benign partial epilepsy in childhood: selective cognitive déficits are related to the location of local spikes determined by combined EEG/MEG. *Epilepsia* 2005; 46 (10): 1661-7.

- You SJ, Kim DS, Ko TS. Benign childhood epilepsy with centrotemporal spikes (BCECTS): early onset of seizures is associated with poorer response to initial treatment. *Epileptic Disord* 2006; 8 (4): 285-8.

- Zhao X, Chi Z, Chi L, *et al.* Clinical and EEG characteristics of benign rolandic epilepsy in Chinese patients. *Brain Dev* 2007; 29 (1): 13-8.

Early-onset benign childhood occipital epilepsy (Panayiotopoulos type)

Natalio Fejerman, Roberto H. Caraballo
Buenos Aires, Argentina

In the first edition of the *Comprehensive text-book on Epilepsy* by J. Engel and T. Pedley, only a few lines mentioned this condition under the heading of "Childhood Epilepsy with Occipital Spikes and other Benign Localization-related Epilepsies" (Gobbi & Guerrini, 1998). At present, Early onset benign childhood occipital epilepsy (Panayiotopoulos type) is not only a clearly recognized syndrome, but it represents the second most frequent benign focal epilepsy syndrome in childhood after benign childhood epilepsy with centrotemporal spikes (BCECTS). The peculiar clinical features of this syndrome should be known not only by epileptologists and neurologists, but also by pediatricians. An early diagnosis would avoid undue interventions and concerns on account of its really benign outcome.

In the still valid ILAE classification of Epilepsy syndromes (Commission on Classification, 1989), besides the well known BCECTS, only the Childhood epilepsy with occipital paroxysms, as described by Gastaut, is recognized (Gastaut, 1982). In comparison with BCECTS with a prevalence of around 15% among children with epilepsies (Panayiotopoulos, 1999a; Engel & Fejerman, 2006; Dalla Bernardina *et al.*, 2005), the Gastaut type of childhood occipital epilepsy (COE) is rare, of uncertain boundaries, and often of unpredictable prognosis (Caraballo *et al.*, 2000). This condition is characterized by brief seizures with mainly visual symptoms such as elementary visual hallucinations, illusions or amaurosis, followed by hemiclonic convulsions. Postictal migraine headaches occur in half of the patients. Age at onset is around 8 to 9 years. EEG shows occipital spike-wave paroxysms that are attenuated or disappear when the eyes are opened (Gastaut, 1982; Panayiotopoulos, 1981; Commission on Classification, 1989; Gastaut *et al.*, 1992)

In 1984 Dalla Bernardina and co-workers found 13 patients with simple or complex focal seizures, rarely associated with visual symptoms, and often accompanied by vomiting but never cephalalgia with occipital spikes on the EEG recordings. At that moment, the patients were not considered to have a distinctive epileptic syndrome, but retrospectively the electroclinical picture seems to be compatible with Panayiotopoulos syndrome (PS).

In 1989, two cardinal papers of Panayiotopoulos based on an already long follow-up of his patients called attention to the particular cluster of symptoms present in what he called

"Benign nocturnal childhood occipital epilepsy" (Panayiotopoulos, 1989a, 1989b). Vomiting as ictal symptom in Epileptic seizures in children had already been emphasized by the same author one year earlier (Panayiotopoulos, 1988). Another peculiar clinical feature of Early onset benign childhood occipital epilepsy (Panayiotopoulos type) was the "cerebral insult-like" partial status epilepticus including autonomic symptoms (Panayiotopoulos & Igoe, 1992; Kivity & Lerman, 1992; Vigevano & Ricci, 1993). In order to stress the variable phenotypes of benign focal epileptic syndromes in childhood, Panayiotopoulos and co-workers used the term "Benign childhood seizure susceptibility syndromes" (Panayiotopoulos, 1993, 1999a). After 1996, Fejerman and co-workers proposed to name this syndrome as Early onset benign childhood occipital epilepsy (Panayiotopoulos type) as opposed to the Late-onset childhood occipital epilepsy (Gastaut type) (Fejerman, 1996, 1997, 2002, 2003; Caraballo et al., 1997, 2000). Three important series of children with this syndrome were published around those years (Ferrie et al., 1997; Oguni et al., 1999; Kivity et al., 2000). Retrospective analysis of their clinical histories allowed the authors to study the variants of childhood epilepsies with occipital paroxysms and to recognize this early-onset variant. In the same year 2000, the first prospective study of 66 children with the Panayiotopoulos type was published (Caraballo et al., 2000).

The Task Force on Classification and Terminology of ILAE published in 2001 a Proposed diagnostic scheme for people with epilepsy (Engel, 2001). It adopted the names proposed by Fejerman including eponymic contents to emphasize the differentiation between the Gastaut type and the Panayiotopoulos type of Childhood epilepsies with occipital paroxysms, keeping intentionally the term "Benign" only for this early-onset form (Fejerman, 1996, 1997). Thereafter, several authors preferred the eponymic nomenclature of "Panayiotopoulos syndrome" (PS) in order to include patients with and without occipital spikes or occipital ictal origins (Caraballo et al., 2000; Berg & Panayiotopoulos, 2000; Ferrie & Grunewald, 2001; Panayiotopoulos, 2002; Martinovic, 2002; Ferrie et al., 2002; Lada et al., 2003; Covanis et al., 2003; Demirbilek & Dervent, 2004; Sanders et al., 2004; Covanis et al., 2005; Panayiotopoulos, 2005; Kanazawa et al., 2005; Koutromanidis et al., 2005; Ferrie et al., 2006; Fejerman & Panayiotopoulos, 2007; Caraballo et al., 2007). Considering the emphasis given in the last years to the presence of autonomic seizures and autonomic status epilepticus in this condition, that occipital EEG abnormalities are not found in a certain proportion of the cases, and that there is no clear documentation of an occipital origin of seizures, we agree here that the name PS might be more appropriate. As a practical tool in this presentation, we will continue to refer to Early onset benign childhood occipital epilepsy (Panayiotopoulos type) as PS.

Types of seizures, age of onset, normal neurological status of patients, and spontaneous evolution allow us to define the PS as a benign age-related focal epilepsy syndrome occurring in early and mid-childhood. The analysis of several large series of published cases and our own present series, clearly demonstrates the significant frequency of PS which is seen in a relation of 1 to 2 or 3, compared to BCECTS.

Epidemiology

We are talking about an epilepsy syndrome which has been seen only in children with a peak incidence between 4 and 5 years of age. Considering that the official recognition of PS took place in 2001, it is very difficult to find epidemiological studies in childhood population including PS among the diagnosis. Besides, unfortunately, most of the studies are based more in seizure types than in syndromes. One study included a mix of seizures and syndromes for the recognition of epilepsies in 440 consecutive pediatric patients. Thirty-six (8%) of the cases were diagnosed as having Benign rolandic epilepsy of childhood and 8 cases (2%) with Benign occipital epilepsy of childhood (Kramer et al., 1998). We may assume that this last group was subevaluated and we don't know how many of the cases corresponded to PS. A cohort of 407 children with their first unprovoked seizure were followed for a mean of 9.4 years and distribution of epilepsy syndromes was reported: of 114 children with localization-related epilepsy syndromes, 26 were idiopathic, 24 of them were rolandic and only 2 occipital (Shinnar et al., 1999). Another study of a population-based active-prevalence cohort in children under 16 years of age was able to classify syndromes in 235 (96%) of the 245 patients followed-up for many years. However, no specific data about PS was included in any of this 3 studies because they were based on the 1989 ILAE's Classification (Sillanpaa et al., 1999). The most comprehensive epidemiologic study of newly diagnosed unprovoked epileptic seizures covering 1942 patients from 1 month to 95 years was done with data provided by 243 child and adult neurologists in France (Jallon et al., 2001). The whole sample was divided in two groups, one with a single seizure at diagnosis and the other with more than one seizure at diagnosis. All patients with idiopathic (localization-related or generalized epilepsies) had at least one EEG. Among 80 patients with idiopathic localization-related epilepsy within the 926 cases of the single seizure group, 14 (17.5%) had Childhood epilepsy with occipital paroxysms, and among the 48 cases within the 1016 of the more than one seizure group, 8 (16.6%) had COE (Jallon et al., 2001). Considering that this study was performed between 1995 and 1996, it is understandable that at the time there was not discrimination between the Gastaut type and the Panayiotopoulos type of COE, but we know well that the latter syndrome is 4 to 8 times more frequent than the Gastaut type of COE.

Therefore, we have to give credit to the daily experience of active epileptologists caring for children who became aware of this condition in the last few years (Berg & Panayiotopoulos, 2000):

- Oguni et al., 1999: among 649 children with localization-related epilepsy selected from their database, 62 met the criteria for diagnosis of PS.
- Kivity et al., 2000: a file review of patients with occipital EEG paroxysms disclosed 72 children with typical PS.
- Caraballo et al., 2000: prospective study of 66 patients with PS selected with strict criteria for inclusion.
- Lada et al., 2003: retrospective analysis of clinical and EEG records of 1,340 children with focal seizures: 43 with PS and more than 2 years since they were seizure free were followed-up.
- Tedrus & Fonseca 2005, 2006: In another file review of 63 children with occipital epileptiform activity in the EEG, with epileptic seizures and no evidence of brain damage, the diagnosis of

idiopathic occipital epilepsy syndrome was possible in 40% of the cases, of which 32 belonged to PS and 8 to the Gastaut type of COE. More recently, the same authors reported on 36 children with diagnosis of PS emphasizing that 14 of them had autonomic status epilepticus.

- Panayiotopoulos 2005: in an on-going hospital based prospective study at the end of 3 years, 228 children aged 1 through 14 years with one or more seizures had one or more EEG. Fourteen of them (again 6.1%) had Panayiotopoulos syndrome.
- Specchio *et al.*, 2006: this series of the group of Vigevano reviewed the clinical and EEG data of 98 children with PS consecutively referred to their lab for first seizure between 1992 and 2005. The follow-up was between 1-14 years (mean 4 years).
- Caraballo *et al.*, 2007: adding new cases after the 66 reported in 2000, they amount now 192 children with typical PS prospectively followed up (see our report of cases).

Clinical features

Panayiotopoulos syndrome occurs in children who are otherwise normal and is not associated with neurodevelopmental problems. Although it has been described as starting as early as one year of age and as late as fourteen years of age, a notable feature is that a large majority of subjects have their first seizure around the age of 4-5 years (Chahine & Mikati 2006). Three quarters of patients have their first seizure between the ages of 3 and 6 years. It affects boys and girls almost equally. Seizures occur predominantly during sleep and in 2/3 of patients occur only in sleep. In seizures occurring while awake, the onset may be inconspicuous with pallor, agitation, feeling seek, and vomiting. At this stage of a first seizure, the epileptic nature of the event can hardly be suspected as ictal, prior to motor convulsive symptoms that may be rightly considered as secondary to an ongoing serious brain insult. It is only the normal post-ictal state of the child that should be reassuring.

The duration of the seizures is usually long, commonly lasting for more than 5 minutes, and in around 40% of the cases for more than 30 minutes constituting then a focal or secondarily generalized status epilepticus. Three groups of symptoms are recognized as seen in *Table I*.

Core clinical features

Ictal emetic symptoms and other autonomic manifestations: ictal vomiting which is considered to be exceptional in other epilepsies, occurs in around 80% of the cases with PS (Panayiotopoulos 1988, Panayiotopoulos 1989a, Panayiotopoulos 1989b, Panayiotopoulos 2002, Panayiotopoulos 1999/2005, Ferrie *et al.*, 1997, Oguni *et al.*, 1999, Caraballo *et al.*, 2000, Lada *et al.*, 2003, Covanis *et al.*, 2003). In one of these series, the prospective study considered vomiting as a criteria for inclusion, although we now know that vomiting is not present in 100% of the cases (Caraballo *et al.*, 2000). In nocturnal seizures, it is usually the first apparent symptom, whereas in seizures occurring while awake, other symptoms of the emetic spectrum such as nausea or retching may appear along or before vomiting (Covanis *et al.*, 2003). Vomiting may occur repetitively or only once during the seizure.

Table I. Frequency of seizure types in children with Panayiotopoulos syndrome

Core clinical features • Ictal emetic symptoms and other autonomic manifestations • Deviation of the eyes • Impairment of consciousness **Frequent types of seizures** • Unilateral clonic or tonic-clonic seizures • Secondary generalized tonic-clonic seizures • Encephalopathy-like status epilepticus (focal motor – unilateral or generalized– and autonomic) **Less frequent – but not rare – symptoms and signs** • Visual symptoms • Migraine-like headaches • Incontinence of urine and faeces • Syncope-like symptoms • Other

Pallor is the most frequent autonomic manifestation. It mainly occurs at onset and commonly together with vomiting. In seizures starting while awake, pallor, nausea and "feeling seek" are frequent symptoms.

Deviation of the eyes: unilateral deviation of the eyes is as common as vomiting and also occurs in around 80% of the patients (Panayiotopoulos 1988, Panayiotopoulos 1989a, Panayiotopoulos 2002, Panayiotopoulos 2005, Ferrie et al., 1997, Oguni et al., 1999, Caraballo et al., 2000). The eye deviation may be brief or prolonged and is frequently accompanied by head-deviation. It may be continuous, or less often intermittent. Consciousness is often but not invariably impaired at this stage. It should be noted that exact details of this symptoms are rarely witnessed because seizures occur mostly at night.

Impairment of Consciousness: Consciousness is usually intact at seizure onset but becomes impaired in 80-90% of cases in the progress of seizures. Impairment of consciousness may be mild or moderate, with the child retaining some ability to respond to verbal commands, but often talking out of context. In seizures with motor components occurring during sleep, complete loss of consciousness may be seen, especially in all those which are prolonged into status. In diurnal seizures, cloudiness of consciousness usually starts after the appearance of autonomic and behavioural symptoms. Awareness may be preserved throughout the ictal state in 10% to 20% of the seizures (Panayiotopoulos 1989b, Panayiotopoulos 2002, Panayiotopoulos 2005, Ferrie et al., 1997, Oguni et al., 1999, Ohtsu et al., 2003).

Frequent features of seizures

Unilateral clonic or tonic-clonic seizures: unilateral clonic convulsions in face and extremities at onset or following vomiting and eye-deviation are seen in 25-30% of the cases (Caraballo et al., 2000, Panayiotopoulos 2002, Panayiotopoulos 1999/2005).

Secondarily generalized tonic-clonic seizures: these types of seizures rarely appear at onset and usually follow seizures starting with focal motor manifestation. In one series of patients, this course was seen in near 40% of the cases (Caraballo *et al.*, 2000).

Status epilepticus: is usually non-convulsive, lasts more than 30 minutes and occurs in around 30% of cases, in all series (Panayiotopoulos 1989a, 2002, 2005, Ferrie *et al.*, 1997, Oguni *et al.*, 1999, Caraballo *et al.*, 2000). This "encephalopathy-like" status epilepticus may progress to hemi-convulsions. Autonomic status epilepticus has been repeatedly reported in the last years (Covanis *et al.*, 2005; Ferrie *et al.*, 2006; Tedrus & Fonseca 2006) Moreover, the prevalence of this phenomenon in children with PS merited a quite recent consensus view of 24 experts around the world (Ferrie *et al.*, 2007). Autonomic status epilepticus (Aut SE) was defined as a lasting seizure or series of seizures in which altered autonomic functions are prominent even if not present at seizure onset. In children, Aut SE is seen almost only in PS, and its more typical presentation is: "if awake, the child begins to complain of feeling sick. Initially they are fully aware and responsive. Retching and/or vomiting frequently follow and these emetic symptoms are usually accompanied by other autonomic features, such as pallor, tachycardia/bradycardia, mydriasis and thermoregulatory disturbances. After a variable time awareness and responsiveness become impaired, often with aversion of the eyes and/or head. Then follows a prolonged period characterized by fluctuating consciousness, interspersed with retching and vomiting with continuing pallor, mydriasis, etc." (Ferrie *et al.*, 2007). We'll see under the heading of "Differential diagnosis" how important it is to recognize PS when it may mimic other pathologies due to true cerebral insult.

Less frequent – but not rare – symptoms

Visual symptoms: are typical of the Gastaut type of COE. However, in less than 10% of patients with PS elementary visual hallucinations, illusions, and blindness were registered in children that were able to describe them when having seizures, mainly while awake (Maher *et al.*, 1995). There is an ongoing debate regarding ictal visual symptoms in PS (Panayiotopoulos 1999a,c). These were not initially reported (Panayiotopoulos 1989b), but were later described as a rare symptom (Ferrie et al 1997, Yalcin et al 1997, Caraballo et al 2000). Twenty of our patients (10.4%) had visual symptoms associated with ictal autonomic manifestations and deviation of the eyes. One child only presented visual symptoms. Ferrie and co-workers (Ferrie *et al.*, 1997) regarded 12 patients with visual symptoms as an overlapping subgroup between Gastaut and Panayiotopoulos type of COE.

Migraine-like headaches: are rarely present, and in older children may sometimes cast doubts about differential diagnosis with the Gastaut type of COE.

Incontinence of urine and faeces may occur when consciousness is impaired.

The occurrence of syncope-like symptoms is another autonomic manifestation that was more recently emphasized. Children becoming completely irresponsive and flaccid, often without convulsions, are reported as not rare by many authors (Panayiotopulos 2002, Panayiotopoulos 2005, Covanis *et al.*, 2003, Covanis *et al.*, 2005, Ferrie *et al.*, 2006).

Atypical evolutions in children with PS are dealt in chapter 10. Nevertheless, cases with atypical features may occur (Panayiotopoulos 2002, Covanis et al., 2005). A recently reported 8 years old boy started at 3 years of age with nocturnal attacks with pallor, vomiting and mild impairment of consciousness followed by severe headache. The child also had monthly episodes of migraine while awake. From the age of seven years the boy experienced diurnal visual seizures lasting 10 to 30 seconds. An ictal video polysomnography was done showing a 14 minutes episode including tachycardia, left tonic eye deviation, and repetitive ictal vomiting (Parisi et al., 2005). These features seemed to be typical of PS, although the presence of severe headache in the nocturnal seizures and of pure visual hallucinations while awake may suggest that it was an intermediate form between PS and the Gastaut type of COE. Another recently reported case started with typical PS seizure at 3 years of age, but between 7 and 10 years of age the girl presented frequent absences, atonic seizures, generalized tonic-clonic convulsions and clonic seizures of the eye lids, associated with much more frequent and diffuse EEG abnormalities. Nevertheless, neuropsychologic impairment or behaviour problems were absent (Saitoh et al., 2006)

Neuropsychological impairments

In 2002 Panayiotopoulos stated that there is no evidence of neuropsychological impairment even after lengthy seizures in children with PS and said that "many of these children have excellent school performance and many of those with long follow-up have excellent professional records". However, systematic evaluations of children with PS including neuropsychological tests are scarce, mainly because the universal recognition of this syndrome is quite recent and many authors still do not disaggregate PS from the Gastaut type of COE in their studies. For instance, in a prospective comprehensive study of 21 children with idiopathic occipital lobe epilepsy diagnosed on the basis of relevant clinical and EEG criteria in children with normal neurologic examination and psychomotor development, the authors disclose one patient with idiopathic photosensitive occipital lobe epilepsy, while the other 20 presented a mix of clinical and EEG features belonging both to PS and the Gastaut type of COE. All of them were compared to 21 normal children matched for age and socioeconomic status. The patients were receiving AED, but no Phenobarbital, Primidone or Phenitoin, although blood levels were not studied. Their conclusions were: a) children with epilepsy performed more poorly than controls in intellectual functioning, in attention, in memory, in all verbal tests combined and in all visual tests combined; b) these differences were not due to intelligence; c) epilepsy and control group did not differ with respect to academic achievement, visomotor, and executive functioning (Gülgönen et al., 2000). The same group included also children with BCECTS in another report and focused on mathematical disability. Overall, no significant differences were found in neuropsychological functioning of children with PS, Gastaut type of COE and BCECTS (Hande Sart et al., 2006). These results contrast with a further study of 22 children, this time identified as having PS, showing that even when IQs were within normal limits, selective dysfunctions related to visual-motor integration global abilities, reading and writing, and arithmetic ability were found (Germano et al., 2005). In a more recent report based on the review of clinical charts of 22 patients with idiopathic occipital lobe epilepsies, 11 of them were considered not to have scholastic difficulties and therefore formal neuropsychological testing was performed only in the other

11 cases. Six of these were diagnosed as idiopathic photosensitive occipital lobe epilepsy, and the other 5 included patients with PS and the Gastaut type of COE. It was suggested that children with these syndromes were at risk for lower intellectual performance, poor scholastic achievement, specific deficit in visuo perceptual domain and psychiatric disorders (Chilosi et al., 2006). Due to the selection of the presented patients probably only 2 or 3 of these studied children had PS.

On account of the significant series of studies of neuropsychological impairments in children with BCECTS (see Chapters 6 & 10) it seems logical to suspect that the same problems might be found in children with PS, but up to now there are not enough studies to support this view. As shown later in our present series of cases, atypical evolutions including transient neuropsychological impairments occurred in only 5 of the 192 followed up patients with PS. This incidence appears to be lower and less severe than the 39 cases with atypical evolutions among the 398 children with BCECTS which we saw in the same length of time.

EEG and other neurophysiological studies

Electroencephalographic findings: the most useful laboratory test is EEG. Ictal EEG reports are rare because of the infrequency of seizures.

a) Interictal EEG findings: We must be aware that most of the patients with PS are first seen between ages 3 and 6 years, and therefore, many of these EEGs are obtained under sleep. Even more, sleep activates the appearance of occipital spikes in these children *(Fig. 1)* (Caraballo et al., 2000). Occipital spikes are bilateral and synchronous, often with voltage asymmetry, or unilateral *(Fig. 2)*. In awake EEGs occipital paroxysms of high amplitude with sharp and slow-wave complexes that occur immediately after closing the eyes are often registered *(Figs. 3, 4)*. These paroxysms are eliminated, or markedly attenuated, when the eyes are opened, phenomenon due to fixation-of-sensitivity *(Fig. 5)* (Panayiotopoulos, 1981, 2002). This phenomenon, which should be sought in every EEG laboratory, was considered pathognomonic of the Gastaut type of COE, but it is not. Not only was it reported in patients with PS but also in other conditions (Newton & Aicardi 1983, Cooper & Lee 1991, Maher et al., 1995).

Even when occipital spikes and spike-wave paroxysms are the main EEG feature, their absence is not against the diagnosis of PS. It has been emphasized that extra-occipital spikes (centrotemporal, frontal, parietal) may also be found in children with PS *(Figs. 6, 7)* (Panayiotopoulos 1999a, Oguni et al., 1999, Covanis et al., 2005). Generalized spike and wave discharges are not seen in PS as frequently as they are in children with BCECTS *(Fig. 8)* (Engel & Fejerman, 2006). A peculiar feature of EEG discharges named "cloned-like", repetitive, multifocal spike-wave complexes has been reported in 19% of the cases (Panayiotopoulos 2002, Covanis et al., 2005). Normal EEGs during sleep are exceptional according to a recent consensus report (Ferrie et al., 2006).

Early-onset benign childhood occipital epilepsy (Panayiotopoulos type)

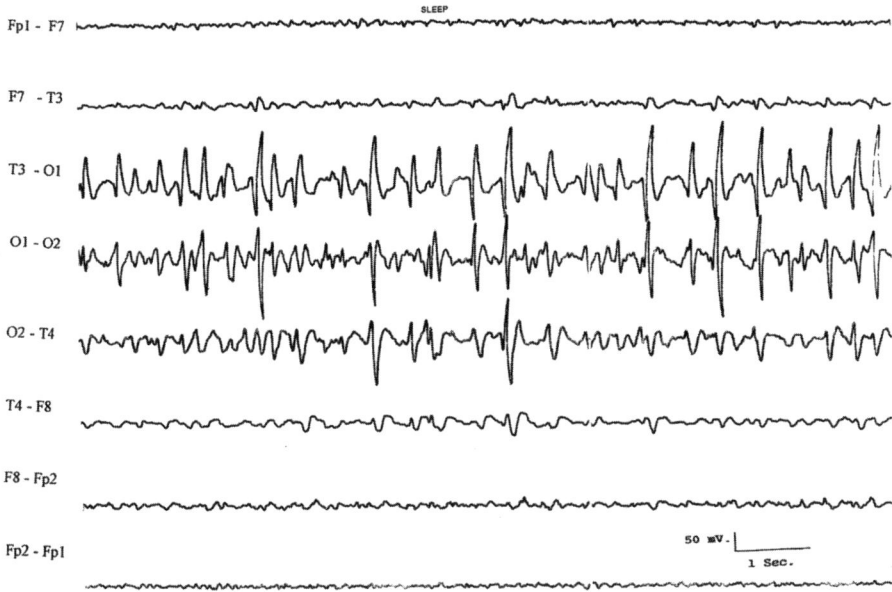

Figure 1. Four years old boy. Sleep EEG with frequent left occipital spikes.

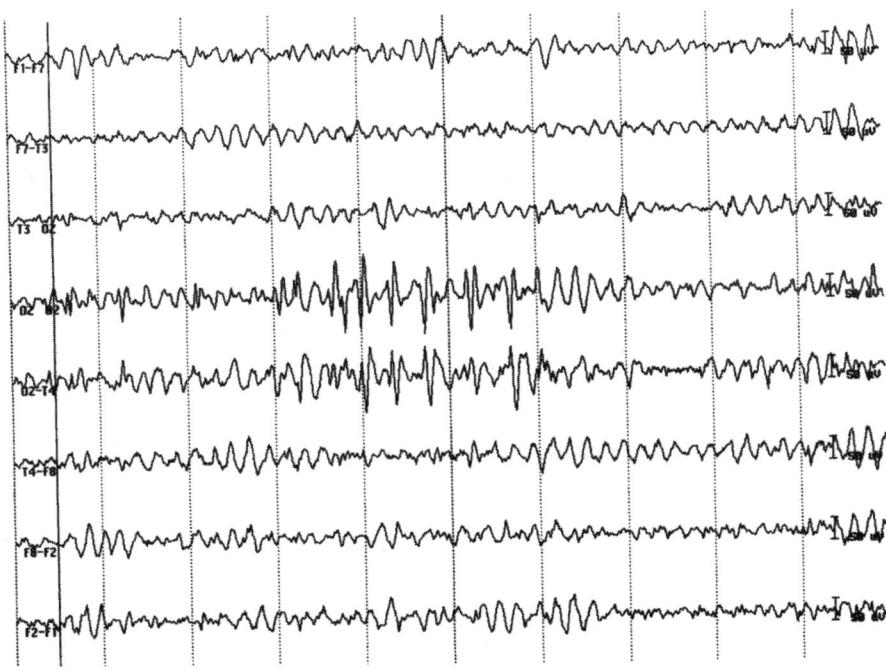

Figure 2. Six years old boy. EEG while awake with a cluster of right occipital spikes.

The evolution of EEG discharges in 76 children with PS followed-up with repeated sleep EEG examinations showed that the occipital spike pattern was prevalent in the first few years of the diagnosis and it became later associated with frontal or centrotemporal spikes (Ohtsu *et al.*, 2003).

An interesting paper related to EEG in PS recently showed that a group of EEG technologists trained on clinical features of PS were able to diagnose the condition in 14 children, and in 9 of them their information was crucial to achieve diagnosis (Sanders *et al.*, 2004).

In a recent study of 8 children with PS dipole analysis of the interictal spike discharges was performed. The various types of spikes observed in PS had similar and stable dipole locations. The dipoles showing high stability were located in the mesial occipital area, and were accompanied by dipoles located in the rolandic area, suggesting a possible pathogenetic link between PS and BCECTS (Yoshinaga *et al.*, 2005).

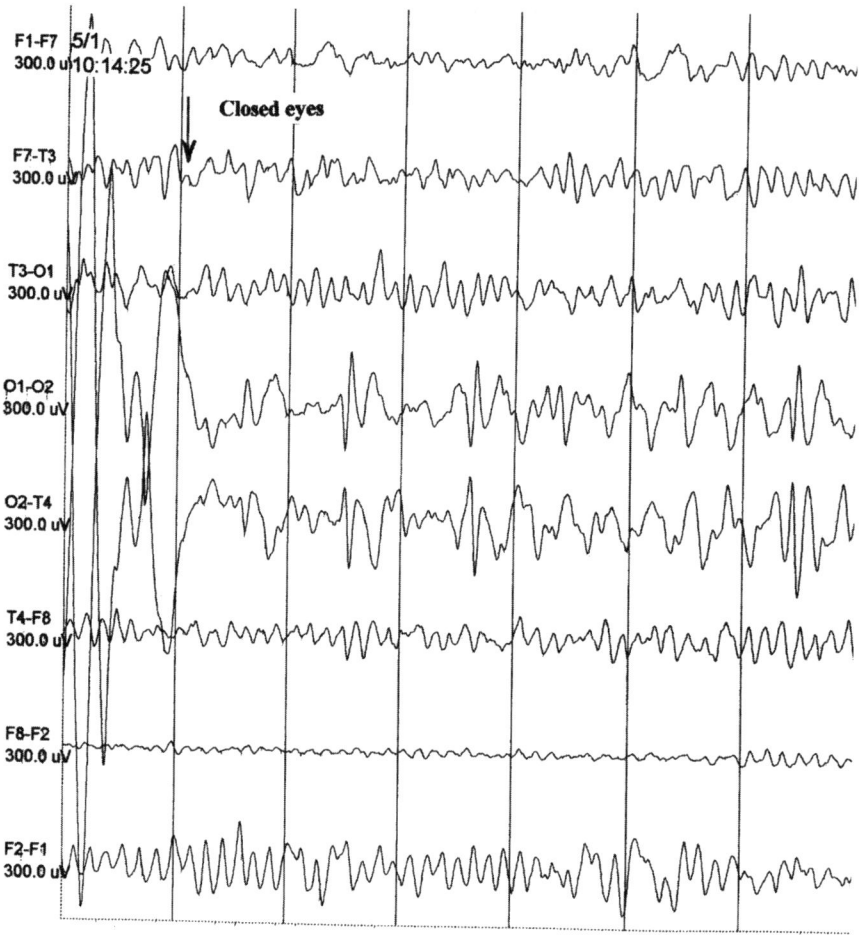

Figure 3. Seven years old boy. EEG while awake. Closing of eyes provokes the appearance of frequent right occipital spikes.

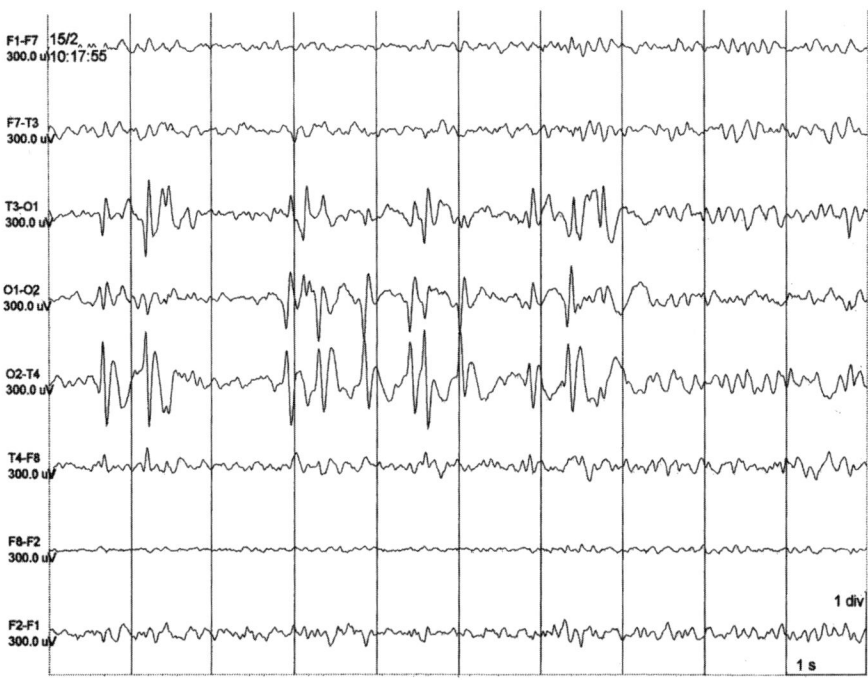

Figure 4. Sleep EEG in the same patient of Fig3. Bilateral occipital spikes dominant on right hemisphere.

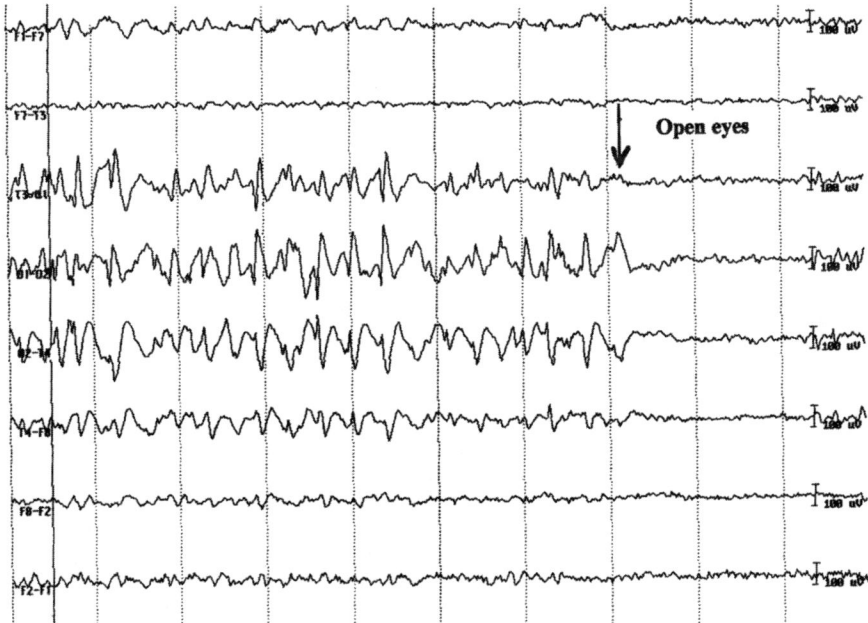

Figure 5. Five years old girl with typical clinical features of PS. Interictal EEG while awake shows bilateral asymmetrical occipital spike wave discharges which disappear after eye-opening.

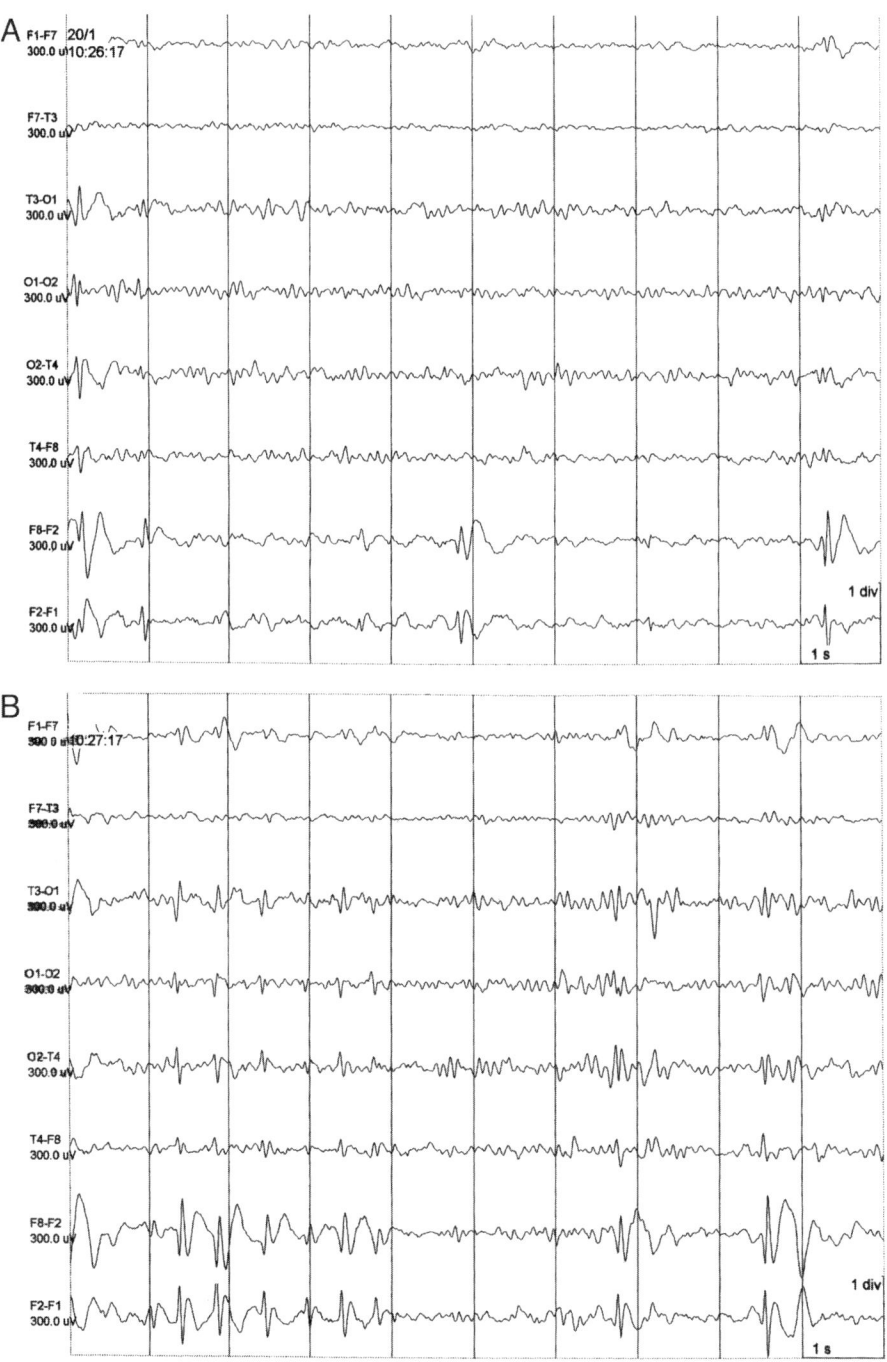

Figure 6. Five years old boy. A: EEG while awake shows right frontal spikes. B: EEG during drowsiness shows more frequent frontal spikes and synchronic spikes in occipital regions.

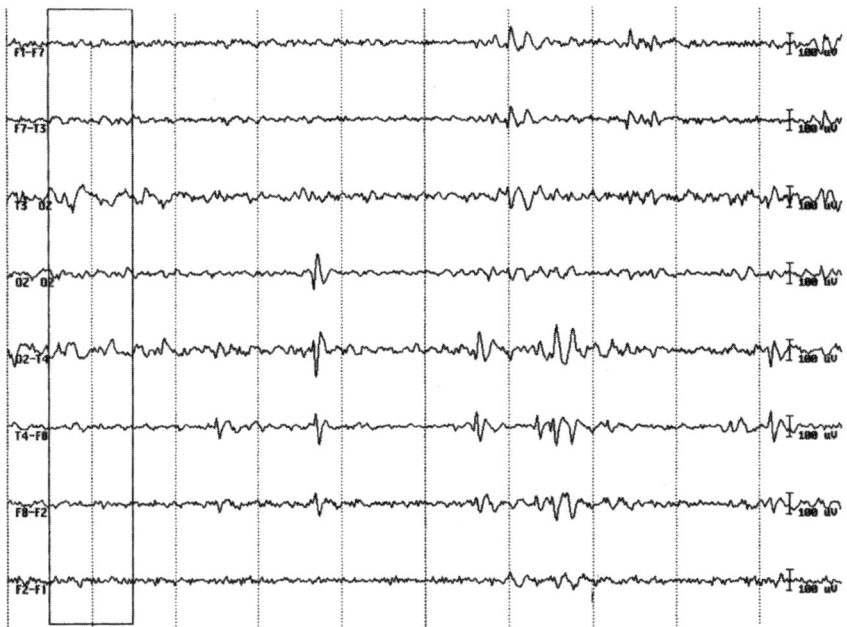

Figure 7. Four years old girl. Sleep EEG shows right occipital spikes and bilateral independent centrotemporal spikes.

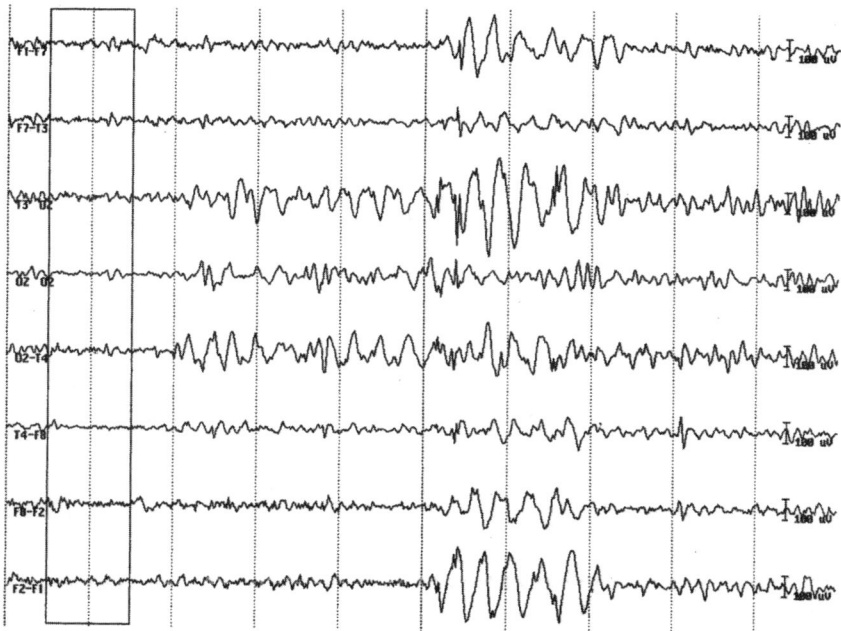

Figure 8. Six years old boy. EEG while awake shows occipital slow waves followed by an irregular generalized spike wave discharge. Isolated right centrotemporal spikes are also seen.

b) Ictal EEGs and video-polysomnography. Typical autonomic seizures and autonomic status epilepticus of PS had been documented by ictal EEG in several patients (Beaumanoir 1993, Oguni et al., 1999, Vigevano et al., 2000, Demirbilek & Dervent 2004, Koutromanidis et al., 2005). The ictal discharge in PS is characterized by rhythmic monomorphic decelerating theta or delta activity which is markedly different than the episodic fast activity of visual seizures of the Gastaut type COE and starts either from the posterior regions (Beaumanoir 1993, Vigevano & Ricci 1993, Oguni et al., 1999, Vigevano et al., 2000, Demirbilek & Dervent 2004) or frontal regions (Covanis et al., 2005). We recently had the opportunity to register an ictal EEG in a 4 year old girl with a seizure consisting on vomiting, pallor and loss of consciousness, and we can see the rhythmic slow-wave with superimposed spike discharges starting in right occipital regions and propagating to frontal areas *(Fig. 9)*. An ictal video polysomnography performed in an 8 years old boy with a form rather severe of PS showed: a run of fast spikes (7 Hz) mainly involving the right occipital region associated with tachycardia; during this 10 minutes the EEG then showed persisting spike-wave activity at 3 Hz initially located in the right occipital region and later involving all the other EEG derivations; 10 minutes after the onset of the seizure the EEG showed numerous high-amplitude slow-waves intermittent with more rapid activity accompanied with tonic deviation of the eyes to the left. Vomiting occurred during the last 2 minutes of the seizure while the same EEG activity was evident in right occipital region but ended after repetitive vomiting. The mentioned low amplitude components disappeared and only post-ictal low frequency components prevalent in the frontal region remained (Parisi et al., 2005).

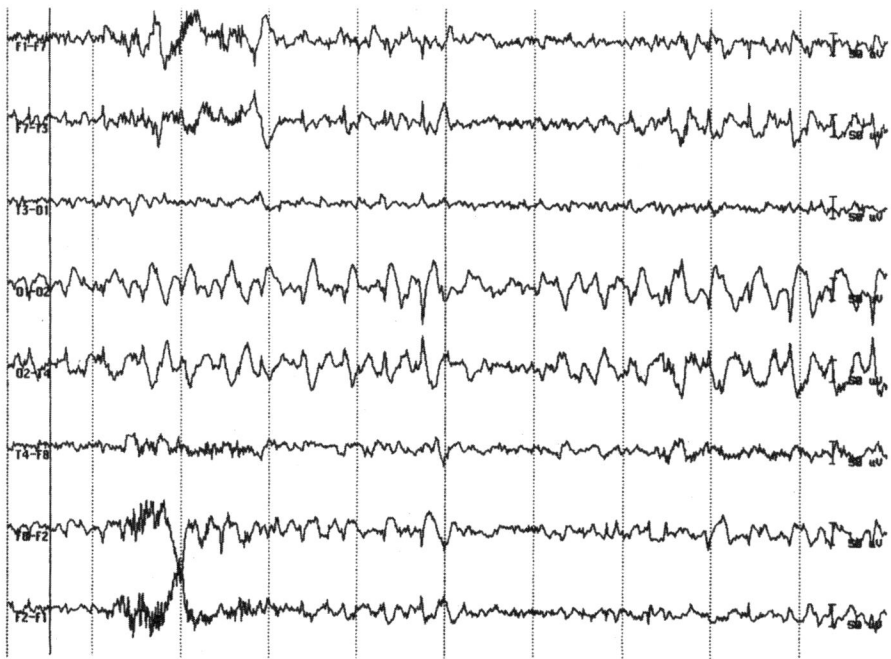

Figure 9. Four years old girl. Ictal EEG shows slow-wave activity with interspersed spikes in right occipital region, propagated to left frontal region.

Other neurophysiological studies: in 13 children with PS and a range of ages from 3 to 14 years, the localizations of equivalent current dipoles (ECDs) of spike-discharges by magnetoencephalography were examined. Eleven patients (84.6%) showed clustered ECDs in the areas alongside the parieto occipital sulcus and/or the calcarine sulcus. Five of the children who also presented Rolandic seizures showed besides clustered ECDs in Rolandic areas (Kanazawa *et al.*, 2005). In a case previously mentioned with some atypical clinical and EEG features during evolution, magnetoencephalography (MEG) revealed the calculated dipoles of the preceding bifrontal spike-wave discharges to be on the frontal areas, while those of the following generalized spike-wave burst were in the bilateral mid-temporal area. Since the reported dipoles in PS patients with multifocal epileptic discharges are usually located in the occipital and rolandic areas, the authors concluded that the unique clinical evolution in their case might have been associated with the unusual frontal localization of dipoles detected by MEG (Saitoh *et al.*, 2006).

Studies of visual evoked potential (VEP) have been performed in 9 children with PS and in 10 children with the Gastaut type of COE. High amplitude VEP responses most attributed to hyperexcitability of the occipital cortical structures were present in the 19 patients (Gokcay *et al.*, 2003).

Aetiology

As an idiopathic epilepsy syndrome, PS is by definition not associated to remote symptomatic or acute symptomatic aetiology. Most probably, it is genetically determined, although neither a gene nor a chromosomic locus has been found in PS. Linkage with chromosome 15 has been reported in BCECTS (Neubauer *et al.*, 1998), although in another study the mentioned locus was not found (Pruna *et al.*, 2000). In one series, one affected sibling with PS was reported (Ferrie *et al.*, 1997) and 2 pairs of affected siblings were seen in each of two other series (Caraballo *et al.*, 2000, Lada *et al.*, 2003). Curiously enough, 3 siblings were reported in 1987 as having Benign occipital epilepsy as described by Gastaut, although reading the paper, those 3 siblings showed seizures starting at ages 4 and 5 years, and the clinical features were quite compatible with PS (Kuzniecky & Rosemblatt 1987).

There is a high prevalence of febrile seizures in children with PS, ranging from 16% to 45% (Vigevano & Ricci 1993, Ferrie *et al.*, 1997, Oguni *et al.*, 1999, Caraballo *et al.*, 2000, Covanis *et al.*, 2003, Covanis *et al.*, 2005). A family history of epilepsy was found in 30.3% of the cases (Caraballo *et al.*, 2000). The finding of several children with PS who had at the same time or later Rolandic seizures and centrotemporal spikes typical of BCECTS (Caraballo *et al.* 1998) as well as siblings having either Rolandic epilepsy or PS speaks in favour of a genetic linkage of these two syndromes, perhaps expressed as a reversible functional derangement of the brain cortical maturation (Panayiotopoulos 1989b, Panayiotopoulos 1999a, Panayiotopoulos 2002, Panayiotopoulos 2005, Ferraro *et al.* 1997, Caraballo *et al.*, 1998, Caraballo *et al.*, 2000, Covanis *et al.*, 2003, Covanis *et al.*, 2005).

Pathophysiology

Basic mechanisms and pathophysiology of PS are largely unknown. Clinical findings indicate that there is a diffuse cortical hyperexcitability which is maturation-related (Panayiotopoulos 2002, Covanis *et al.*, 2005, Ferrie *et al.*, 2006). On account of EEG findings, even when the majority of cases show occipital spikes, a significant number of patients presents spikes in other areas, and according to the mentioned reference of PS and BCECTS in the same children, spikes may appear in two areas at the same time or with the course of time (Caraballo *et al.*, 1998, Covanis *et al.*, 2003). Besides, the high frequency of ictal vomiting indicates that epileptic discharges are generated at various cortical locations. The same concept is valid for other autonomic manifestations. As mentioned earlier, different cortical locations in patients with PS were also documented with magnetoencephalography (Kanazawa *et al.*, 2005).

Diagnostic work-up

Neuroimaging and other laboratory examinations: by definition of an idiopathic epilepsy syndrome, neurologic and neuropsychologic evaluations of children with PS are normal. Some of the initial symptoms may mislead the pediatrician regarding the nature of the condition, mainly when vomiting and other autonomic symptoms are present. Excessive laboratory examinations may then be undertaken. When syncope-like manifestations occur, cardiologic consultation is required.

Brain imaging studies are normal. However, the spectacularity of ictal features, and specially the frequency of status epilepticus, makes MRI necessary to rule out the several brain insulting conditions that may provoke focal, unilateral or generalized seizures.

Differential diagnosis and relation with other epilepsy syndromes

Despite sound clinico-EEG manifestations, Panayiotopoulos syndrome escaped recognition for many years, for many reasons. Ictal vomiting is rarely considered as a seizure event. When this is associated with deteriorating level of consciousness followed by convulsions, the prevailing diagnoses at the acute stage are encephalitis, acute toxic encephalopathy or other acute cerebral insults. If the seizures are hemigeneralized, a more focal cerebral insult is always looked for. If the child is seen after complete recovery, atypical migraine, gastroenteritis, or even syncope are likely diagnoses (Covanis 2006). In *Table II* the main differential diagnosis of PS are listed. The presence of prolonged seizures in a previously healthy child, inevitably leads to think on acute cerebral insults due to encephalitis, intoxication, acute disseminated encephalomyelitis, MELAS or acute cerebro-vascular event. Complete recovery after one or more hours of seizures makes

Table II. Differential diagnosis of Panayiotopoulos syndrome

- **With other neurological conditions**
  - Encephalitis
  - Acute toxic encephalopathy
  - Acute disseminated encephalomyelitis (ADEM)
  - Mitochondrial encephalopathy with lactic acidosis and stroke (MELAS)
  - Acute cerebrovascular event
  - Migraine (basilar artery migraine)
  - Diseases of the autonomic nervous system
- **With other epilepsy syndromes**
  - With other idiopathic epilepsy syndromes
    - Childhood epilepsy with occipital paroxysms (Gastaut type)
    - Benign childhood epilepsy with centrotemporal spikes
    - Idiopathic photosensitive occipital epilepsy
  - With symptomatic occipital epilepsies
    - Celiac disease, occipital calcifications and epilepsy
    - Occipital epilepsy after neonatal hypoglycemia
    - Other symptomatic occipital epilepsies

not probable the mentioned diagnosis, although, as stated before, brain imaging studies are usually obtained. Basilar or other infrequent forms of atypical migraine are one of the main differential diagnoses in cases with prolonged or repeated vomiting with other autonomic system symptoms. Both conditions may appear abruptly, and in both, full recovery is seen. Consciousness impairment does not rule out the diagnosis of migraine (Panayiotopoulos 1999b). However, it is extremely rare for migraine to start with vomiting interrupting sleep in young children.

The syncope-like episodes, with pallor, irresponsiveness and flaccidity may lead to think in real syncopal attacks and to ask for cardiological examination. Of course, the common syncope in children does not appear during sleep, but nausea, pallor and sick feeling of an awake child are not rarely first symptoms of syncopal attacks in children.

The differential diagnosis between PS and the Gastaut type of COE is detailed in *Table III*. We previously proposed (Fejerman 1996, Caraballo et al 1997) that the syndrome of childhood epilepsy with occipital spikes described by Gastaut (1982) is markedly different from the syndrome described by Panayiotopoulos (Panayiotopoulos 1989a, b), despite similar interictal EEG abnormalities. No matter how enthusiastic we may be to recognise each of these syndromes, we must admit that there are intermediate cases presenting visual symptoms in patients with PS and vomiting or other autonomic symptoms in patients with the Gastaut type of COE. A good example is the case of a 4 years old girl whose seizures started with visual symptoms followed by migraine-like headache and vomiting. On account of age of onset and EEG features *(Fig. 10)* we diagnosed PS, although the ictal symptoms were compatible with COE "Gastaut type" syndrome.

The mean age of onset of BCECTS is around 7-8 years of age and its typical features differ clearly from those of PS. However, we'll see later that it is not so rare to see children presenting at the same time ictal symptoms of both syndromes. As for the idiopathic photosensitive occipital lobe epilepsy, its mean age of onset is around 11 years and all ictal events are preceded by the exposure

Table III. Differential diagnosis between Panayiotopoulos syndrome and Gastaut type Childhood occipital epilepsy

	Panayiotopoulos syndrome	Gastaut type Childhood Occipital Epilepsy
Prevalence amongst benign focal epilepsies in childhood	25-30%*	3-5%
Age at onset	1-14 years (mean: 4-5 years)	3-16 years (mean 8-9 years)
Duration of seizures:		
• Less than 4 minutes	rare	as a rule
• 5 or more minutes	as a rule	rare
High seizure frequency	rare	as a rule
Seizures during sleep	more than 2/3 of cases	less than 1/3 of cases
Features of seizures:		
• Ictal vomiting	frequent	rare
• Deviation of the eyes	frequent	rare
• Impairment of consciousness	frequent	rare
• Visual hallucinations	rare	as a rule
• Loss of vision	rare	frequent
• Autonomic disturbances	common	rare
• Migraine-like headache	rare	frequent
Seizures evolving into status	frequent	rare
Interictal EEG	Frequent occipital spikes. Less frequent spikes in other areas	Spike-wave occipital paroxysms reactive to eye opening
Prognosis:		
• Remission within 1-3 years from 1st seizure	As a rule	rare
• Evolution into CSWS	rare (3 cases reported)**	rare (2 cases reported)
• Overall prognosis	excellent	uncertain

* *Prevalence of PS in the series of cases presented here is 31,21% and 4,06% for the Gastaut type of Childhood Occipital Epilepsy.*
** *In the new series of cases presented in this Chapter, 5 cases showed evolution into CSWS.*

to photic stimulation, either intermittent lights, or TV and computer games screens (Tassinari *et al.*, 1989, Guerrini *et al.*, 1995). Besides, this condition is quite rare and less frequent than the other reflex epilepsies secondary to visual stimuli (see Chapter 8).

Symptomatic occipital epilepsies may present clinical features similar to the idiopathic occipital epilepsies. Even the EEG may show the occipital spike-and-wave discharges disappearing after eye opening which characterize the Gastaut type of COE and may also be seen in PS (Newton &

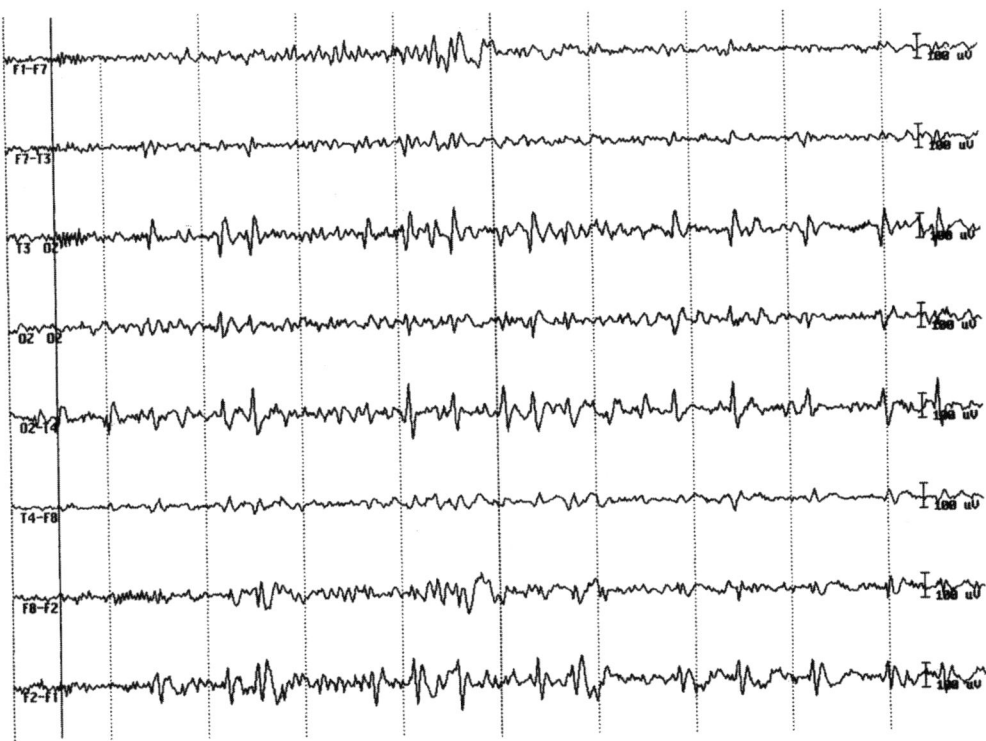

Figure 10. Four years old girl. Sleep EEG shows temporooccipital spikes with less frequent synchronic frontal spikes.

Aicardi 1983, Cooper & Lee 1991). There are two particular conditions to think about in children with seizures including visual symptomatology and occipital spikes or spike-waves. One is Celiac disease with occipital calcifications and epilepsy. The majority of the patients with this condition do not refer overt symptoms of Celiac disease in their personal history. That is why, upon the presence of occipital discharges and seizures, posterior cerebral calcifications have to be discarded. If present, specific studies for Celiac disease are mandatory because in these children their epilepsy improves with gluten free diet (Gobbi et al., 1997, Arroyo et al., 1997). Silent Celiac disease was investigated in a study of 72 patients observed consecutively over a 5-year period with an initial diagnosis of idiopathic partial epilepsy. In the 47 children with BCECTS, specific antibodies were not found, but in 2 of the 25 cases with childhood partial epilepsy with occipital paroxysms (COE), the results were positive and later confirmed by jejunal biopsy (Labate et al., 2001). No intention to discriminate between the Gastaut type and the Panayiotopoulos type of COE was shown in this study.

In a recent series of 12 patients, we showed the clear association between history of neonatal hypoglycemia and posterior cerebral lesions provoking seizures. Epileptic seizures in these children wee usually well controlled by antiepileptic drugs (AED), but most of the cases presented intellectual impairment (Caraballo et al., 2004a).

Association of PS with other idiopathic epilepsy syndromes

Occasional findings of isolated cases with electroclinical features of BCECTS in children with idiopathic occipital epilepsies were reported in some series (Panayiotopoulos 1989a, Panayiotopoulos 2002, Kivity & Lerman 1992, Ferraro et al., 1997). In 1998, Idiopathic partial epilepsies with Rolandic and Occipital spikes appearing in the same patients were reported in ten cases. Five of them had first PS and after 2 or more years presented hemifacial motor seizures with anarthria typical of BCECTS. The other five patients presented anarthria and hemifacial contractions with sialorrhea and ictal vomiting with head deviation as typical seizures of PS and BCECTS in the same epoch and even in the same episodes *(Fig. 11)* (Caraballo et al., 1998). This finding was later ratified by another group of authors (Covanis et al., 2003). This coexistence and/or contiguous expression of PS and BCECTS in the same children is even more clear in our new series of patients presented in this chapter, because 24 out of 192 children with PS had seizures characteristic of BCECTS either concomitantly with typical PS seizures or in the course of the disease. Ten of them had ictal manifestations combining autonomic or occipital and Rolandic features, 6 had both type of seizures independently and 8 children developed Rolandic seizures after a seizure free period ranging from 2.5 to 4 years.

Another small series of cases reporting the presence of 2 idiopathic epilepsy syndromes in the same children, showed that absence epilepsy was associated with the Gastaut type of COE in five patients and with PS in one child (Caraballo et al., 2004b).

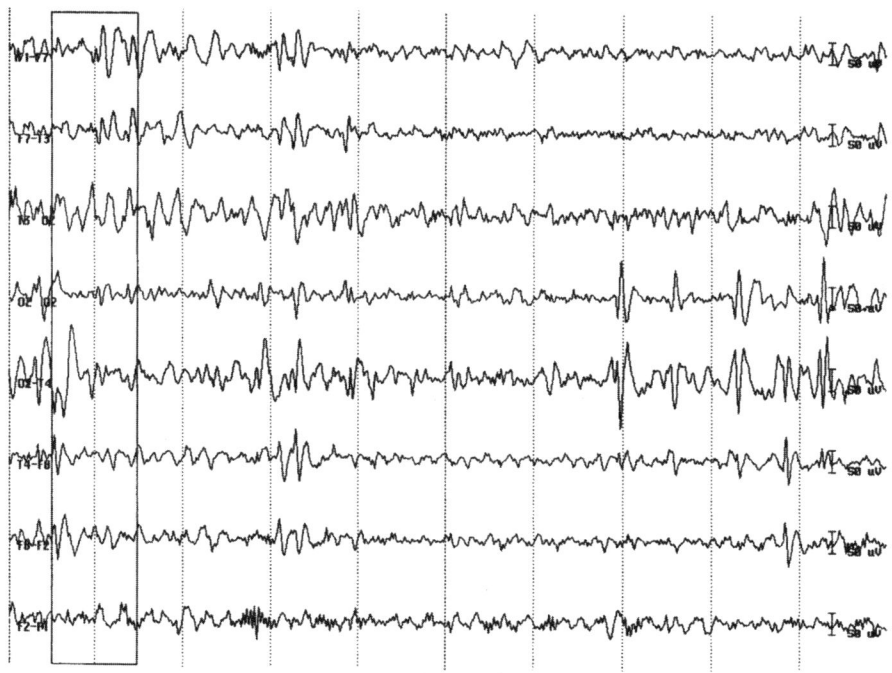

Figure 11. Seven years old boy with typical Rolandic seizures and autonomic seizures followed by eye-deviation in the same epoch. Sleep EEG shows spikes in right centrotemporal and right occipital regions.

Treatment

There is no clear position about treatment in PS. Since around 1/3 of the patients only have one seizure, either brief or prolonged, many authors recommend not to start with AED treatment (Panayiotopoulos 2005, Covanis et al., 2005). However, it is not so easy for pediatric neurologists to advise parents after a prolonged seizure that there is no need to prevent the repetition of the event using medication. We agree about the good outcome in patients without medication, but we prefer to medicate after the first seizure when it was prolonged. Carbamazepine or Valproic acid are the drugs of choice, and the latter is preferred when the EEG shows spike-and-wave discharges instead of spikes. As it was demonstrated in BCECTS, Carbamazepine may induce seizure exacerbation in PS (Kikumoto et al., 2006). One has to be always aware of the EEG effects of AEDs (Clemens et al., 2006). Levetiracetam showed to be well tolerated by children as adjunctive treatment in pediatric partial seizures (Glauser et al., 2006), and even was suggested as useful to treat patients within the spectrum of ESES (Aebi et al., 2005). If this finding is ratified, Levetiracetam would become a good alternative of treatment for benign focal epilepsies in childhood. At any rate, clear instructions should be given to parents of how to use rectal Diazepam immediately after onset of a new seizure.

Prognosis and long-term evolution

Despite the high incidence of seizures prolonged into status epilepticus, PS is a remarkably benign epilepsy syndrome (Panayiotopoulos 1999c, Caraballo et al., 2000, Verrotti et al., 2000, Panayiotopoulos 2002, Panayiotopoulos 2005, Covanis et al., 2005). One third of the patients have only a single seizure and most of the cases present 2 to 5 seizures in total. Remission usually occurs 1 or 2 years after the first seizure, and there are no comparable data to know if there is a significant difference in cases treated with AEDs.

Regarding the risk of persistence of seizures or of developing other types of epilepsy in adult life, except the personal experience of Dr. Panayiotopoulos, the other series did not reach yet such a long term follow-up of their patients to obtain information.

A retrospective study to evaluate prognostic factors in 46 patients with PS considered mainly the frequency of seizures presented by the children during a follow-up of 5 years and concluded that a low seizure frequency in the first months could have prognostic value, proposing to delay for 6 months after epilepsy onset the introduction of AEDs (Lanzi et al., 2003).

As stated before, a number of cases presenting BCECTS after the onset of PS are well documented and even one case with typical absence epilepsy, following PS was recently reported. The concept is that even when these associations occur, long-term prognosis is almost always benign. We say "almost" because nothing is absolute in medicine.

We have presented evidence of 3 cases with typical features of PS that presented atypical evolutions quite like what it was described in BCECTS (Fejerman et al., 2000). The 3 children started with inhibitory seizures and drops, atypical absences, and language and behavioural impairment associated with continuous spike-and-waves discharges in the sleep EEG. They were well managed with appropriate changes in AEDs, but we don't know what could have been the natural evolution of this complication (Caraballo et al., 2001, Ferrie et al., 2002).

Regarding the few cases with PS who presented atypical evolutions, as detailed in our present series of cases, we are aware of only one case that remained with neuropsychologic impairments. Finally, ictal cardiorrespiratory arrest was recently reported in a patient with PS (Verrotti et al., 2005), as an exception confirming the rule of very good long-term prognosis.

Data about our present series of cases

The study was initiated in February 1990 at the department of neurology of our hospital. This is the main pediatric neurology unit in the city of Buenos Aires, covering a population of 1.350.000 children.

This may be considered a prospective study, although we must clarify that the first 66 patients published by our group (Caraballo et al., 2000) had been selected under somewhat different inclusion criteria and were re-evaluated for this study.

The following inclusion criteria for PS were applied:

a. Autonomic manifestations, visual symptoms and/or simple motor focal seizures followed or not by impairment of consciousness with or without secondary generalization;
b. Functional occipital and extraoccipital spikes alone or combined on the interictal EEG, or a normal EEG;
c. Normal neurological and mental status;
d. Normal brain imaging.

Patients with known mental or neurological deficits, or patients with typical electroclinical pictures of BCECTS or Gastaut type COE from onset were excluded from the study, but followed closely to see whether they showed signs and symptoms of PS in the course of the disease.

We analyzed gender, age at onset, personal and family history of epilepsy, febrile seizures and migraine; duration and seizure manifestations, circadian distribution and frequency of seizures, therapeutic response and final outcome.

EEGs were performed while awake and asleep. Electrodes were placed according to the international 10-20 system. The morphology, topography and the reactivity of interictal paroxysms to eye closing and opening were studied; the latter only in children who collaborated while awake.

All patients underwent brain CT scans, and 120 had MRIs that were normal.

Between February 1990 and February 2004, 192 patients met the inclusion criteria, and they have been followed up to the present time. All patients were evaluated longitudinally, clinically and with EEGs for 2 to 16 years (mean: 8.5 years). A mean of 10 ± 4 EEGs were obtained for each patient. Clinical and EEG details of all patients were reviewed and unanimously agreed upon by all authors. The results were as follows:

Number of patients and gender

There were 192 children, 108 boys and 84 girls, which met the inclusion criteria of PS in a 15-year period. In the same period, we also registered a). 25 children with Gastaut type COE with visual seizures and occipital paroxysms blocking on eye opening and b). 398 children with BCECTS.

Age at onset

Age at first afebrile seizure ranged from 1.7 to 12.5 years, with a mean age of 5 and a median of 4.5 years.

Personal and family history of febrile convulsions, epilepsy, or migraine

A family history of epilepsy was found in 60 cases (31.3%). Details about the type of epileptic syndromes in close relatives are lacking, but four pairs of siblings with PS are included in this series. Febrile seizures were reported in 26 (13.5%) and migraine in 30 (15,6%). Fifty-five (28.5%) patients had had febrile convulsions and 15 migraine (7.8%).

Ictal manifestations

Pallor was an ictal manifestation in 180 children (93.7%). Ictal vomiting was found in 160 children (82.3%). Forty (20.8%) and 30 (15.6%) patients also had nausea and retching, respectively, that either appeared along with or before vomiting. Ten patients (5.2%) presented nausea and/or retching without vomiting. Five children (2.5%) had incontinence of urine and two (1%) syncope-like symptoms, all associated with impairment of consciousness. These autonomic signs or symptoms could occur at onset or during the course of the seizure. Eye and head deviation occurred in 170 (88.0%), clonic partial seizures in 59 (30.7%), visual symptoms in 20 (10.4%), and secondarily generalized seizures in 70 (36.4%). One-hundred-and-fifty (78.1%) patients who did not present secondary generalization had partial impairment of consciousness at the end of the seizures.

According to parents' report, the duration of seizures was rarely less than 5 minutes. Seventy patients (36.4%) had partial status epilepticus, lasting more than 30 minutes. In all patients, partial status epilepticus was characterized by pallor and/or vomiting, eye deviation and impairment of consciousness, followed by unilateral or generalized motor seizures in 35 children (50%). In 14 patients (20%), partial status epilepticus was the first manifestation of the syndrome.

Circadian distribution

All 192 children except five (2.6%) had seizures during sleep, but 59 (30.7%) also had seizures while awake.

Frequency of seizures

Eighty-five children (44.2%) had a single seizure, and 79 (41.2%) had infrequent and sporadic seizures (2-5) with seizure-free intervals of 6 months or longer. However, 18 patients (9.3%) had seizures every 1 to 5 months and 10 (5.2%) several times per month.

Rolandic seizures

Twenty-four (12.5%) patients with PS also had seizures with speech arrest and hemifacial motor symptoms characteristic of BCECTS, either in the course of the disease or concomitantly with otherwise typical PS seizures. Eight of these 24 children developed Rolandic seizures after a seizure-free period ranging from 2.5 to 4 years. Of the other 16 children, 10 had ictal manifestations combining occipital and Rolandic features and six had occipital and Rolandic seizures, independently. None of the cases with BCECTS evolved into PS.

Electroencephalographic findings

Occipital spikes were observed in 144 children (75%) *(Fig. 1a)*. In 60%, spikes were bilateral and synchronous, often with voltage asymmetry *(Fig. 1b)*. In the other 40%, spikes were unilateral and mainly on the right side (70%). Fifty patients (26%) also had temporal spikes and 20 (10.4%) had frontal spikes *(Figs. 2a, 2b, 3)*. Forty-five children (23.4%) only had extraoccipital spikes, 29 had temporal spikes, and 10 had frontal spikes and six fronto-temporal spikes. Spikes were activated by sleep in 90.9%, and their pattern remained unchanged. Of 130 patients with awake EEGs, 120 (92.3%) had occipital spikes or spike-wave paroxysms and these were blocked by opening of the eyes in 99 (82.5%). Three children (1.6%) had a normal EEG recording.

Of the 16 patients who concomitantly presented Rolandic seizures, 12 had occipital and Rolandic spikes and four had only Rolandic spikes. Four of the eight children who developed Rolandic seizures after a seizure-free period had occipital spikes only.

Three patients had generalized spike-wave discharges when awake and during sleep *(Fig. 4)*. Intermittent photic stimulation was normal in all patients.

Ictal EEG recordings showed rhythmic spikes or spike waves in the occipital region in two patients, propagating to the frontal region in one *(Fig. 5)*. In both children, the seizure was characterized by pallor, vomiting and eye deviation followed by impairment of consciousness.

Treatment

Antiepileptic treatment was started in 172 patients (89.5%), with single drugs, such as carbamazepine (112 patients), phenobarbital (20), valproic acid (20), ox-carbazepine (10) or clobazam (10), either after the first or after subsequent seizures. Phenobarbital was chosen in families who attended our public hospital but had serious difficulties to buy medications. Obviously, the cost of Phenobarbital is quite low. Twenty children (10.5%) never received any antiepileptic drugs. Of these 172 patients, 152 (88.3%) became seizure free after treatment; 71 of them had had only a single fit before treatment. Ten patients (6%) presented infrequent seizures, and the remaining 10 patients (6%) continued having frequent seizures.

Evolution

Approximately half of the children only had a single seizure. In all others, seizures remitted within 1 to 6 years (mean: 3 years) after onset, despite persistent EEG abnormalities in 50 (52%) of 96 patients.

Antiepileptic treatment was discontinued after 1 or 2 years of treatment in 95 patients (55.2%) who remained seizure free during 2.5 to 12.5 years of follow-up. In the evolution we did not find any electroclinical differences between treated patients and non-treated patients.

One patient developed an electroclinical picture compatible with epilepsy with typical absences after a seizure-free period of three years (Caraballo et al., 2004b).

Five patients developed an atypical evolution characterized by negative myoclonus, absences and frequent simple focal seizures associated with frequent or continuous bilateral spikes and waves during slow sleep. All presented transient neuropsychological impairment. Two of these cases were previously reported (Caraballo et al., 2001). One of them presented rolandic seizures and ictal vomiting followed by eye deviation and consciousness impairment before the onset of these particular electroclinical features. Four of these five patients had a good evolution, but one presented cognitive impairment at the last control at seventeen years of age (see Chapter 10).

References

- Aebi A, Poznanski N, Verheulpen D, et al. Levetiracetam efficacy in epileptic syndromes with continuous spikes and waves during slow sleep: experience in 12 cases. *Epilepsia* 2005; 46 (12): 1937-42.

- Arroyo HA, De Rosa S, Fejerman N. Epilepsy, cerebral calcifications and coeliac disease: Argentine multicentre experience. In: Gobbi G, Andermann F, Naccarato S, Banchini G (Eds). *Epilepsy and other neurological disorders in coeliac disease*. London: John Libbey, 1997: 93-101.

- Beaumanoir A. Semiology of occipital seizures in infants and children. In: Andermann F., Beaumanoir A., Mira L., Roger J., Tassinari CA (Eds). *Occipital seizures and epilepsies in children*. London: John Libbey, 1993: 71-86.

- Berg AT, Panayiotopoulos CP. Diversity in epilepsy and a newly recognized benign childhood syndrome (Editorial). *Neurology* 2000; 55: 1073-4.

- Caraballo RH, Cersosimo RO, Medina CS, Tenembaum S, Fejerman N. Epilepsias parciales idiopáticas con paroxismos occipitales. *Revista de Neurologia* 1997; 25: 1052-8.

- Caraballo RH, Cersosimo R, Fejerman N. Idiopathic partial epilepsies with Rolandic and occipital spikes appearing in the same children. *J Epilepsy* 1998; 11: 261-4.

- Caraballo R, Cersosimo R, Medina C, Fejerman N. Panayiotopoulos-type benign childhood occipital epilepsy: a prospective study. *Neurology* 2000; 55: 1096-100.

- Caraballo RH, Astorino F, Cersosimo R, Soprano AM, Fejerman N. Atypical evolution in childhood epilepsy with occipital paroxysms (Panayiotopoulos type). *Epileptic Disorders* 2001; 3: 157-62.

- Caraballo RH, Sakr D, Mozzi M, *et al.* (2004a) Symptomatic occipital lobe epilepsy following neonatal hypoglycemia. *Pediatr Neurol* 2004; 31 (1): 24-9.

- Caraballo RH, Sologuestua A, Grañana N, *et al.* (2004b) Idiopathic occipital and absence epilepsies appearing in the same children. *Pediatric Neurology* 2004; 30 (1): 24-8.

- Caraballo RH, Cersosimo R, Fejerman N. Panayiotopoulos syndrome: a prospective study of 192 patients. *Epilepsia* 2007; In press.

- Chahine L, Mikati M. Benign pediatric localization-related epilepsies. Part II. Syndromes in childhood. *Epileptic Disord* 2006; 8 (4): 243-58.

- Chilosi AM, Brovedani P, Moscatelli M, *et al.* Neuropsychological findings in idiopathic occipital lobe epilepsies. *Epilepsia* 2006, 47 (Suppl 2): 76-8.

- Clemens B, Menes A, Piros P, *et al.* Quantitative EEG effects of carbamazepine, oxcarbazepine, valproate, lamotrigine, and possible clinical relevance of the findings. *Epilepsy Res* 2006; 70 (2-3): 190-9.

- Commission on Classification and Terminology of the International League Against Epilepsy. Proposal for revised classification of epilepsies and epileptic syndromes. *Epilepsia* 1989; 30: 389-99.

- Cooper GW, Lee SI. Reactive occipital epileptiform activity: is it benign? *Epilepsia* 1991; 32: 63-8.

- Covanis A, Lada C, Skiadas K. Children with rolandic spikes and ictus emeticus: Rolandic epilepsy or Panayiotopoulos syndrome? *Epileptic Disorders* 2003; 5: 139-43.

- Covanis A, Ferrie CD, Koutroumanidis M, *et al.* Panayiotopoulos syndrome and Gastaut type idiopathic childhood occipital epilepsy. In: Roger J, Bureau M, Dravet CH, *et al.* (Eds). *Epileptic syndromes in infancy, childhood and adolescence* (4th Ed.). Montrouge: John Libbey Eurotext, 2005: 227-53.

- Covanis A. A benign childhood autonomic epilepsy frequently imitating encephalitis, syncope, migraine, sleep disorder, or gastroenteritis. *Pediatrics* 2006; 118: 1237e-43e.

- Dalla Bernardina B, Colamaria V, Capovilla G, Bondavalli S. Sleep and benign partial epilepsias of childhood. In: Degen R, Niedermeyer E (Eds). *Epilepsy, sleep and sleep deprivation*. Amsterdam: Elsevier Science publishers, 1984: 119-33.

- Dalla Bernardina B, Fontana E, Caraballo R, Zullini E, Darra F, Collamaria V. The partial occipital epilepsies in childhood. In: Andermann F, Beaumanoir A, Mira L, Roger J, Tassinari CA (Eds). *Occipital seizures and epilepsies in children*. London: John Libbey, 1993: 173-81.

- Dalla Bernardina B, Sgrò V, Fejerman N. Epilepsy with centrotemporal spikes and related syndromes. In: Roger J, Bureau M, Dravet CH, *et al.* (Eds). *Epileptic syndromes in infancy, childhood and adolescence* (4th Ed.). Montrouge: John Libbey Eurotext, 2005: 203-25.

- Demirbilek V, Dervent A. Panayiotopoulos syndrome: video-EEG illustration of a typical seizure. *Epileptic Disorders* 2004; 6: 121-4.

- Engel J, Jr. A proposed diagnostic scheme for people with epileptic seizures and with epilepsy: Report of the ILAE Task Force on Classification and Terminology. *Epilepsia* 2001; 42: 796-803.

- Engel J., Fejerman N. Benign childhood epilepsy with centrotemporal spikes. In: Engel J, Fejerman N. (Eds). *MedLink Neurology* (Section of Epilepsy). San Diego: MedLink Corporation, 1999-2006. Available at www.medlink.com.

- Fejerman N. Atypical evolutions of benign partial epilepsies in children. *Int Pediatrics* 1996; 11: 351-6.

- Fejerman N. New idiopathic partial epilepsies. *Epilepsia* 1997; 38 (Suppl. 7): 26.

- Fejerman N, Caraballo RH, Tenembaum S. Atypical evolutions of Benign Localization-related Epilepsies in Children. Are they predictable? *Epilepsia* 2000; 41: 380-90.

- Fejerman N. Benign focal epilepsies in infancy, childhood and adolescence. *Rev Neurol* 2002; 34: 7-18.

- Fejerman N. Epileptic syndromes and diseases. In: Aminoff M, Daroff RB (Eds). *Encyclopedia of the Neurological Sciences*. San Diego: Academic Press, 2003: 264-88.

- Fejerman N, Panayiotopoulos T. Early-onset benign childhood occipital epilepsy (Panayiotopoulos type). In: Engel J, Pedley TA (Eds). *Epilepsy: a comprehensive textbook*. Philadelphia: Lippincott Williams & Wilkins, 2007, In Press.

- Ferraro SM, Daraio MC, Mazzola ME, et al. Coexistence of two forms of Benign childhood partial epilepsias. *Epilepsia* 1997; 38 (Suppl. 7): 38.

- Ferrie CD, Beaumanoir A, Guerrini R, et al. Early-onset benign occipital seizure susceptibility syndrome. *Epilepsia* 1997; 38: 285-93.

- Ferrie CD, Grunewald RA. Panayiotopoulos syndrome: a common and benign childhood epilepsy (Commentary). *Lancet* 2001; 357: 821-3.

- Ferrie CD, Koutroumanidis M, Rowlinson S, Sanders S, Panayiotopoulos CP. Atypical evolution of Panayiotopoulos syndrome: a case report (published with video-sequences). *Epileptic Disorders* 2002; 4: 35-42.

- Ferrie CD, Caraballo RH, Covanis A, et al. Panayiotopoulos syndrome: a consensus view. *Develop Med Child Neurol* Mar 2006; 48 (3): 236-40.

- Ferrie CD, Caraballo R, Covanis A, et al. Autonomic status epilepticus in Panayiotopoulos síndrome and other childhood and adult epilepsius: a consensus view. *Epilepsia* 2007; in press.

- Gastaut H. A new type of epilepsy: benign partial epilepsy of childhood with occipital spike-waves. *Clin Electroencephalog* 1982; 13: 13-22.

- Gastaut H, Roger J, Bureau M. Benign epilepsy of childhood with occipital paroxysms. Up-date. In: Roger J, Bureau M, Dravet C, Dreifuss FE, Perret A, Wolf P (Eds). *Epileptic syndromes in infancy, childhood and adolescence*. London: John Libbey, 1992: 201-17.

- Germano E, Gagliano A, Magazu A, et al. Benign childhood epilepsy with occipital paroxysms: neuropsychological findings. *Epilepsy Res* 2005; 64 (3): 137-50.

- Glauser T, Ben-Menachem E, Bourgeois B, et al. ILAE treatment guidelines: evidence-based analysis of antiepileptic drug efficacy and effectiveness as initial monotherapy for epileptic seizures and syndromes. *Epilepsia* 2006; 47 (7): 1094-120.

- Gobbi G, Bertani G and the Italian working group on coeliac disease and epilepsy. Coeliac disease and epilepsy. In: Gobbi G, Andermann F, Naccarato S, Banchini G (Eds). *Epilepsy and other neurological disorders in coeliac disease*. London: John Libbey, 1997: 65-80.

- Gobbi G, Guerrini R. Childhood epilepsy with occipital spikes and other benign localization-related epilepsias. In: Engel J, Pedley TA (Eds). *Epilepsy. A comprehensive textbook*. Philadelphia: Lippincott-Raven, 1998: 2315-26.

- Gokcay A, Celebisoy N, Gokcay F, Ekmekci O, Ulku A. Visual evoked potentials in children with occipital epilepsies. *Brain Dev* 2003; 25 (4): 268-71.

- Guerrini R, Dravet C, Genton P, *et al*. Idiopathic photosensitive occipital lobe epilepsy. *Epilepsia* 1995; 36: 883-91.

- Gülgönen S, Demirbilek V, Korkmaz B, *et al*. Neuropsychological functions in idiopathic occipital lobe epilepsy. *Epilepsia* 2000; 41 (4): 405-11.

- Hande Sart Z, Demirbilek V, Korkmaz B, *et al*. The consequences of idiopathic partial epilepsies in relation to neuropsychological functioning: a closer look at the associated mathematical disability. *Epileptic Disorders* 2006; 8 (1): 24-31.

- Jallon P, Loiseau P, Loiseau J. Newly diagnosed unprovoked epileptic seizures: presentation at diagnosis in CAROLE study. Coordination active du réseau observatoire longitudinal de l'épilepsie. *Epilepsia* 2001; 42 (4): 464-75.

- Kanazawa O, Tohyama J, Akasaka N, Kamimura T. A magnetoencephalographic study of patients with Panayiotopoulos syndrome. *Epilepsia* 2005; 46 (7): 1106-13.

- Kikumoto K, Yoshinaga H, Oka M, *et al*. EEG and seizure exacerbation induced by carbamazepine in Panayiotopoulos syndrome. *Epileptic Disord* 2006; 8 (1): 53-6.

- Kivity S, Lerman P. Stormy onset with prolonged loss of consciousness in benign childhood epilepsy with occipital paroxysms. *J Neurol Neurosurg Psychiatr* 1992; 55: 45-8.

- Kivity S, Ephraim T, Weitz R, Tamir A. Childhood epilepsy with occipital paroxysms: Clinical variants in 134 patients. *Epilepsia* 2000; 41: 1522-3.

- Koutroumanidis M, Rowlinson S, Sanders S. Recurrent autonomic status epilepticus in Panayiotopoulos syndrome: video/EEG studies. *Epilepsy Behav* 2005; 7 (3): 543-7.

- Kramer U, Nevo Y, Neufeld Y, *et al*. Epidemiology of Epilepsy in Childhood: A cohort of 440 consecutive patients. *Pediatric Neurology* 1998; 18 (1): 46-50.

- Kuzniecky R, Rosenblatt B. Benign occipital epilepsy: a family study. *Epilepsia* 1987; 28: 346-50.

- Labate A, Gambardella A, Messina D, *et al*. Silent celiac disease in patients with childhood localization related epilepsias. *Epilepsia* 2001; 42 (9): 1153-5.

- Lanzi G, Longaretti F, Romeo A, *et al*. Early-onset occipital idiopathic epilepsy: a syndrome to be treated? *J Child Neurol* 2003; 18 (1): 72-4.

- Lada C, Skiadas K, Theodorou V, Covanis A. A study of 43 patients with Panayiotopoulos syndrome: A common and benign childhood seizure susceptibility. *Epilepsia* 2003; 44: 81-8.

- Maher J, Ronen GM, Ogunyemi AO, Goulden KJ. Occipital paroxysmal discharges suppressed by eye opening: variability in clinical and seizure manifestations in childhood. *Epilepsia* 1995; 36: 52-7.

- Martinovic Z. Panayiotopoulos syndrome or Early-onset Benign Childhood Occipital Epilepsy? *Epilepsia* 2002; 43: 1268-72.

- Neubauer BA, Fiedler B, Himmelein B, *et al*. Centrotemporal spikes in families with Rolandic epilepsy: linkage to chromosome 15q14. *Neurology* 1998; 51: 1608-12.

- Newton R, Aicardi J. Clinical findings in children with occipital spike-wave complexes suppressed by eye-opening. *Neurology* 1983; 33: 1526-9.

- Oguni H, Hayashi K, Imai K, Hirano Y, Mutoh A, Osawa M. Study on the early-onset variant of benign childhood epilepsy with occipital paroxysms otherwise described as early-onset benign occipital seizure susceptibility syndrome. *Epilepsia* 1999; 40: 1020-30.

- Ohtsu M, Oguni H, Hayashi K, Funatsuka M, Imai K, Osawa M. EEG in Children with Early-onset Benign Occipital Seizure Susceptibility Syndrome: Panayiotopoulos Syndrome. *Epilepsia* 2003; 44: 435-42.

- Panayiotopoulos CP. Inhibitory effect of central vision on occipital lobe seizures. *Neurology* 1981; 31: 1330-3.

- Panayiotopoulos CP. Vomiting as an ictal manifestation of epileptic seizures and syndromes. *J Neurol Neurosurg Psychiatr* 1988; 51: 1448-51.

- Panayiotopoulos CP. (1989a) Benign childhood epilepsy with occipital paroxysms: a 15-year prospective study. *Ann Neurol* 1989; 26: 51-6.

- Panayiotopoulos CP. (1989b) Benign nocturnal childhood occipital epilepsy: a new syndrome with nocturnal seizures, tonic deviation of the eyes, and vomiting. *J Child Neurol* 1989; 4: 43-9.

- Panayiotopoulos CP, Igoe DM. Cerebral insult-like partial status epilepticus in the early-onset variant of benign childhood epilepsy with occipital paroxysms. *Seizure* 1992; 1: 99-102.

- Panayiotopoulos CP. Benign childhood epilepsy with occipital paroxysms. In: Andermann F, Beaumanoir A, Mira L, Roger J, Tassinari CA (Eds). *Occipital seizures and epilepsies in children*. London: John Libbey, 1993: 151-64.

- Panayiotopoulos CP. (1999a) *Benign childhood partial seizures and related epileptic syndromes*. London: John Libbey, 1999.

- Panayiotopoulos CP. (1999b) Elementary visual hallucinations, blindness, and headache in idiopathic occipital epilepsy: differentiation from migraine. *J Neurol Neurosurg Psychiatry* 1999; 66: 536-40.

- Panayiotopoulos CP. (1999c) Extra-occipital benign childhood seizures with ictal vomiting and excellent prognosis. *J Neurol Neurosurg Psychiatr* 1999; 66: 82-5.

- Panayiotopoulos CP. *Panayiotopoulos syndrome: A common and benign childhood epileptic syndrome*. London: John Libbey, 2002.

- Panayiotopoulos CP. Early onset benign childhood occipital epilepsy (Panayiotopoulos syndrome). In: Engel J, Fejerman N (Eds). *MedLink Neurology* (Section of Epilepsy). San Diego: MedLink Corporation, 1999/2005. Available at www.medlink.com.

- Panayiotopoulos CP. Benign childhood focal seizures and related epileptic syndromes. In: Panayiotopoulos CP (Ed). *The epilepsies: Seizures, syndromes and management*. Oxford: Bladon Medical Publishing, 2005: 223-69.

- Parisi P, Ferri R, Pagani J, Cecili M, Montemitro E, Villa MP. Ictal Video-polysomnography and EEG spectral análisis in a child with severe Panayiotopoulos syndrome. *Epileptic Disor* 2005; 7 (41): 333-9.

- Pruna D, Persico I, Serra D, *et al*. Lack of association with the 15q14 candidate region for benign epilepsy of childhood with centrotemporal spikes in a Sardinian population. *Epilepsia* 2000; Suppl Florence: 164.

- Saitoh M, Kubota M, Kimura I, *et al*. A case of Panayiotopoulos syndrome showing an atypical course. *Seizure* 2006; 15 (8): 643-8.

- Sanders S, Rowlinson S, Manidakis I, Ferrie CD, Koutroumanidis M. The contribution of the EEG technologists in the diagnosis of Panayiotopoulos syndrome (susceptibility to early onset benign childhood autonomic seizures). *Seizure* 2004; 13: 565-73.

- Shinnar S, O'Dell C, Berg AT. Distribution of Epilepsy syndromes in a cohort of children prospectively monitored from the time of their first unprovoked seizure. *Epilepsia* 1999; 40 (10): 1378-83.

- Sillanpaa M, Jalava M, Shinnar S. Epilepsy syndromes in patients with childhood-onset seizures in Finland. *Pediatr Neurol* 1999; 21 (2): 533-7.

- Specchio N, Fusco L, Volkov J, Vigevano F. Panayiotopoulos syndrome: clinical and EEG characteristics of children. *Epilepsia* 2006; 47 (suppl 3): 29.

- Tassinari CA, Rubboli G, Plasmati R, *et al*. Television-induced epilepsy with occipital seizures: a variety of idiopathic partial occipital epilepsy. In: Beaumanoir A, Gastaut H, Naquet R (Eds). *Reflex seizures and reflex epilepsies*. Geneva: Editions Medicine & Hygiene, 1989: 241-3.

- Tedrus GM, Fonseca LC. Idiopathic childhood occipital epilepsies: clinical and electroencephalographic features in 63 children. *Arq Neuropsiquiatr* 2005; 63 (1): 61-7.

- Tedrus GM, Fonseca LC. Autonomic seizures and autonomic status epilepticus in early onset benign childhood occipital epilepsy (Panayiotopoulos syndrome). *Arq Neuropsiquiatr* 2006; 44 (3): 723-6.

- Tenembaum S, Deonna T, Fejerman N, Medina C, Ingvar-Maeder M, Gubser-Mercati D. Continuous spike-waves and dementia in childhood epilepsy with occipital paroxysms. *J Epilepsy* 1997; 10: 139-45.

- Verrotti A, Domizio S, Guerra M, *et al*. Childhood epilepsy with occipital paroxysms and benign nocturnal childhood occipital epilepsy. *J Child Neurol* 2000; 15: 218-21.

- Verrotti A, Salladini C, Trotta D, di Corcia G, Chiarelli F. Ictal cardiorespiratory arrest in Panayiotopoulos syndrome: a case report. *Neurology* 2005; 64: 1816-7.

- Vigevano F, Ricci S. Benign occipital epilepsy of childhood with prolonged seizures and autonomic symptoms. In: Andermann F, Beaumanoir A, Mira L, Roger J, Tassinari CA (Eds) *Occipital seizures and epilepsies in children*. London: John Libbey, 1993: 133-40.

- Vigevano F, Lispi ML, Ricci S. Early onset benign occipital susceptibility syndrome: video-EEG documentation of an illustrative case. *Clin Neurophysiol* 2000; 111 (Suppl 2): S81-S86.

- Yalcin AD, Kaymaz A, Forta H. Childhood occipital epilepsy: seizure manifestations and electroencephalographic features. *Brain Dev* 1997; 19: 408-13.

- Yoshinaga H, Koutroumanidis M, Shirasawa A, Kikumoto K, Ohtsuka Y, Oka E. Dipole analysis in Panayiotopoulos syndrome. *Brain Dev* 2005; 27: 46-52.

Late-onset childhood occipital epilepsy (Gastaut type)

Roberto H. Caraballo, Natalio Fejerman
Buenos Aires, Argentina

This childhood occipital epilepsy (COE) "Gastaut type" is a rare manifestation of a focal idiopathic epilepsy that has an age-related onset and is often age limited. COE "Gastaut type" is characterized by brief seizures with mainly visual symptoms such as elementary visual hallucinations, illusions, or amaurosis, followed by hemiclonic seizures while awake. Ictal or postictal migraine headache occurs in half of the patients, and mean age at onset is 8.9 years. The interictal EEGs reveal occipital spike-wave paroxysms that attenuate when the eyes are opened (Gastaut, 1982; Gastaut et al., 1992).

Long time ago Gastaut (1950) observed an epilepsy with ictal symptoms of occipital origin and an interictal EEG recording showing occipital spike-waves discharges reactive to eye opening. Gibb and Gibbs (1952) described pediatric patients with age-dependent seizures associated with occipital spikes.

Part of the story of the COE Gastaut type started with a publication originated in F. Andermann's group (Camfield et al., 1978) reporting four adolescents with episodes of what they called basilar migraine, plus seizures and temporo-occipital spike-wave discharges attenuated upon eye opening in the interictal EEGs. They assumed a basilar artery compromise on account of the loss of vision during the attacks. Age of onset was 4 years in one case and 9 to 11 years in the other 3. Prolonged vomiting or consciousness impairment was seen in two of them. Outcome was benign in the four cases in terms of response to AED and normalization of EEGs. A few years later Gastaut (1982) presented a series of 36 patients with seizures pointing to occipital lobe origin, associated migraine like symptoms and occipital paroxysms of spike-waves. Based on the well defined electroclinical features of the patients, he suggested the entity as a new epileptic syndrome in childhood. The 1989 ILAE Commission named this syndrome "childhood epilepsy with occipital paroxysms" and included it in the group of localization-related idiopathic epilepsies together with the benign childhood epilepsy with centrotemporal spikes (BCECTS) (Commission..., 1989). Fejerman and co-workers proposed designating this syndrome as "Gastaut type of benign childhood occipital epilepsy" in order to distinguish it from the "Panayiotopoulos type of benign childhood occipital epilepsy" or Panayiotopoulos syndrome (PS), which also manifests with occipital paroxysms (Fejerman, 1996, 2002; Caraballo *et al.*, 1997, 2000). This COE Gastaut type epileptic syndrome has been recognized in the 2001 ILAE's proposed diagnostic scheme as Late-onset childhood occipital epilepsy "Gastaut type" (Engel, 2001).

Several series of patients and chapters of books have been published with emphasis on electro-clinical features and evolution of this syndrome (Gastaut, 1985; Gastaut *et al.*, 1992; Panayioto-poulos, 1980, 1981, 1999a, b, c, 2005a; Beaumanoir, 1983, 1993a, b; Aso *et al.*, 1987; Terasaki *et al.*, 1987; De Romanis *et al.*, 1993; Genton & Guerrini, 1994; Maher *et al.*, 1995; Gobbi & Guerrini, 1997; Caraballo *et al.*, 1997; Watanabe, 2004, Covanis *et al.*, 2005). Over the last years, this syndrome has been loosing recognition. In the last report of the ILAE Classification Core Group this syndrome is listed in the group of epilepsies that start in childhood, but its score as a confirmed epileptic syndrome was lowest (Engel, 2006).

We believe, however, that COE "Gastaut type" presents enough clinical and EEG features, that even not being pathognomonic, cluster themselves in a significant number of children to allow us to consider it as a definite epileptic syndrome within the group of idiopathic focal epilepsies in childhood.

Epidemiology

COE "Gastaut type" is a rare condition with a probable prevalence of 0.2-0.9 per cent of all epilepsies, and 2-7 per cent of benign childhood focal seizures (Covanis *et al.*, 2005). It has been estimated in 0,15% of all focal epilepsies in childhood (Oguni *et al.*, 1999a; Chahine & Mikati, 2006).

In a 15-year period we registered 398 cases with benign childhood epilepsy with centrotemporal spikes, 192 cases of PS, and 29 with COE "Gastaut type" (Caraballo *et al.*, 2007). According to this experience in a tertiary level neuropediatric center, 29 (4.7%) of the 615 children with benign focal epilepsies seen in 15 years were diagnosed as COE Gastaut type (see "Data of our present series of cases"). However, as stated in the chapter on PS, the exact prevalence of idiopathic childhood occipital epilepsies will be known only with epidemiological studies acknowledging the different variants of COE now recognized.

Clinical features

The seizures of COE Gastaut type are always of occipital lobe onset and primarily manifest with visual seizures, which are the most typical and usually the first ictal symptom, but others type of seizures may be associated. The main type of seizures recognized in patients with COE "Gastaut type" are visual manifestations, motor seizures, migraine like symptoms and less frequently autonomic manifestations.

Visual seizures

Visual seizures occurred predominantly during the day at no particular time, but they may appear during sleep causing the patients to awake. They consist of elementary and complex visual hallucinations, visual illusions, blindness or partial visual loss and sensory hallucinations.

a) The elementary visual hallucinations occur as an initial seizure symptom in the majority of the patients. These hallucinations are brief developing rapidly, and last for 5-15 seconds, seldom exceeding 1-2 minutes. In rare cases, they last more than 15 minutes or even longer. The hallucinations are usually multicoloured and circular, appearing either in the periphery of a hemifield or centrally. They may multiply in number or size or both, move horizontally to the other side, and they may be flashing or static. They often may be the only ictal manifestation or they may progress to other seizures symptoms. The elementary visual hallucinations are almost always stereotyped in morphology, colours, location, movement, and other specific features for each patient. The patients often know well when during the visual hallucinations, impairment of consciousness and secondarily generalized tonic-clonic seizures are likely to occur. It is interesting to note that the features of the visual ictal symptomatology are clearly different from the visual aura of migraine (Gastaut, 1982; Gastaut *et al.*, 1992; Caraballo *et al.*, 1997; Panayiotopoulos, 1999a; Covanis *et al.*, 2005). In cases with migraine episodes the visual manifestations are characterized mainly by achromatic or black and white linear patterns, expanding from the centre to the periphery of a visual hemifield. In *Table I* we describe the differential diagnosis between COE Gastaut type and migraine.

b) Complex visual hallucinations are less frequent occurring approximately in 10 per cent of patients and usually develop from elementary visual hallucinations. The patient may see a face or figures, which often have the same location and movement sequence as that of the elementary visual hallucinations. They do not have the same emotional characteristics or complicated character as those associated with temporal lobe seizures.

c) Ictal visual illusions such as micropsia, metamorphopsia, palinopsia and polyopia are probably generated from the non-dominant parietal regions. This type of visual manifestations are extremely rare and they are probably only associated with symptomatic occipital seizures (Panayiotopoulos, 1999b, 2005a; Covanis *et al.*, 2005; Zakaria *et al.*, 2006).

Table I. Differential diagnosis between COE "Gastaut type" and symptomatic occipital lobe epilepsies

– MELAS disease
– Lafora disease
– Coeliac disease and epilepsy
– Occipital lobe epilepsy after neonatal hypoglycemia
– Sturge-Weber disease (without facial angioma)
– Periventricular leukomalacia and epilepsy
– Posterior periventricular nodular heterotopia
– Reversible posterior encephalopathy
– Chemotherapy, radiotherapy, occipital tumours, vasculitis, demyelination, others

d) Acute transient blindness is the second most common ictal symptom. It often occurs alone and may be the only ictal symptom in patients who experience visual hallucinations without blindness during other seizures. Blindness is sudden and total, and generally lasts longer than the visual hallucinations. If occurring alone, without visual hallucinations, it may persist 2-5 minutes (Covanis et al., 2005). In a report on epileptic blindness occurring in 14 children, four of them presented the full spectrum of clinico-EEG features of COE Gastaut type (Sahar & Barak, 2003).

Blurring of vision at onset of occipital seizures, with or without visual hallucinations, is probably fairly common (Panayiotopoulos 1999a, b, c, 2005a; Covanis et al., 2005). Postictal blindness, hemianopsia, and other partial visual loss after visual seizures with or without secondarily generalization have often been described.

A sensation of ocular movement in the absence of detectable motion is not frequent, but mainly occurs as a progression during elementary visual hallucinations (Covanis et al., 2005).

Motor seizures and other types of seizures

Deviation of the eyes, often associated with ipsilateral turning of the head, is the most common nonvisual symptom, occurring in around 70 per cent of patients. It may start after or also during visual hallucinations, is sometimes mild, but often more severe and progresses to hemiconvulsions and generalized tonic-clonic seizures (Gastaut, 1982,1985; Gastaut et al., 1992; Caraballo et al., 1997; Panayiotopoulos, 1999a; Covanis et al., 2005).

Forced eyelid closure and eyelid blinking – an interesting ictal clinical symptom of occipital seizures – occur in around 10% of patients, usually at a stage in which consciousness is impaired, and may be followed by secondarily secondarily generalized tonic-clonic seizures ("GTCS") (Covanis et al., 2005).

Elementary visual hallucinations or other ictal symptoms may evolve into hemi or generalized convulsions. Visual seizures are often followed by other nonvisual seizure symptoms such as hemiconvulsions (43%), complex focal seizures (14%), dysphasia, dysaesthesia, versive convulsions (25%), and generalized tonic-clonic seizures (13%) (Gastaut & Zifkin, 1987). Typical complex focal seizures of temporal lobe origin are rarely present, and then we should think in a symptomatic cause (Panayiotopoulos, 1999a).

Ictal vomiting, is extremely rare in COE "Gastaut type" and probably represents overlapping between the PS syndrome and COE "Gastaut type" (Aso et al., 1987; Caraballo et al., 1997). Other autonomic manifestations such as syncope, mydriasis, pallor are exceptional as well (Panayiotopoulos, 1999a; Caraballo et al., 1997).

Consciousness in not impaired during the elementary or complex visual hallucinations, blindness and other occipital seizure symptoms (simple focal seizures), but may be diminished or lost in the course of the seizure, usually preceding eye deviation or convulsions.

Migraine-like symptoms

Ictal or postictal headache is a common symptom in a 30-50% of the patients, even in episodes which don't present motor convulsions. As in migraine, the headache occurs immediately or within 5-10 minutes of the end of the visual hallucinations. Its duration and severity appear to be proportional to the duration and severity of the preceding seizures. The headache is often mild to moderate and diffuse, but may be severe and pulsating, and associated with nausea, vomiting, photophobia, and phonophobia, which may make it indistinguishable from migraine (Panayiotopoulos, 1987; Andermann & Zifkin, 1998). In several papers on COE Gastaut type headaches are considered as post-ictal (Gastaut, 1985; Gastaut et al., 1992; Covanis et al., 2005), although we are not quite sure about it because in many patients, either the headache or the autonomic migraine-like manifestations are present before the end of the attack. We have to remember that postictal headache is also common in other cryptogenic or symptomatic occipital seizures (Panayiotopoulos 1999a, 1999b; Caraballo et al., 1997).

Even when migraine and epilepsy are distinct conditions with specific and separate pathophysiologic mechanisms, they are associated in a number of patients and a causal relationship between both conditions has been debated to the point that a whole book was devoted to the subject (Andermann & Lugaresi, 1987). Comorbidity of migraine and epilepsy has been clearly demonstrated (Andermann & Andermann, 1987; Andermann, 2000). Between 8 and 50% of patients with epilepsy also have migraine and similar results have been found in adults as in children (Marks & Erhemberg, 1993; Yamane et al., 2004). The connection between migraine an epilepsy gave rise to speculations about common genetic susceptibility (Ottman & Lipton, 1996).

A reported case of "Migralepsy" (Milligan & Bromfield, 2005) prompted a response on the significance of differentiating occipital seizures from migraine (Panayiotopoulos, 2006). Migralepsy is an old term that is reintroduced every once on a while, but we think that it may be confusing (Di Blasi et al., 2007).

Andermann and Zifkin (1998) reviewed the subject and listed a number of what they called "migraine epilepsy syndromes" including even alternating hemiplegia of childhood.

EEG features

In COE "Gastaut type" the EEG shows occipital paroxysms, which, in routine recordings, occur when the eyes are closed and disappear or attenuate upon eye opening, reflecting fixation-off sensitivity *(Fig. 1a, b, c)*. EEGs with random occipital spikes, sometimes occurring only during sleep, are frequent *(Fig. 2)*. EEG abnormalities may be disproportional to the clinical severity *(Fig. 3)*. Spikes in other areas are also registered in patients with COE Gastaut type *(Fig. 4)*. Although less frequent than in BCETCTS, generalized spike-waves discharges may be seen in these patients *(Fig. 5)*. In patients with COE "Gastaut type" the disappearance of the EEG abnormality usually coincides with cessation of the seizures (Gibbs & Gibbs, 1952).

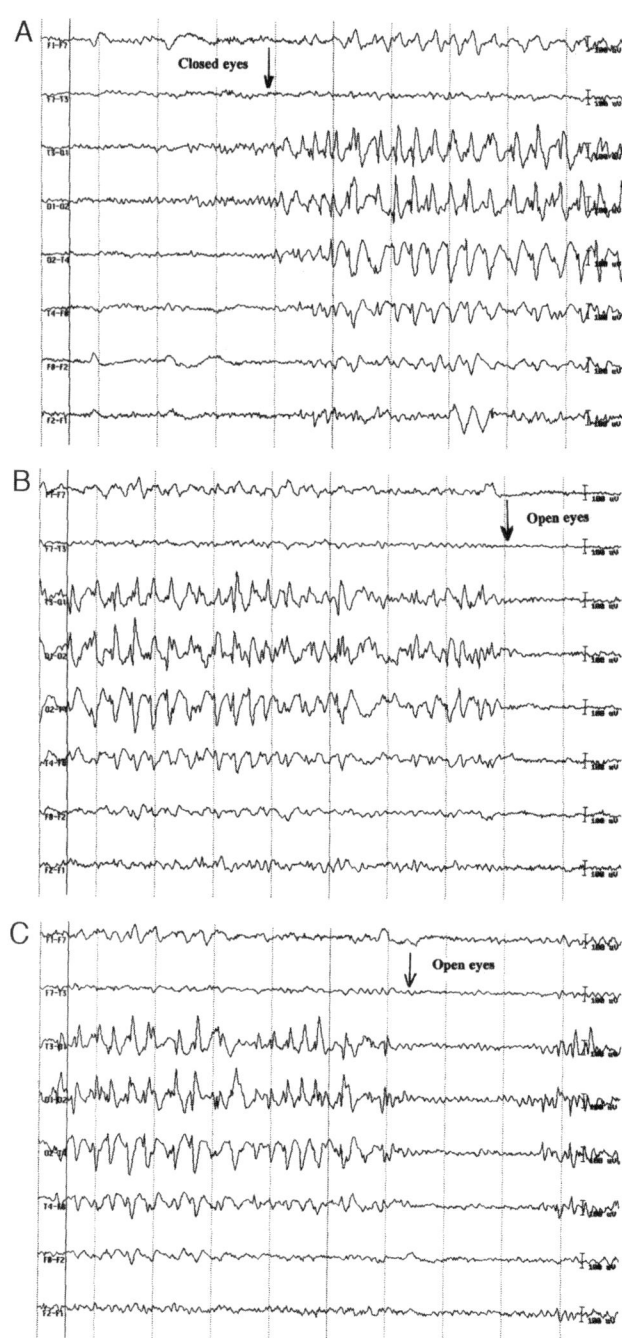

Figure 1. Nine years old boy. **A**: EEG while awake shows onset of occipital spike-wave discharges after eye closure. **B**: Spike-wave discharges disappear after eye opening. **C**: Spike-wave discharges attenuate after eye opening but reappear later.

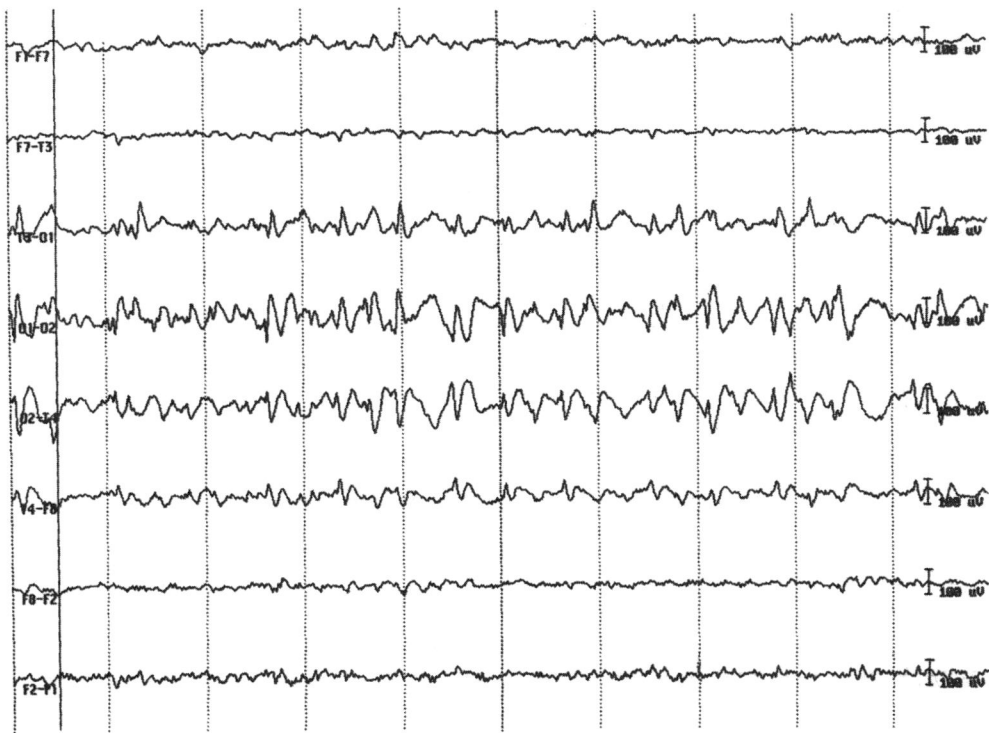

Figure 2. Ten years old boy. Sleep EEG shows spikes in posterior areas, dominant in right occipital.

Occipital spikes are not a specific finding of any epilepsy syndrome (Gibbs & Gibbs, 1952). Occipital spikes occur with organic brain disease with or without seizures in children with congenital or early onset visual and ocular deficit, and in 0.5-1.2 per cent of normal pre-school age children (Gibbs & Gibbs, 1952; Kellaway, 1980). They are common in young children with a peak age at first discovery of 4-5 years and tend to disappear in adult life.

Even when occipital spike-wave paroxysms are always present in the EEGs of patients with COE Gastaut type, they are also seen in non-idiopathic occipital lobe epilepsies. Several cases with occipital spike-waves which disappear after opening the eyes have been reported in children with symptomatic epilepsy (Newton & Aicardi, 1983; Cooper & Lee, 1991).

Only a few patients with COE "Gastaut type" have consistently normal EEGs. Centrotemporal, frontal and giant somatosensory spikes may occur but less often than in PS.

During visual seizures, the ictal EEG recordings show a discharge of rapid focal occipital spikes, which become progressively higher in amplitude and slower in frequency. Elementary visual hallucinations are related to a fast spike activity, which may spread to the other hemisphere (Fig. 6). Complex visual hallucinations appear to be related to slower discharges. In oculoclonic seizures, spikes and spikes and waves, which are slower than those seen during elementary visual

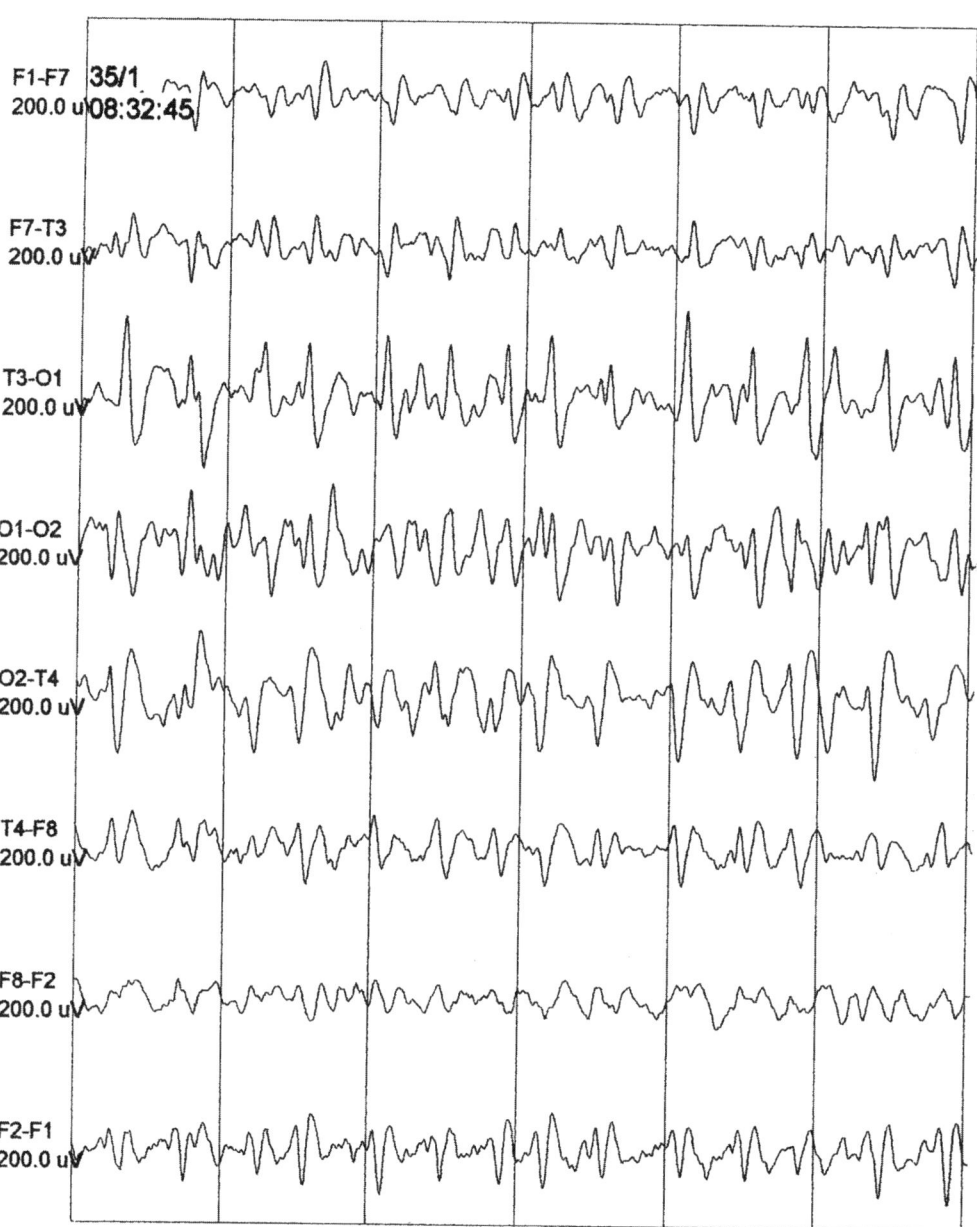

Figure 3. Eight years old boy with typical visual seizures. At the time of the present EEG while awake the child was medicated and seizure free. His evolution was excellent. EEG while awake shows frequent spike discharges dominant on occipital and frontal areas.

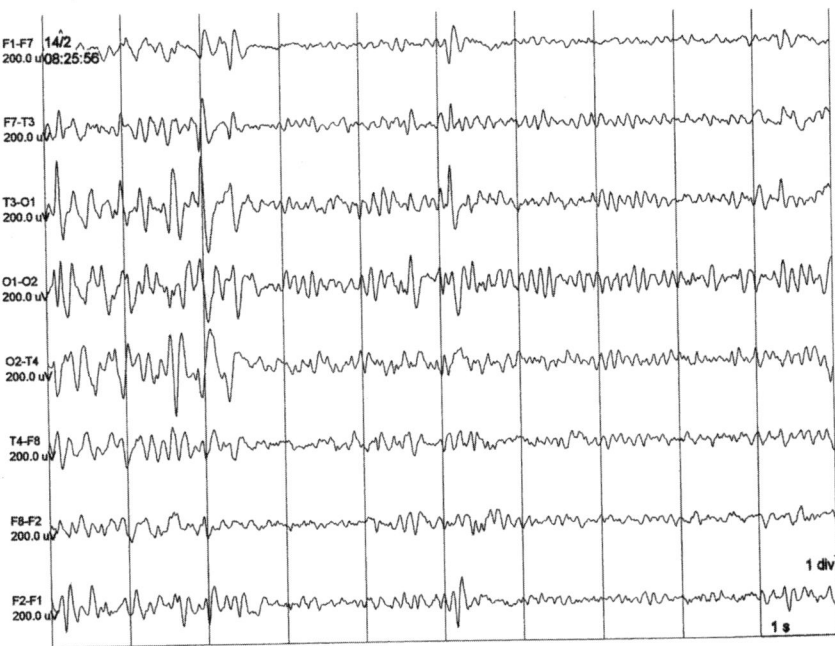

Figure 4. Ten years old boy. EEG while awake shows the typical posterior spike-wave discharges and independent centrotemporal spikes.

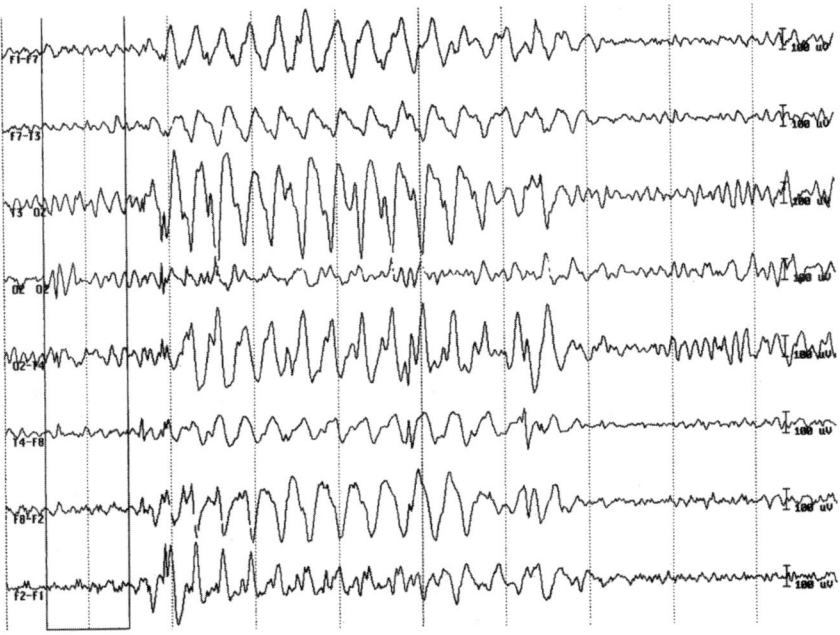

Figure 5. Ten years old girl. EEG while awake with generalized 3-3.5 Hz spike-wave discharges without evidence of absence.

hallucinations, and a localized ictal fast spike rhythm may occur prior to the deviation of the eyes. There are usually no postictal abnormalities. During blindness, the ictal EEG is characterized by pseudoperiodic slow waves and spikes, different from the EEG during ictal visual hallucinations.

The postictal EEG of occipital seizures generally returns quickly to the preictal state, whereas in the migrainous attacks the postictal EEG recordings are prolonged (Beaumanoir, 1993b).

Gastaut and Zifkin (1987) recorded spontaneous electroclinical seizures and electrical seizures during sleep. Some seizures showed particular ictal EEG manifestations characterized by bilateral fast activity, focal fast occipital spikes followed by bilateral fast activity in the posterior region, or high amplitude single generalized sharp slow waves. Similar ictal EEG findings have been published (Beaumanoir, 1983; Aso et al., 1987; Terasaki et al., 1987; De Romanis et al., 1993; Thomas et al., 2003).

Oguni and co-workers (1999b) confirmed the age-specific localization of spike foci, and additionally they demonstrated a frequent shifting in localization of spike foci with age advancing in most of patients with idiopathic and symptomatic childhood focal epilepsies. Occipital foci identified in the youngest age group tended to shift in localization frequently within a short period, and finally disappeared around the adolescent age. This finding suggests an underlying multifocal nature of epileptogenesis in patients with childhood focal epilepsy regardless of aetiology (Oguni et al., 1999b).

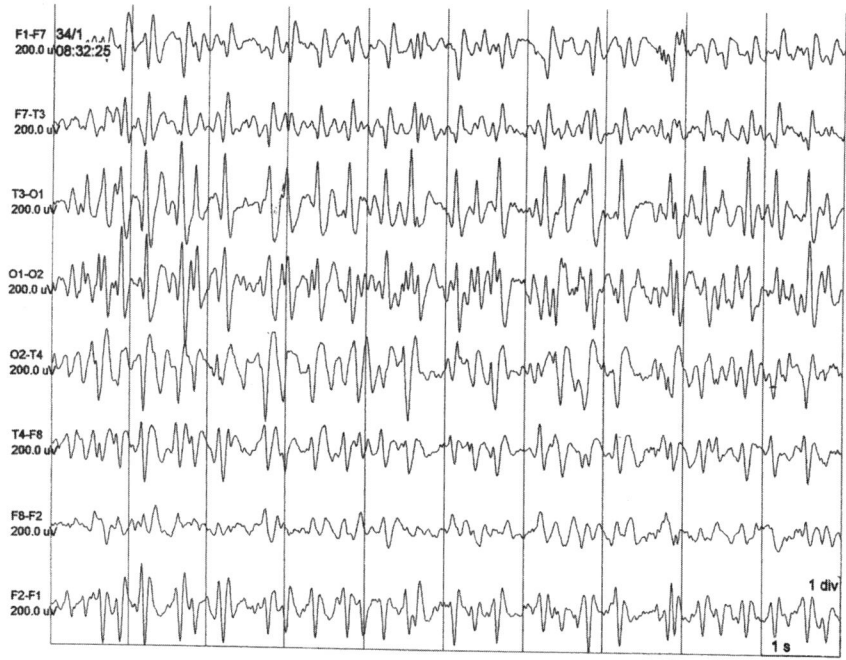

Figure 6. Nine years old boy. Ictal EEG during visual hallucinations shows onset with left occipital spikes which propagate bilaterally, but dominant on posterior regions. Impairment of consciousness occurred after initial visual symptoms.

Aetiology

Family history of epilepsy is found in 20-30% of cases and family history of migraine in 15%, approximately (Gastaut & Zifkin, 1987; Caraballo *et al.*, 1997). Family history of similar seizures is exceptional (Nagendran *et al.*, 1989). A personal history of febrile seizures has been reported in 14% of cases with COE Gastaut type (Caraballo *et al.*, 1997). No attempt to relate this syndrome to a particular loci has been apparently published. Nevertheless, being an idiopathic epileptic syndrome, the possibility of some type of genetic influence is always open.

Pathophysiology

Scalp and deep ictal EEG recording findings clearly show that elementary visual hallucinations arise from the visual cortex.

The mechanisms of ictal or postictal headache are unknown. It is possible that the occipital seizure discharge triggers a genuine migraine headache through a trigeminovascular or brain stem mechanism (Panayiotopouos, 1999a). The postictal migrainous symptoms of some attacks may be explained by a persistence in the posterior cerebral and basilar arteries of the initial vasodilation accompanying the occipital ictal activity in children with impaired or labile cerebrovascular autoregulation who are predisposed to migraines.

The postictal migraine may also be related to an epileptic phenomenon. Study of the ictal EEG recordings of postictal manifestations may clarify the exact mechanisms involved (Andermann & Zifkin, 1998).

The whole sequence of signs and symptoms might be interpreted as epileptic seizures induced by classical migraine occipital aura (Andermann & Zifkin, 1998) or as intercalated seizures attacks in the course of a migraneous episode (Terzano *et al.*, 1987).

Diagnostic work-up

By definition of an idiopathic syndrome, neurological examination, mental status, and high resolution MRI are normal. Ideally, all patients should have high resolution MRI to rule out static or progressive occipital lesions because of the high incidence of symptomatic occipital epilepsies with similar clinical and EEG manifestations.

Even when we already dealt with all the features of EEG in COE "Gastaut type", we must insist here on the need to check the changes in the EEG after eye opening in order to detect the peculiar phenomenon of disappearance of the occipital spike-wave discharges, even when it is not pathognomonic of this syndrome.

Differential diagnosis and relation with other epilepsy syndromes

The differential diagnosis of COE "Gastaut type" is mainly from probably symptomatic (cryptogenic)/symptomatic occipital epilepsy, migraine with aura, and basilar migraine. Symptomatic occipital epilepsy often imitates COE "Gastaut type" including the interictal electroencephalographic findings. There are many conditions that may manifest with symptomatic occipital seizures. It is important to differentiate mitochondrial encephalomyopathy with lactic acidosis and stroke-like episodes (MELAS) syndrome (Montagna et al., 1988) These patients present with occipital seizures, which at first are infrequent and easy to control, and they also have migraneous attacks. However, as the disease progresses, stroke-like episodes with frequent bouts of epilepsia partialis continua, quite difficult to control, usually occur (Andermann, 1993).

Lafora disease may begin in 50% of the patients with visual seizures involving simple or more complex hallucinations or scotomas associated with tonic-clonic seizures. A severe resting and action myoclonus then progresses along with neuropsychologic deterioration (Genton et al., 2005).

Coeliac disease, posterior cerebral calcifications and epilepsy with visual seizures should be also considered (Gobbi et al., 1997). Our group published a series of patients who responded well to a correct diet (Arroyo et al., 2002). In a search of silent Coeliac disease in 47 children with BCECTS and 25 patients with childhood epilepsy with occipital paroxysms, two cases of the latter group had antiendomysium IgA antibodies and presented features of Coeliac disease in the jejunal biopsy. In one of them occipital calcifications were found in the computed tomography. No data to know whether these two patients had PS or COE Gastaut type were given (Labate et al., 2001).

Epilepsy with occipital seizures in patients with Sturge-Weber syndrome without a port-wine facial nevus have been described (Arzimanoglou & Aicardi, 1993).

Recently, our group published a series of patients with occipital lobe epilepsy in children with history of neonatal hypoglycemia generally with benign course (Caraballo et al., 2004a). Reversible posterior leukoencephalopathy secondary to hypertension is associated with occipital seizures (Arroyo et al., 2003). Two adults with this syndrome associated with renal failure were reported in whom occipital onset seizures were present without other clinical signs or symptoms of hypertensive encephalopathy (Bakshi et al., 1998). Other differential diagnoses are described in *Table I*.

The differentiation of occipital seizures with elementary visual hallucinations from migraine should not be difficult if all of their features are properly evaluated *(Table II)*.

The differential diagnosis of COE "Gastaut type" with other idiopathic focal epilepsies in childhood includes in first place Panayiotopoulos Syndrome (PS). In fact the story went in the other way because COE "Gastaut type" was the only idiopathic occipital epilepsy included in the still valid ILAE's 1989 Classification and it took several years until PS was almost officially recognized (Engel, 2001). In one of the studies which helped to reinforce the existence of the PS, the records

Table II. Differential diagnosis between COE Gastaut type and migraine

	COE Gastaut type	Migraine
Daily attacks	As a rule	Rare
Visual hallucinations		
Duration		
Brief duration	As a rule	Rare
Moderate duration	Frequent	Rare
Prolonged duration	Rare	As a rule
Types of hallucinations		
Mainly coloured circular patterns	As a rule	Rare
Mainly achromatic or black and white linear patterns	Rare	As a rule
Moving to the opposite side of the visual field	As a rule	None
Expanding from the center to the periphery of a visual hemifield	Rare	As a rule
Loss of vision	Frequent	Rare
Episodes including tonic deviation of eyes	As a rule	None
Episodes evolving to impairment of consciousness with convulsions	Frequent	Very rare
Other neurological symptoms during attacks		
Ictal – postictal vomiting	Rare	Frequent
Severe headache	Frequent	As a rule
Brainstem symptoms	None	As a rule in basilar migraine

of 134 patients who met the criteria for idiopathic childhood occipital epilepsy disclosed 24 of them as belonging to the Gastaut type and 72 to the Panayiotopoulos type, while the rest of the patients did not fit to any of both types (Kivity et al., 2000). In this year 2000 we published our first prospective study with a large series of children with PS (Caraballo et al., 2000) (See Chapter 7).

Visual and purely occipital seizures may progress to autonomic symptoms, mainly retching and ictal vomiting, like those occurring in Panayiotopoulos syndrome (Guerrini et al., 1995; Panayiotopoulos, 1999a). We have seen an 11-years old girl with typical occipital spike-wave discharges appearing after eye-closure, who had seizures with clear autonomic features (vomiting and pallor) right after visual symptoms. According to age of onset and EEG features she was classified as COE Gastaut type, although the seizures were compatible with PS.

It has been repeatedly stated that all the idiopathic focal epilepsies in childhood may represent variable phenotypes of an only condition which has in common a cortical excitability recognized as benign childhood seizure susceptibility syndrome (Panayiotopoulos, 1999a, 2005a). We are not sure about it, but the fact that COE "Gastaut type" and PS have so many features in common is striking and that was the reason for the delay in the recognition of PS. Whatever the truth might be, we think that the concept of differentiating particular syndromes is quite useful for pediatric neurologists and epileptologists. Decision about therapy, for instance, is much helped by this possibility.

Idiopathic photosensitive occipital epilepsy is an interesting and still developing epilepsy syndrome that was first described by Tassinari *et al.* (1989), and should also be considered as a differential diagnosis. Occipital seizures may be induced by television, video games, and intermittent photic stimulation and can manifest with multicoloured circular visual hallucinations that are often associated with blindness. Tonic deviation of the eyes, epigastric discomfort and vomiting, headache and generalized convulsions may follow (Panayiotopoulos, 1999a, 2005a; Guerrini *et al.*, 2005) Duration varies from 2-5 minutes or up to 2 hours. Some patients may have only one or two seizures, but others have many and without remission. Interictal EEG shows spontaneous and photically induced occipital spikes. Centrotemporal spikes may coexist. The ictal EEGs show the occipital origin and subsequent spread of the discharges to the temporal regions (Guerrini *et al.*, 1995; Panayiotopoulos, 2005b; Gobbi & Guerrini, 1997). In COE "Gastaut type" some patients have positive photosensitivity. Gastaut included photosensitive patients with COE in his syndrome. These overlapping electroclinical manifestations between COE "Gastaut type" and idiopathic photosensitive occipital epilepsy may suggest that the latter is not an independent epilepsy syndrome, but a variant of COE with particularly high photosensitivity. A similar criterion was adopted regarding the babies with reflex myoclonic seizures in relation to benign myoclonus epilepsy in infancy (Dravet *et al.*, 2005).

Association of COE Gastaut type with other idiopathic epilepsy syndromes

We already mentioned in chapter 6 our report of 10 children who presented BCECTS and PS either at the same time or one syndrome after the other (Caraballo *et al.*, 1998).

Two girls with typical BCECTS starting at 4 and 5 years of age and easily controlled with AED, presented at age 12 years, after several years seizures free, clinical and EEG features of occipital lobe epilepsy with clear photosensitivity, reinforcing the concept of existence of different idiopathic epilepsy syndromes one after the other in the same children (Guerrini *et al.*, 1997). Whether we consider the presence of photosensitivity triggering occipital seizures as part of a different syndrome or as a variant of COE Gastaut type is irrelevant in comparison to the fact that a focal idiopathic epileptic syndrome appeared in these two girls a time after remission of BCECTS. Incidentally, in our series of 29 cases detailed at the end of this chapter, two girls of 14 and 16 years with photosensitive seizures also had had typical BCETS at ages 7 and 9 respectively. An interval of 3 and 4 years without seizures respectively elapsed between both syndromes.

An association between COE "Gastaut type" and typical absence seizures in children has been reported by our group. Typical absences appeared at the same time as visual seizures in two patients, and after one year in three patients. All patients had occipital paroxysms and 3 Hz generalized spike-wave discharges on the EEG (Caraballo *et al.*, 2004b) *(Fig. 7)*. Recently, we published three patients with COE "Gastaut type" and a particular evolution. The patients had ictal events that were characterized by visual symptoms followed by typical absences. In two of them, the seizures continued despite AED treatment (Caraballo *et al.*, 2005). One may interpret that the appearance of typical absences in these 3 patients might be due to the phenomenon of secondary bilateral synchronies.

Treatment

Patients with COE "Gastaut type" often suffer from frequent seizures and therefore medical treatment is mandatory. Currently there are no control studies that had demonstrated which is the drug of first choice. It has been stated that seizures usually stop or dramatically reduce within days after appropriate treatment with Carbamazepine (Panayiotopoulos, 1999a, c; Covanis *et al.*, 2005). We have used Valproic acid in the cases with clear spike-wave activities in occipital areas with good results. However, we think that carbamazepine, oxcarbazepine, valproic acid, levetiracetam and other AEDs, are equally indicated.

A slow reduction in the dose of medication 2-3 years after the last visual or other minor or major seizure may be advised, but treatment should be reinitiated if visual seizures reappear.

Prognosis and long-term evolution

Some controversies in the diagnosis of idiopathic occipital epilepsies in childhood and adolescence (Parra, 2006) may also shed doubts about prognosis and long term evolution. Therefore, the prognosis of "COE" Gastaut type is not as clear as in PS. Available data indicate that remission occurs in 50-60% of patients within 2-4 years from onset (Gastaut *et al.*, 1992; Covanis *et al.*, 2005). Seizures show a fairly good response to AEDs in more than 90% of patients.

There are cases of symptomatic occipital epilepsy presenting the same clinical and EEG features, and they probably influence the number of not so good results of treatment supposedly seen in patients with COE Gastaut type.

In a study of neuropsychological functions in 21 children with idiopathic occipital lobe epilepsy compared to controls, lower scores in attention, memory and IQ were found in the patients (Gülgönen *et al.*, 2000). According to the age of onset of seizures and the clinical manifestations, we assume that the majority of the cases presented corresponded to the COE "Gastaut type" syndrome, although at the time the authors talked about 20 of the children having childhood epilepsy with occipital paroxysms and 1 case with the idiopathic photosensitive occipital lobe

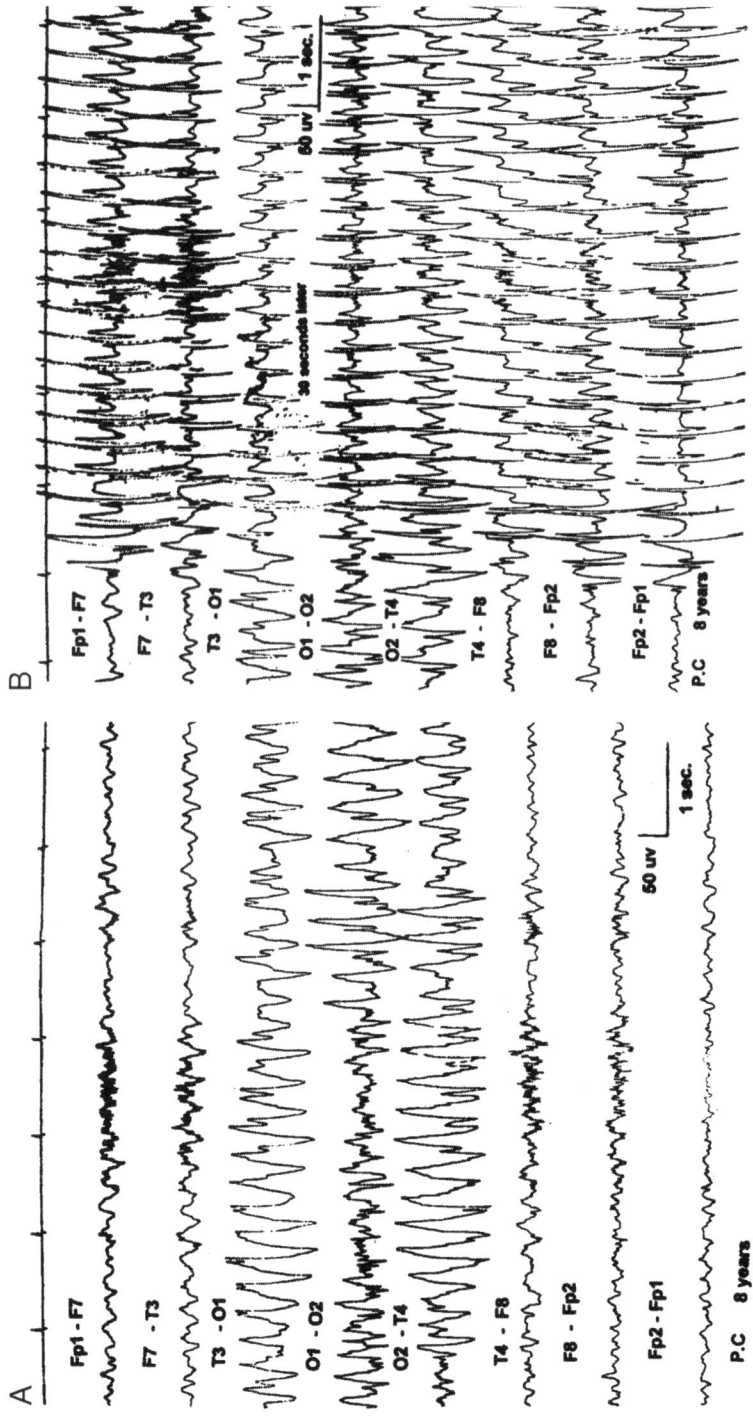

Figure 7. Nine years old boy. A: Ictal EEG while awake: irregular bilateral occipital spike-wave discharges during simple visual hallucinations. B: thirty seconds after onset, the ictal EEG shows that the previous occipital paroxysms are followed by generalized spike-wave activity coincident with a typical absence.

epilepsy without discriminating the Gastaut type from PS. In a neuropsychologic study of 30 children with idiopathic partial epilepsies compared to controls, 17 of them were diagnosed as idiopathic childhood occipital epilepsy syndromes including 6 children with PS, 8 with COE "Gastaut type" and 3 with the photosensitive variant. Results showed isolated deficits. The mean performance in the patients group was significantly lower than in the control group in 6 out of 12 neuropsychological measures, but no difference was found between the patient irrespectively of the syndrome diagnosed (Hande Sart *et al.*, 2006). Curiously, in a recent review on the spectrum of idiopathic focal epilepsies including the occipital epilepsies and their natural history, no mention on the evolution of the Gastaut type is made (Gobbi *et al.*, 2006).

Our group described the first 2 cases with COE "Gastaut type" presenting atypical evolutions. One of them was a patient followed-up in the group of Thierry Deonna in Switzerland. These patients had severe cognitive deterioration associated with continuous spike waves during slow-wave sleep (See Chapter 10). Our case had a good response to intravenous gamma-globulin with excellent evolution on cognitive abilities, and the other child did not have any response to AEDs nor to intravenous gammaglobulin and severe cognitive impairment persisted (Fejerman *et al.*, 1991; Tenembaum *et al.*, 1997). These atypical evolutions in patients with COE "Gastaut type" are similar to atypical evolutions in patients with Rolandic epilepsy and Panayiotopoulos syndrome (Fejerman *et al.*, 2000; Caraballo *et al.*, 2001).

Data about our present series of cases

Number of patients and gender

Between February 1990 and February 2004, 29 patients (15 girls and 14 boys) met the inclusion criteria of COE "Gastaut type"; they have been followed up to the present time. Patients presented already in previous reports are included (Caraballo *et al.*, 1997, 2004b).

Age at onset

Age at first afebrile seizure ranged from 4 to 16 years, with a mean age of 8.5 and a median of 8 years.

Personal and family history of febrile seizures, epilepsy, or migraine

A family history of epilepsy was found in 6 cases (21%). Details about the type of epileptic syndromes in close relatives are lacking. Febrile seizures were reported in 6 (21%) and migraine in 3 (10.5%). Four patients (13.5%) had had febrile seizures and 2 migraine (7%).

Clinical features

Elementary visual hallucinations occurred as an initial seizure symptom in 24 patients (82.5%). Ictal elementary visual hallucinations consisted of small multicoloured circular patterns that often appear in the periphery of a visual field, frequently moving horizontally towards the other side.

Complex visual hallucinations occurred in two patients (7%) and were characterized by the appearance of figures with the same location and movement sequence as in elementary visual hallucinations.

Blindness and/or blurring of vision occurred in 14 patients (51.5%), and were the only clinical manifestations in five patients. Post-ictal blindness and hemianopsia occurred in six patients (21%). Fifteen patients (62.5%) had deviation of the eyes associated with ipsilateral turning of the head, occurring after the visual hallucinations. Hemiconvulsions, secondarily GTCS and complex focal seizures occurred in 13 (44%), 6 (21%) and 4 (13%), respectively. Migraine manifestations were present in 13 patients (44%).

According to parent reports, the duration of seizures was brief, less than 1-2 minutes, but in nine cases the duration of the seizures was 10-15 minutes.

All 29 children had seizures when awake, but nine (34.5%) also had seizures during sleep.

Five patients had many seizures per week, 10 had many seizures per month, 10 had seizures every 1-5 months, and 4 had seizures every 6 or more months.

EEG features

The EEG showed occipital paroxysms, which occurred when the eyes were closed and attenuate when the eyes were opened in all patients. EEGs with occipital paroxysms during sleep also occurred in all cases. Occipital paroxysms were bilateral in 18 patients (62%) and unilateral in the other 11 (38%). Eight patients (24%) had centrotemporal spikes as well, and four (13%) had generalized spike-waves discharges. Intermittent photic stimulation was positive in five patients. Ictal EEG recording in one patient showed left occipital spikes rapidly followed by rhythmic bilateral spikes.

Treatment

Antiepileptic treatment was started in all patients, with single drugs, such as valproic acid (13 patients), carbamazepine (5 patients), ox-carbazepine (3 patients) and with multiple antiepileptic drugs (valproic acid and clobazan) (5 patients).

Evolution

In approximately 80% of the patients, seizures remitted within 2 to 7 years (mean: 4 years) after onset, despite persistent EEG abnormalities in 10 (50%) of 20 patients. Antiepileptic treatment was discontinued after 2 or 4 years of treatment in 16 patients (55%) who remained seizure free during 3 to 10 years of follow-up. Three patients (10.5%) continued having frequent seizures and 2 patients (7%) presented infrequent seizures.

One case presented an atypical evolution. This patient had severe cognitive deterioration associated with continuous spike waves during slow-wave sleep and had a good response to intravenous gamma-globulin with excellent evolution on cognitive abilities.

Typical absences appeared at the same time as visual seizures in two patients, and after one year in three patients. All patients had occipital paroxysms and 3 Hz generalized spike-wave discharges on the EEG. One of them had ictal events that were characterized by visual symptoms followed by typical absences.

References

- Andermann E, Andermann F. Migraine-Epilepsy relationships: epidemiological and genetic aspects. In: Andermann F, Lugaresi E (Eds). *Migraine and Epilepsy*. Boston: Butterworths, 1987: 281-92.

- Andermann F, Lugaresi E (Eds). *Migraine and Epilepsy*. Boston: Butterworths, 1987.

- Andermann F. Occipital epileptic abnormalities in mitochondrial disorders. In: Anderman F, Beaumanoir A, Mira L, et al. (Eds). Occipital seizures and epilepsies in children. London: John Libbey, 1993: 111-20.

- Andermann F, Zikfin B. The benign occipital epilepsies of childhood: an overview of the idiopathic syndromes and of the relationship to migraine. *Epilepsia* 1998; 39 (Suppl 4): S9-S23.

- Andermann F. Migraine and the benign partial epilepsies of childhood evidence for an association. *Epileptic Disorders* 2000; 2 (Suppl 1): S37-S39.

- Arzimanoglou A, Aicardi J. The epilepsy of Sturge-Weber syndrome: clinical features and treatment in 23 patients. *Acta Neurol Scand* 1993; Suppl; 140: 18-22.

- Arroyo HA, De Rosa S, Ruggieri V, De Dávila M, Fejerman N and the Argentinean Epilepsy and celiac disease group. "Epilepsy, occipital calcifications and oligosymptomatic celiac disease in childhood". *J Child Neurol* 2002; 17 (11): 800-6.

- Arroyo HA, Gañez L, Fejerman N. Encefalopatía posterior reversible en la infancia. *Rev Neurol* (Barc) 2003; 37 (6): 506-10.

- Aso K, Watanabe K, Negoro T, *et al*. Visual seizures in children. *Epilepsy Res* 1987; 1: 246-53.

- Bakshi R, Bates VE, Mechtler LL, *et al*. Occipital lobe seizures as the major clinical manifestation of reversible posterior leukoencephalopathy syndrome: magnetic resonance imaging findings. *Epilepsia* 1998; 39 (3): 295-9.

- Beaumanoir A. Infantile epilepsy with occipital focus and good prognosis. *European Neurology* 1983; 22: 43-52.

- Beaumanoir A. (1993a) Semiology of occipital seizures in infants and children. In: Andermann F, Beaumanoir A, Mira L, Roger J, Tassinari CA (Eds). *Occipital seizures and epilepsy in children*. London: John Libbey, 1993: 71-86.

- Beaumanoir A. (1993b) An EEG contribution to the study of migraine and of the association between migraine and epilepsy in childhood. In: Andermann F, Beaumanoir A, Mira L, Roger J, Tassinari CA (Eds). *Occipital seizures and epilepsy in children*. London: John Libbey, 1993: 101-10.

- Camfield PR, Metrakos K, Anderman F. Basilar migraine, seizures, and severe epileptiform EEG abnormalities. *Neurology* 1978; 28: 584-8.

- Caraballo RH, Cersósimo RO, Medina C, Tenembaum S, Fejerman N. Epilepsias parciales idiopáticas con paroxismos occipitales. *Rev Neurol* (Barc) 1997; 25: 1052-8.

- Caraballo R, Cersósimo R, Fejerman N. Idiopathic partial epilepsies with Rolandic and occipital spikes appearing in the same children. *J Epilepsy* 1998; 11: 261-4.

- Caraballo R, Cersósimo R, Medina C, Fejerman N. Panayiotopoulos-type benign childhood occipital epilepsy. A prospective study. *Neurology* 2000; 55: 1096-100.

- Caraballo RH, Astorino F, Cersósimo RO, Soprano AM, Fejerman N. Atypical evolution in childhood epilepsy with occipital paroxysms (Panayiotopoulos type). *Epileptic Disord* 2001; 3: 157-62.

- Caraballo R, Sakr D, Mozzi M, *et al.* (2004a) Symptomatic occipital lobe epilepsy following neonatal hypoglicemia. *Pediatr Neurol* 2004; 31: 24-9.

- Caraballo RH, Sologuestua A, Granana N, *et al.* (2004b) Idiopathic occipital and absence epilepsies appearing in the same children. *Pediatr Neurol* 2004; 30: 24-8.

- Caraballo R, Cersósimo R, Fejerman N. Late-onset, "Gastaut type", childhood occipital epilepsy: an unusual evolution. *Epileptic Disorders* 2005; 7: 341-6.

- Caraballo R, Cersósimo R, Fejerman N. Panayiotopoulos syndrome: a prospective study of 192 patients. *Epilepsia* 2007; In Press.

- Chahine LM, Mikati MA. Benign pediatric localization-related epilepsies Part II. Syndromes in childhood. *Epileptic Disord* 2006; 8 (4): 243-58.

- Commission on Classification and Terminology of the International League Against epilepsy. Proposal for Revised Classification of Epilepsy and Epileptic Syndromes. *Epilepsia* 1989; 30: 389-99.

- Cooper GW, Lee SI. Reactive occipital epileptiform activity: is it benign? *Epilepsia* 1991; 32 (1): 63-8.

- Covanis A, Ferrie CD, Koutroumanidis M, Oguni H, Panayiotopoulos K. Panayiotopoulos syndrome and Gastaut type idiopathic childhood occipital epilepsy. In: Roger J, Bureau M, Dravet Ch, Genton P, Tassinari CA, Wolf P (Eds). *Epileptic syndromes in Infancy, childhood and adolescence* (4th Ed.). Montrouge: John Libbey, 2005: 227-53.

- De Romanis F, Buzzi MG, Assenza S, Brusa L, Cerbo R. Basilar migraine with electroencephalographic findings of occipital spike-wave complexes: a long-term study in seven children. *Cephalalgia* 1993; 13: 192-6.

- Di Blasi M, Arroyo HA, Fejerman N. Cefaleas y migrañas. In: Fejerman N, Fernandez Alvares E (Eds). *Neurología Pediátrica* (3rd Ed.). Buenos Aires: Editorial Panamericana, 2007: 675-90.

- Dravet CH, Bureau M, Oguni H, Fukuyama Y, Cokar O. Severe myoclonic epilepsy in infancy (Dravet syndrome). In: Roger J, Bureau M, Dravet CH, Genton P, Tassinari C, Wolf P (Eds). *Epileptic syndromes in infancy, childhood and adolescence* (4th Ed.). Montrouge: John Libbey, 2005: 89-114.

- Engel J. A proposed diagnostic scheme for people with epileptic seizures and with epilepsy: report of the ILAE Task Force on Classification and Terminology. *Epilepsia* 2001; 42: 796-803.

- Engel J. Report of the ILAE Classification Core Group. *Epilepsia* 2006; 47 (9): 1558-68.

- Fejerman N, Tenembaum S, Medina C, Caraballo R, Soprano AM. Continuous spike-waves during slow-wave sleep and awake in a case of childhood epilepsy with occipital paroxysms. *Epilepsia* 1991; 32: 16 (abstract).

- Fejerman N. Evoluciones atípicas de las epilepsias parciales benignas en los niños. *Rev Neurol* (Barc) 1996; 24 (135): 1415-20.

- Fejerman N, Caraballo R, Tenembaum S. Atypical evolutions of benign localization-related epilepsies in children: Are they Predictable? *Epilepsia* 2000; 41: 380-90.

- Fejerman N. Epilepsias focales benignas del lactante, niño y adolescente. *Rev Neurol* (Barc) 2002; 34: 7-18.

Late-onset childhood occipital epilepsy (Gastaut type)

- Gastaut H. Évidences électrographiques d'un mécanisme sous-cortical dans certaines épilepsies partielles. La signification clinique des "secteurs aréo-thalamiques". *Rev Neurol* (Paris) 1950; 83: 396-401.

- Gastaut H. A new type of epilepsy: Benign partial epilepsy of childhood with occipital spikes-waves. *Clin Electroencephalogr* 1982; 13: 13-22.

- Gastaut H. Benign epilepsy of childhood with occipital paroxysms. In: Roger J, Dravet CH, Bureau M, Dreiffus FE, Wolf P (Eds). *Epileptic syndromes in infancy, childhood and adolescence.* London: John Libbey, 1985: 150-70.

- Gastaut H, Zifkin BG. Benign epilepsy of childhood with occipital spike and wave complexes. In: Andermann F, Lugaresi E (Eds). *Migraine and epilepsy.* Boston, MA: Butterworths, 1987: 47-81.

- Gastaut H, Roger J, Bureau M. Benign epilepsy of childhood with occipital paroxysms Up-date. In: Roger J, Bureau M, Dravet CH, Dreiffus FE, Perret A, Wolf P (Eds). *Epileptic syndromes in infancy, childhood and adolescence.* London: John Libbey, 1992: 201-17.

- Genton P, Guerrini R. Idiopathic localization-related epilepsies: the non-rolandic types. In: Wolf P (Ed). *Epileptic seizures and syndromes.* London: John Libbey, 1994: 241-56.

- Genton PP, Malafosse A, Moulard B, *et al.* Progressive myoclonus epilepsies. In: Roger J, Bureau M, Dravet CH, Genton P, Tassinari C, Wolf P. *Epileptic syndromes in infancy, childhood and adolescence* (4th ed.). Montrouge: John Libbey, 2005: 441-66.

- Gibbs FA, Gibbs EL. *Atlas of Electroencephalographia, Vol 2 Epilepsy (2) Reading.* MA: Addison-Wesley, 1952: 214-90.

- Gobbi G, Andermann F, Naccarato S, Banchini G (Eds). *Epilepsy and other neurological disorders in coeliac disease.* London: John Libbey, 1997.

- Gobbi G, Guerrini R. Childhood epilepsy with occipital spikes and other benign localization-related epilepsies. In: Engel J, Pedley T (Eds). *Epilepsy: a comprehensive textbook.* Philadelphia: Lippincott-Raven, 1997: 2315-26.

- Gobbi G, Boni A, Filippini M. The spectrum of idiopathic Rolandic epilepsy syndromes and idiopathic occipital epilepsies: from the benign to the disabling. *Epilepsia* 2006; 47 (Suppl 2): 62-6.

- Guerrini R, Dravet C, Genton P, *et al.* Idiopathic photosensitive occipital lobe epilepsy. *Epilepsia* 1995; 36: 883-91.

- Guerrini R, Bonanni P, Parmeggiani L, Belmonte A. Adolescent onset of idiopathic photosensitive occipital epilepsy after remission of benign rolandic epilepsy. *Epilepsia* 1997; 38: 777-81.

- Guerrini R, Bonanni P, Parmeggiani A. Idiopathic photosensitive occipital lobe epilepsy. In: Gilman S (Ed). *Medlink Neurology.* San Diego SA: Arbor Publishing, 2005.

- Gülgönen S, Demirbilek V, Korkmaz B, Dervent A, Townes BD. Neuropsychological functions in idiopathic occipital lobe epilepsy. *Epilepsia* 2000; 41: 405-11.

- Hande Sart Z, Demirbilek V, Korkmaz B, *et al.* The consequences of idiopathic partial epilepsies in relation to neuropsychological functioning: a closer look at the associated mathematical disability. *Epileptic Disorders* 2006; 8 (1): 24-31.

- Kellaway P. The incidence, significance and natural history of spike foci in children. In: Henry CE (Ed). *Current clinical neurophysiology. Update on EEG and Evoked Potentials.* New York: Elsevier/New Holland, 1980: 151-75.

- Kivity S, Ephraim T, Weitz R, Tamir A. Childhood epilepsy with occipital paroxysms: Clinical variants in 134 patients. *Epilepsia* 2000; 41: 1522-3.

- Labate A, Gambardella A, Messina D, *et al.* Silent celiac disease in patients with childhood localization related epilepsies. *Epilepsia* 2001; 42 (9): 1153-5.

- Maher J, Ronen GM, Ogunyemi AO, Goulden KJ. Occipital paroxysmal discharges suppressed by eye opening: variability in clinical and seizure manifestations in childhood. *Epilepsia* 1995; 36: 52-7.

- Marks DA, Ehrenberg BL. Migraine-related seizures in adults with epilepsy, with EEG correlation. *Neurology* 1993; 43 (12): 2476-83.

- Milligan TA, Bromfield E. A case of "migralepsy". *Epilepsia* 2005; 46 (Suppl 10): 2-6.

- Montagna P, Sacquegna T, Martinelli P, *et al*. Mitochondrial abnormalities in migraine. Preliminary findings. *Headache* 1988; 28 (7): 477-80.

- Nagendran K, Prior PF, Rossiter MA. Benign occipital epilepsy of childhood: a family study. *J Roy Soc Med* 1989; 82: 684-5.

- Newton R, Aicardi J. Clinical findings in children with occipital spike-wave complexes suppressed by eye-opening. *Neurology* 1983; 33 (11): 1526-9.

- Oguni H, Hayashi K, Imai K, *et al*. (1999a) Study on the early-onset variant of benign childhood epilepsy with occipital paroxysms otherwise described as early-onset benign occipital seizures susceptibility syndrome. *Epilepsia* 1999; 40: 1020-30.

- Oguni H, Hayashi K, Osawa M. (1999b) Migration of epileptic foci in children. *Adv Neurol* 1999; 81: 131-43.

- Ottman R, Lipton RB. Is the comorbidity of epilepsy and migraine due to a shared genetic susceptibility? *Neurology* 1996; 47 (4): 918-24.

- Panayiotopoulos CP. Basilar migraine? Seizures, and severe epileptic EEG abnormalities. *Neurology* 1980; 30: 1122-5.

- Panayiotopoulos CP. Inhibitory effect of central vision on occipital lobe seizures. *Neurology* 1981; 31: 1330-3.

- Panayiotopoulos CP. Difficulties in differentiating migraine and epilepsy based on clinical and EEG findings. In: Andermann F, Lugaresi E (Eds). *Migraine and epilepsy*. London: Butterworths, 1987: 31-46.

- Panayiotopoulos CP. (1999a) *Benign childhood partial seizures and related epileptic syndromes*. London: John Libbey, 1999.

- Panayitopoulos CP. (1999b) Elementary visual hallucinations, blindness, and headache in idiopathic occipital epilepsy: differentiation from migraine. *J Neurol Neurosurg Psychiatry* 1999; 66: 536-40.

- Panayiotopoulos CP. (1999c) Visual phenomena and headache in occipital epilepsy: a review, a systematic study and differentiation from migraine. *Epileptic Disorders* 1999; 1: 205-16.

- Panayiotopoulos CP. (2005a) Benign childhood focal seizures and related epileptic syndromes. In: Panayiotopoulos CP (Ed). *The epilepsies; seizures, syndromes and management*. Oxford: Bladon Medical Publishing, 2005: 223-69.

- Panayiotopoulos CP. (2005b) Idiopathic photosensitive occipital epilepsy. In: Panayiotopoulos CP (Ed). *The epilepsies; seizures, syndromes and management*. Oxford: Bladon Medical Publishing, 2005: 469-74.

- Panayiotopoulos CP. "Migralepsy" and the significance of differentiating occipital seizures from migraine. *Epilepsia* 2006; 47 (4): 806-8.

- Parra J. Controversies and problems in the diagnosis of benign occipital epilepsies in infancy, childhood and adolescence. *Rev Neurol* 2006; 10 (43) (suppl 1): S51-S56.

- Sahar E, Barak S. Favorable outcome of epileptic blindness in children. *Journal of Child Neurology* 2003; 18 (1): 12-6.

- Tassinari CA, Rubboli G, Pasmati R, *et al*. Television-induced epilepsy with occipital seizures: a variety of idiopathic partial occipital epilepsy. In: Beaumanoir A, Gastaut H, Naquet R (Eds). *Reflex seizures and reflex epilepsies*. Geneva: Éditions Médecine & Hygiène, 1989: 241-3.

- Tenembaum S, Deonna TW, Fejerman N, Medina C, Ingvar-Maeder M, Gubser-Mercati D. Continuous spike-waves and dementia in childhood epilepsy with occipital paroxysms. *J Epilepsy* 1997; 10: 139-45.

- Terasaki T, Yamatogi Y, Ohtahara S. Electroclinical delineation of occipital lobe epilepsies in childhood. In: Andermann F, Lugaresi E (Eds). *Migraine and epilepsy*. Boston: Butterworths, 1987: 125-37.

- Terzano MG, Manzoni GC, Parrino L. Benign epilepsy with occipital paroxysms and migraine: the question of intercalated attacks. In: Andermann F, Lugaresi E (Eds). *Migraine and epilepsy*. Boston: Butterworths, 1987: 83-96.

- Thomas P, Arzimanoglou A, Aicardi J. Benign idiopathic occipital epilepsy: report of a case of the late (Gastaut type). *Epileptic Disorders* 2003; 5: 57-9.

- Watanabe K. Benign partial epilepsies. In: Wallace SJ, Farrell K (Eds). *Epilepsy in children*. London: Arnold, 2004: 199-220.

- Yamane LE, Montenegro MA, Guerreiro MM. Comorbidity headache and epilepsy in childhood. *Neuropediatrics* 2004; 35 (2): 99-102.

- Zakaria A, Lalani I, Belorgey L, Foreman PL. Focal occipital seizures with cerebral polyopia. *Epileptic disorders* 2006; 8 (4): 295-7.

Are there other types of benign focal epilepsies in childhood?

Bernardo Dalla Bernardina, Elena Fontana, Francesca Darra
Verona, Italy

Following the recognition of benign epilepsy with centrotemporal spikes (BECTS) (Nayrac & Beaussart, 1958), many efforts have been done to find other idiopathic benign focal epileptic syndromes. Two of them, "benign infantile seizures" and "early onset benign childhood occipital epilepsy (Panayiotopoulos syndrome PS)" have been recognized by the ILAE Classification Core Group (Engel, 2006). However others, extensively described in this book, such as "benign infantile focal epilepsy with midline spikes and waves during sleep" and "benign focal seizures in adolescence" have not been considered by the ILAE Classification Core Group, because their electroclinical features are not sufficiently suggestive *per se* to be considered a well defined and recognizable syndrome (Engel, 2006).

Other forms, that we will briefly describe in this chapter, have been proposed during the past years in literature, but have not received enough significant confirming contributions.

Benign frontal lobe epilepsy of childhood

This form has been proposed by Beaumanoir and Nahory (1983) and indirectly confirmed only by Loiseau *et al.* (1991) who recognized the existence of this entity in approximately 11% of all personal cases of idiopathic focal epilepsies. The seizures characterizing this form are reported as infrequent and variable in type (absence-like, versive, secondarily generalized during sleep). The EEG interictal pattern varies and is characterized in some cases by focal paroxysms similar to those observed in BECTS and in others only by focal slow activity. The ictal patterns are shifting frontal discharges.

Considering the small population reported by Beaumanoir and Nahory (1983) the electroclinical picture is much too heterogeneous to realize a well defined and recognizable syndrome. No other authors have ever confirmed the existence of a similar electroclinical picture.

Probably as just suggested by Genton and Guerrini (1994) the population described by Beaumanoir and Nahory (1983) includes both particular forms of BECTS and probably forms of symptomatic frontal lobe epilepsies with a mild evolution.

Benign partial epilepsy with extreme somatosensory evoked potentials

It has been described as a benign partial epilepsy characterized by a four stage electroclinical stereotyped evolution (De Marco & Tassinari, 1981; Tassinari & De Marco, 1992).

In the first stage the only abnormal EEG feature is the presence of extreme somatosensory evoked potentials (ESEPs). Such ESEPs constitutes the only EEG finding in patients without seizures or other neurological impairment.

In the second stage spontaneous focal EEG abnormalities appear during sleep.

In the third stage, spontaneous focal abnormalities appear when the subject is awake, generally involving the same regions where the ESEPs were first observed and with a similar morphology.

The fourth stage is characterized by the appearance of electroclinical seizures.

This epilepsy is therefore characterized by the appearance of partial motor seizures with head version in a neurologically normal child showing on the EEG ESEPs evoked by tapping of feet or fingers. The seizures appear between 4 and 8 years, within 5 months and 2 years after ESEPs appearance. They are generally rare but in some cases can be grouped in status. ESEPs and spontaneous associated paroxysmal abnormalities are quite similar to typical centrotemporal spikes even if preferentially located on parietal and parasagittal regions. The seizures usually persist for about 1 year and then subside. In the Tassinari and De Marco population (1992) the fits disappeared before 9 years of age and did not recur during the follow-up period, which lasted an average of 8 years. The spontaneous interictal focal discharges, as well as the ESEPs, sometimes persisted for years after the seizures had stopped. In some patients they disappeared within 1-3 years after seizures stop, and ESEPs were no longer observed.

The evolution of ESEPs is invariably favourable both for epilepsy and mental outcome.

According to Tassinari and De Marco (1992) this form deserves to be distinguished from BECTS by the following clinical aspects:

1) Although in both syndromes the seizures are mainly motor, in patients with ESEPs they usually do not affect the facial muscles, and occur predominantly during day time.

2) Seizures accompanied by ESEPs persist for about 1 year, whereas the fits of BECT may persist for several years.

3) In EEG recordings, the topography of spikes in the latter syndrome is mainly rolandic or mid-temporal, while in cases of ESEPs the spikes are mostly parietal and parasagittal.

The authors conclude that ESEPs is a particular form of benign epilepsy, which expresses primarily with partial motor seizures preceded by ESEPs and associated with focal EEG abnormalities involving mainly the parietal regions.

The phenomenon of ESEPs is frequently observed in other idiopathic benign focal epilepsies (Dalla Bernardina et al., 1990, 1991; Tassinari et al., 1988) and consequently cannot be considered a diagnostic parameter on its own.

In fact the electroclinical features of this entity are so that it can be probably considered as an equally benign variant of BECTS rather than a separate syndrome.

Benign partial epilepsy with affective symptoms ("benign psychomotor epilepsy")

Following the first description of Dalla Bernardina et al. (1980, 1992b) only few other similar observations have been reported (Dulac & Arthuis, 1980; Wakai et al., 1994). It is characterized by the appearance, in a neurologically normal child, of partial complex seizures of which the predominant symptom is a sudden fright or terror expressed by screaming, calling the mother with attempt to cling to her or to anyone nearby. Loss of contact and autonomic manifestations are constantly associated, while tonic or clonic motor manifestations are rare. Lasting from one to a few minutes the seizures appear in clusters recurring several times a day during wakefulness and sleep without any significant postictal disturbance. The most frequent EEG interictal abnormalities are characterized by paroxysms CTS-like involving the fronto-temporal or parieto-temporal areas of one or both hemispheres. Seizure discharges are, in the majority of the cases, located in the fronto-temporal, centrotemporal or parietal areas, whereas in some instances they are more diffuse from the onset. No polymorphic seizures, both during wakefulness and sleep, or significant post-ictal disturbances are observed. The seizures are promptly controlled by treatment and the long-term evolution is invariably favourable. Analysing the follow-up of 21 subjects initially described in 1980 (Dalla Bernardina et al., 1980, 1992b) we observed that 16/21 aged between 15 and 28 years were treatment and seizure free, while 5/16 aged over 18 years were suffering from more or less frequent seizures in spite of treatment. The electroclinical distinctive findings of these 5 patients were:

– The ictal and clinical findings in 4 consisted in seizures characterized at onset by more or less important and variable "subjective" symptoms described by the patients at the end of the seizure; in 1 case seizures were characterized by a significant unilateral deficit following the seizure stopping for several minutes. In one of these the seizures were characterized by a rotatory component too.
– The interictal EEG in four subjects never looked like the typical rolandic spikes paroxysmal abnormalities both during wake and sleep. In one case typical right rolandic spikes were associated with a focus of slow waves on the controlateral parietal region and with brief bursts of generalized spikes and waves elicited by ILS.
– The ictal EEG in three cases was characterized by discharges at onset of brief focal "flattening" of the EEG activity.

Following these observations the Authors outlined that the diagnosis of benign psychomotor epilepsy (BPE) is possible only when no other symptoms, other than affective ones, are present during seizures, and when interictal abnormalities like rolandic spikes are present, in absence of slow abnormalities and of any polymorphism of the ictal discharge. They concluded that BPE does not constitute an independent form of idiopathic partial epilepsy but probably only a relatively rare variant of BECTS.

In fact benign partial epilepsy with affective symptoms can constitute a relatively rare variant of BECTS or a benign form of limbic epilepsy. It is possible to hypothesize the existence, during two periods of life, infancy (Capovilla and Vigevano, 2001) and preschool age (Dalla Bernardina et al., 1992b), of children suffering from an age dependent epilepsy characterized by the abrupt appearance and recurrence of partial complex seizures, strongly suggesting a temporal lobe involvement with a significant or predominant affective ictal component of idiopathic nature: this epilepsy recovers spontaneously and is therefore truly benign (Dalla Bernardina et al., 2001).

Following these brief descriptions it appears that none of the above mentioned electroclinical entities can be considered as a well defined separate syndrome and probably at present there are no well defined and recognizable syndromes other than those accepted by the ILAE Classification Core Group (Engel, 2006). Considering these accepted syndromes we do not agree with the diagnostic scheme recently proposed by Chahine and Mikati (2006) that claims that until the patient is followed-up and epilepsy remits the diagnosis of a benign syndrome is only presumptive.

If the term "benign" is reserved to define age-dependent idiopathic epilepsies of which diagnosis allows the prediction of a likely spontaneous recovery, their clinical and EEG findings must be well defined, coherent and recognizable within a brief-medium time from seizure onset.

To accept the validity for all cases of this diagnostic scheme that Chahine and Mikati (2006) have taken from Okumura et al. (2000, 2006), means to exclude the existence of syndromes for which it is possible to do a correct diagnosis with a foreseeable benign prognosis briefly after seizure onset.

On the other hand it is most probable that, as outlined previously by some Authors (Dalla Bernardina et al., 1985, 1992b), there are a lot of cases of benign idiopathic focal epilepsy that do not show all the electroclinical characteristics that allow diagnostic arrangement in one of the recognised syndromes. For this reason it is probably interesting to outline, as previously attempted by some Authors (Roger et al., 1981, 1990; Roger & Bureau, 1983, 1987; Dalla Bernardina et al., 1985, 1992a, 1992b, 1993, 2002, 2005; Lerman & Kivity, 1991; Genton & Guerrini, 1994), the clinical and EEG findings compatible or incompatible with a diagnostic hypothesis of benign idiopathic focal epilepsy (BIFE) in children.

The compatible and incompatible clinical and EEG findings *(Table I)* are:
– Absence of neurological deficit;
– Absence of intellectual and neuropsychological deficit. A correct diagnostic approach needs a neuropsychological assessment at onset;
– Moreover in any case with anamnestic or clinical doubtful findings a neuroradiological investigation by MRI, in order to exclude possible structured abnormality, is necessary too;
– Obviously in subjects with, for example, a fixed neurological or intellectual deficit the diagnosis of BECTS must not be excluded "a priori" as suggested by Herranz (2002) but as just previously stressed (Dalla Bernardina et al., 2005) it must be considered presumptive. In fact the incorrect

Are there other types of benign focal epilepsies in childhood?

Table I. Clinical and EEG features compatible or incompatible with benign idiopathic focal epilepsy in children

COMPATIBLE	INCOMPATIBLE
Clinical features – Normal development – Normal neurological picture – Normal cognitive and neuropsychological picture – Stereotyped seizures while awake and during sleep – Seizures variable in duration and frequency	**Clinical features** – Development disorder – Neurological deficit – Cognitive and neuropsychological impairment – Polymorphous seizures – Peculiar seizures like tonic, partial complex motor, gelastic, "rotatory", etc. – Very brief seizures – Seizures progressively increasing in frequency
EEG features – Normal background activity while awake and during sleep – Interictal paroxysm as CT-like spikes or focal SW not morphologically modified during sleep	**EEG features** – Background activity abnormalities – Unusual activities – Slow focal paroxysms – Fast spikes or polyspikes – Rhythmic spikes in trains – Ictal flattening – Fast discharges in bursts

habit to include in benign syndromes cases with atypical clinical manifestations like development delay (Wirrel *et al.*, 1995) or underlying neuropsychological impairment (Hahn *et al.*, 2001; Vinayan *et al.*, 2005), has induced, in clinical practice and literature, a significant ambiguity in diagnostic criteria (Bouma *et al.*, 1997) and prognosis of benign idiopathic focal epilepsies;

– Familial antecedents for epilepsy: particularly if characterized by a benign evolution and recovery of seizures before puberty can be helpful to diagnosis;

– Seizures variable in symptomatology but not clinically and electrically truly polymorphous (Dalla Bernardina *et al.*, 1992a, 2002, 2005; Roger & Bureau, 1987). Moreover some kind of seizures like those reported in *Table I* are incompatible with the diagnostic hypothesis of a benign form because never reported in recognized benign syndromes;

– Seizures variable in duration lasting from 1 to several minutes often realizing a long-lasting status; vice versa very brief seizures lasting only a few seconds are to be considered an incompatible element (Dalla Bernardina *et al.*, 1993);

– Seizures variable in frequency (very rare or very frequent) at onset and throughout the evolution. While a stormy onset with a long-lasting seizure or with several a day seizures in clusters is possible in benign forms, a progressive increasing in frequency of seizure recurrence throughout evolution is unlikely;

– EEG background activity must be normal, well organized while awake and during sleep without focal slowing neither unusual activities. The presence of unusual activities even coexisting with interictal paroxysms typically evoking a diagnosis of benign form must induce to retain doubtful a similar diagnosis (Darra *et al.*, 1996);

– Interictal paroxysms can be absent, when present they have centrotemporal spikes-like or focal spike-wave-like morphology, often involving independently the same regions of both hemispheres;

– They can increase in frequency and amplitude during sleep without any significant change in morphology;

– A significant morphological modification during sleep with appearance of fast spikes or polyspikes, is incompatible with a diagnosis of a benign form, analogously incompatible is the following in trains of paroxysms with pseudorhythmic trend;
– Finally as interictal paroxysms can be multifocal, the lateralizing electroclinical ictal symptoms can vary in the same child from one seizure to the next evoking the possible independent involvement of homologous lobes. This lobar involvement appears peculiarly common to all known idiopathic benign focal epilepsies of infancy and childhood. As just outlined (Dalla Bernardina *et al.*, 2005) all these epilepsies represent a peculiar model of focal epilepsy for which the term "focal" rather than referring to a focal cortical epileptogenic area, expresses an age-dependent predisposition to generate epileptic seizures by a definite functional area. This is particularly interesting in order to better study the genetic-epileptogenetic mechanisms supporting these epilepsies and discuss their nosological plan. The frequent bilateral asynchronous expression of seizures and of interictal paroxysms, the tendency to migrate with age from lobe to lobe mostly anteriorly of the interictal paroxysms (Dalla Bernardina *et al.*, 2002, 2005) and the possible occurrence of two different benign forms in the same child at different ages (Fejerman *et al.*, this book), appear in agreement with this hypothesis. A further evidence is given by the "migration" on the EEG of the triggering areas of the ESEPs evoked by tapping of feet or fingers documented by Tassinari *et al.* (1988) (Dalla Bernardina *et al.*, 1990). Finally the tendency to secondary bisynchronism of paroxysms (CSWS) observed in some children, could be triggered too by the contextual age-dependent predisposition to generate epileptic discharges by a functional bilateral area.

While these electroclinical parameters can be helpful in the diagnostic approach, the response to treatment cannot be considered a diagnostic criteria because in some cases, surely benign, seizures can persist until the spontaneous recovery in spite of treatment (Lerman & Kivity, 1975; Loiseau *et al.*, 1992; Dalla Bernardina *et al.*, 1992a, 2002).

Following the above mentioned electroclinical findings it is possible to recognize the cases, that even if without the typical characteristics of one of the forms recognized by the ILAE Classification Core Group (Engel, 2006), could however have a possible or probable idiopathic benign focal epilepsy.

Accepting the idea that there are idiopathic benign focal epilepsies of infancy and childhood other than those "includable" in the recognized forms, in order to recognize them, but keeping them separate to avoid to "pollute" the nosological boundaries of the well defined recognized syndromes, in clinical practice we can use the diagnostic algorithm proposed by Chahine and Mikati (2006) modified as in *Figure 1*.

Obviously any migration from possible to probable and to definite implies a length of time from onset necessary to collect all electroclinical elements that is variable according to type of epilepsy.

As stressed above the response to AED therapy cannot be considered a diagnostic point because in some benign forms the seizures can recur in spite of treatment and, on the other hand, a very good response can be observed in some symptomatic cases.

Are there other types of benign focal epilepsies in childhood?

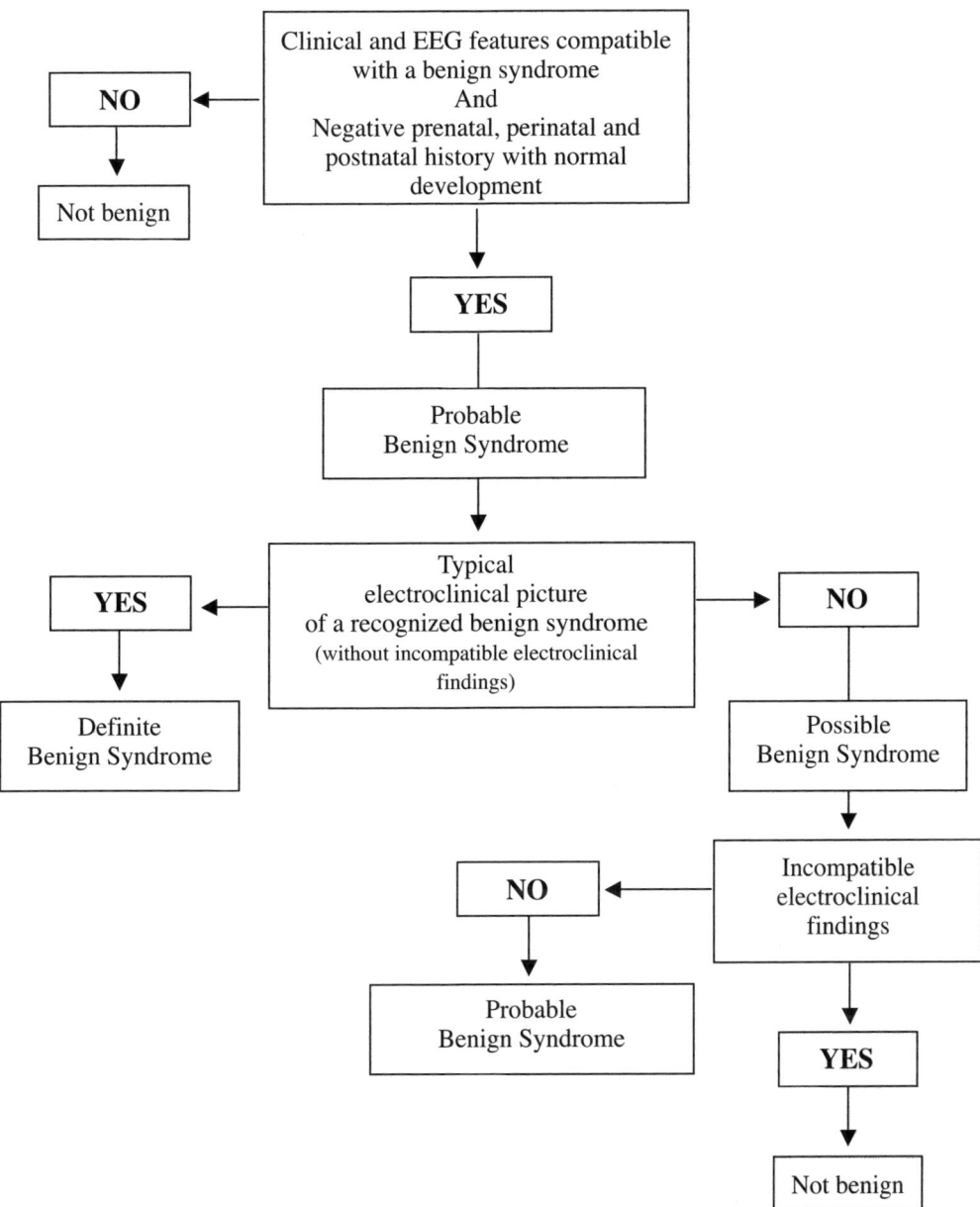

Figure 1. Diagnostic algorithm of benign focal epilepsies in children.

Finally the definite diagnosis of benign syndrome cannot be made only at the end of the evolution for several reasons. Firstly the spontaneous recovery of the seizures is not itself a subsequent demonstration of the idiopathic benign nature of epilepsy. Second we cannot propose to accept in an International Classification a syndromic entity for which diagnosis can be done only after recovery. Last but not least is that the early recognition of benignity of an epilepsy represents a very important issue from a prognostic point of view.

In conclusion in our opinion it could be interesting to continue the effort to better identify the electroclinical findings allowing the recognition of cases that, even if not presenting the typical features of the recognized forms, could however behave as a benign epilepsy avoiding therefore to remain unrecognized or be forcedly included in a recognized form "polluting" unavoidably its nosological boundaries.

An interesting final consideration is the following: in spite of the ILAE Classification Core Group's (Engel, 2006) opinion there is in clinical practice the increasing evidence of the need, other than of the "drawer" for probably symptomatic, even of the "drawer" for "probably idiopathic".

References

- Beaumanoir A, Nahory A. Les epilepsies bénignes partielles: 11 cas d'épilepsie partielle frontale à évolution favorable. *Rev EEG Neurophysiol* 1983 ; 13: 207-11.

- Bouma PA, Bovenkerk AC, Westendorp RG, Brouwer OF. The course of benign partial epilepsy of childhood with centrotemporal spikes: a meta-analysis. *Neurology* 1997; 48: 430-7.

- Capovilla G, Vigevano F. Benign idiopathic partial epilepsies in infancy. *J Child Neurol* 2001; 16: 874-81.

- Chahine LM, Mikati MA. Benign pediatric localization-related epilepsies. Part I. Syndromes in Infancy. *Epil Disord* 2006; 8 (3): 169-83.

- Dalla Bernardina B, Bureau M, Dravet C, Dulac O, Tassinari CA, Roger J. Epilepsie bénigne de l'enfant avec crises à séméiologie affective. *Rev EEG Neurophysiol* 1980 ; 10: 8-18.

- Dalla Bernardina B, Chiamenti C, Capovilla G, Colamaria V. Benign partial epilepsies in childhood. In: Roger J, Dravet C, Bureau M, Dreifuss FE, Wolf P (Eds). *Epileptic syndromes in infancy, childhood and adolescence* (1st ed.). London: John Libbey, 1985: 137-49.

- Dalla Bernardina B, Sgrò V, Fontana E, *et al*. Partial epilepsies in children with rolandic somatosensory evoked spikes (hand tapping): neurophysiological (EEG and SEP) study. *EEG Clin Neurophysiol* 1990; 75: S32.

- Dalla Bernardina B, Sgrò V, Caraballo R, *et al*. Sleep and benign partial epilepsies of childhood: EEG and evoked potentials study. In: Degen R, Rodin EA (Eds). *Epilepsy, sleep and sleep deprivation*. Amsterdam: Elsevier, 1991: 83-96.

- Dalla Bernardina B, Sgrò V, Fontana E, Colamaria V, La Selva L (1992a): Idiopathic partial epilepsies in children. In: Roger J, Bureau M, Dravet C, Dreifuss FE, Perret A, Wolf P (Eds) *Epileptic syndromes in infancy, childhood and adolescence* (2nd ed.). London: John Libbey, 1992: 173-88.

- Dalla Bernardina B, Colamaria V, Chiamenti C, Capovilla G, Trevisan E, Tassinari CA (1992b): Benign partial epilepsy with affective symptoms (benign psychomotor epilepsy). In: Roger J, Bureau M, Dravet C, Dreifuss FE, Perret A, Wolf P (Eds). *Epileptic syndromes in infancy, childhood and adolescence* (2nd ed.). London: John Libbey, 1992: 219-24.

- Dalla Bernardina B, Fontana E, Cappellaro O, *et al*. The partial occipital epilepsies. In: Andermann F, Beaumanoir A, Mira L, Roger J, Tassinari CA (Eds). *Occipital seizures and epilepsies in children*. London: John Libbey, 1993: 173-81.

Are there other types of benign focal epilepsies in childhood?

- Dalla Bernardina B, Darra F, Fontana E, Beaumanoir A. Is there a benign limbic epilepsy in children? In: Avanzini G, Beaumanoir A, Mira L (Eds). *Limbic seizures in children*. London: John Libbey, 2001: 241-7.

- Dalla Bernardina B, Sgrò V, Fejerman N. Epilepsy with centrotemporal spikes and related syndromes. In: Roger J, Bureau M, Dravet C, Genton P, Tassinari CA, Wolf P (Eds). *Epileptic syndromes in infancy, childhood and adolescence* (3rd Ed.). London: John Libbey, 2002: 181-202.

- Dalla Bernardina B, Sgrò V, Fejerman N. Epilepsy with centrotemporal spikes and related syndromes. In: Roger J, Bureau M, Dravet C, Genton P, Tassinari CA, Wolf P (Eds) *Epileptic syndromes in infancy, childhood and adolescence* (4th ed.). Montrouge: John Libbey Eurotext, 2005: 203-25.

- Darra F, Montagnini A, Piardi F, Santorum E, Fenzi V, Dalla Bernardina B. BECT-like epilepsy in subjects with focal gyral anomalies: electroclinical findings for differential diagnosis. *Boll Lega It Epil* 1996; 95/96: 421-2.

- De Marco P, Tassinari CA. Extreme somatosensory evoked potential (ESEP): a EEG sign forecating the possible occurrence of seizures in children. *Epilepsia* 1981; 22: 569-85.

- Dulac O, Arthuis M. Épilepsies psychomotrice bénigne de l'enfant. In: *Journées parisiennes de pédiatrie*. Paris: Flammarion, 1980: 211-20.

- Engel J. Report of the ILAE Classification Core Group. *Epilepsia* 2006; 47 (9): 1558-68.

- Genton P, Guerrini R. idiopathic localization-related epilepsies: the non-rolandic types. In: P Wolf (Ed). *Epileptic seizures and syndromes*. London: John Libbey; 1994: 241-56.

- Hahn A, Pistohl J, Neubauer BA, Stephani U. Atypical "benign" partial epilepsy or pseudo-Lennox syndrome. Part I: Symptomatology and long-term prognosis. *Neuropediatrics* 2001; 32: 1-8.

- Herranz JL. Broad clinical prognostic spectrum of Rolandic epilepsy: agreement, disagreement and open questions. *Rev Neurol* 2002; 35 (1): 79-81.

- Lerman P, Kivity S. Benign focal epilepsy of childhood. A follow-up of 100 recovered patients. *Arch Neurol* 1975; 32: 261-4.

- Lerman P, Kivity S. The benign partial nonrolandic epilepsies. *J Clin Neurophysiol* 1991; 8: 275-87.

- Loiseau P, Duchè B, Loiseau B. Classification of epilepsies and epileptic syndromes in two different samples of patients. *Epilepsia* 1991; 32, 303-9.

- Loiseau P, Duche B, Cohadon S. The prognosis of benign localized epilepsy in early childhood. *Epilepsy Research* 1992; 6 (Suppl): 75-81.

- Nayrac P, Beaussart M. Les pointes-ondes prérolandiques : expression EEG très particulière. *Rev Neurol* 1958; 99: 201-6.

- Okumura A, Hayakawa F, Kato T, Kuno K, Negoro T, Watanabe K. Early recognition of benign partial epilepsy in infancy. *Epilepsia* 2000; 41: 714-7.

- Okumura A, Watanabe K, Negoro T, *et al*. long-term follow-up of patients with benign partial epilepsy in infancy. *Epilepsia* 2006; 47 (1): 181-5.

- Roger J, Bureau M. Facteurs de prognostic et évolution des épilepsies partielles de l'enfant. *Riv Ital EEG Neurofisiol Clin* 1983; Suppl. 1: 171-4.

- Roger J, Bureau M. Les épilepsies partielles idiopathiques de l'enfant (épilepsies partielles bénignes ou primaires). *Rev Neurol* 1987; 143: 381-91.

- Roger J, Dravet C, Menendez P, Bureau M. Les épilepsies partielles de l'enfant. Évolution et facteurs de prognostic. *Rev EEG Neurophysiol* 1981; 11: 431-7.

- Roger J, Bureau M, Genton, P. Idiopathic partial epilepsies. In: Dam M, Gram M (Eds). *Comprehensive epileptology*. New York: Raven Press, 1990: 153-70.

• Tassinari CA, De Marco P, Plasmati R, Pantieri R, Blanco M, Michelucci R. Extreme somato-sensory evoked potentials (ESEPs) elicited by tapping of hands or feet in children: a somatosensory cerebral evoked potentials study. *Neurophysiol Clin* 1988; 18: 123-8.

• Tassinari CA, De Marco P. Benign partial epilepsy with extreme somato-sensory evoked potentials. In: Roger J, Bureau M, Dravet C, Dreifuss FE, Perret A, Wolf P (Eds). *Epileptic syndromes in infancy, childhood and adolescence* (2nd ed.). London: John Libbey, 1992: 225-9.

• Vinayan KP, Biji V, Thomas S. Educational problems with underlying neurpsychological impairment are common in children with benign childhood epilepsy with centrotemporal spikes (BECTS). *Seizure* 2005; 14: 207-12.

• Wakai S, Yoto Y, Higashidate Y, Tachi N, Chiba S. Benign partial epilepsy with affective symptoms: hyperkinetic behaviour during interictal periods. *Epilepsia* 1994; 35: 810-2.

• Wirrel E, Camield P, Gordon K, Dooley J, Camfield C. Benign rolandic epilepsy: atypical features are very common. *J Child Neurol* 1995; 10: 455-8.

Atypical evolutions of benign focal epilepsies in childhood

Natalio Fejerman*, Roberto H. Caraballo*,
Bernardo Dalla Bernardina**
*Buenos Aires, Argentina
**Verona, Italy

Benign childhood epilepsy with centrotemporal spikes (BCECTS) was initially presented as an absolutely benign epilepsy syndrome, but with the course of time a number of investigations showed that a significant number of patients with BCECTS did present some degree of neuropsychological impairment (See chapter 6). Thus, a trend to discriminate between typical and atypical cases of BCECTS appeared in the literature (Wirrell et al., 1995; Weglage et al., 1997; Verrotti et al., 2002). Clinical and/or EEG clues to early diagnosis of this risk were presented (Massa et al., 2001; Kramer et al., 2002). Nevertheless, there is consensus that the recognition of some atypical clinical or EEG features in cases of BCECTS does not mean that those children are going to present severe school failures or behavioural problems (Croona et al., 1999; Fejerman 2007).

When we refer to "atypical evolutions" of benign focal epilepsies in childhood (BFEC) in this chapter, instead, we intend to describe a subset of patients who present severe aggravation of epileptic manifestations and/or marked language, and/or cognitive, and/or behaviour impairments. The first description of this event by Aicardi and Chevrie in 1982, reported on seven children with BCECTS presenting periods with new types of seizures, mainly atonic and myoclonic, associated with continuous spike-and-waves in slow-sleep EEG, and transitory deterioration in school performance. They used the term "atypical benign partial epilepsy of childhood" and commented that the majority of them had been previously diagnosed as Lennox-Gastaut syndrome. In this book we are calling it "Atypical benign focal epilepsy of childhood" (ABFEC). We have provided evidence reporting a series of children who had first typical clinico-EEG features of BCECTS, and years later presented the mentioned severe aggravation, not only under the features of ABFEC (Fejerman et al., 2000). Our initial report included the first two cases with status epilepticus of benign childhood epilepsy with centrotemporal spikes (SEBCECTS) (Fejerman & Di Blasi, 1987). Later, we were able to demonstrate that children with BCECTS may evolve into two other conditions considered as epileptic syndromes in the 1989 ILAE's classification (Commission..., 1989), namely the Landau-Kleffner syndrome (LKS) and the Continuous spike-and-wave during slow sleep syndrome (CSWSS) (Fejerman, 1996; Fejerman et al., 1998, 2000). We also presented the first descriptions of patients with Childhood occipital epilepsies of the

Gastaut type and of the Panayiotopoulos type who showed the same atypical evolutions with continuous spike-and-wave activities in the EEG and severe neuropsychological impairment (Fejerman *et al.*, 1991; Tenembaum *et al.*, 1997; Caraballo *et al.*, 2001).

The question is: are these four conditions – ABFEC, SEBCECTS, LKS, CSWSS – independent syndromes, syndromes related to BCECTS (or other BFEC) as part of a continuum, or atypical evolutions appearing in a minority of patients with BCECTS? Obviously, evidence of these situations registered during the follow-up of a significant number of patients with BCECTS is not enough to generalize it to all the cases.

Another question is: how do we explain the fact that children with definite CNS lesions, acquired or genetically determined, may also present the same kind of epileptic encephalopathy course under the form of ABFEC, as described in a significant group of children with congenital hemiparesis associated with unilateral polymichrogyria, with symptoms of LKS as seen in a few cases, or featuring the complex clinical spectrum of the CSWSS in a larger number of patients with different types (and different aetiologies) of cerebral lesions? (Caraballo *et al.*, 1999a; Fejerman *et al.*, 2000). We intend to analyze first the pathophysiology underlying the appearance of electrical status epilepticus during sleep (ESES); second, to describe in more detail the clinical-EEG features of the four mentioned conditions, and third, to present a new series of cases of each of these entities, be they real epileptic syndromes or atypical evolutions of BCECTS. We also include data about our cases with the Gastaut type of childhood occipital epilepsy and with Panayiotopoulos syndrome (PS) who showed the same atypical clinico-EEG course.

EEG findings and pathophysiology

ABFEC, SEBCECTS, LKS and CSWSS have in common the presence of electrical status epilepticus during slow sleep (ESES). There is strong evidence to support the hypothesis that spike-and-wave status is the result of secondary bilateral synchrony (SBS) (Dalla Bernardina *et al.*, 1989, 2002, 2005; Kobayashi *et al.*, 1994; Tassinari *et al.*, 2000). SBS refers to bilateral and synchronic EEG discharges generated by a unilateral cortical focus (Lombroso & Erba, 1970; Panayiotopoulos, 2005). The triggering spikes of SBS may be at any brain location, but for symptomatic epilepsies are mainly in the frontal lobe. SBS consist of high amplitude bilateral spike-wave discharges which appear symmetrical and synchronous, but in particular cases these discharges may show a significant asymmetry in amplitude, clearly related to the damaged hemisphere in the symptomatic focal epilepsies. Focal epilepsies with SBS are often severe and usually of frontal or temporal lobe origin. They manifest with a mix of focal and secondarily generalized seizures including atonic seizures which may cause sudden falls, myoclonic seizures, absences and generalized tonic-clonic seizures. It is well known that due to the presence of the mentioned seizures and bilateral spike-wave discharges in the EEG, many of these patients are erroneously diagnosed as having Lennox Gastaut syndrome (Panayiotopoulos, 2005). What we are considering now, instead, is the role of SBS in the pathogenesis of certain epileptic encephalopathies in childhood. First, we have to recognize that bilateral spike-wave discharges do appear in severely injured children. A series of 29 children with prenatal or perinatal unilateral thalamic injuries associated with symptomatic CSWSS or sleep SW overactivation was reported (Guzzetta et al., 2005). CSWSS was also detected in children with shunted hydrocephalus, suggesting involvement of thalamo-cortical circuitries (Veggiotti et al., 1998). The third and most typical example of CSWSS associated with a prenatal brain malformation is given by the large series of children with unilateral polymichrogyria who present typical seizures, EEG, and course of ABFEC (see Chapter 11). Hence, we have to recognize that the phenomenon of SBS may have variable intensities. When it appears mainly in slow-sleep and covers a high proportion of the EEG activity during that period of sleep, we call it ESES or Continuous spike-waves during slow sleep (CSWS). The presence of CSWS is usually responsible of a real epileptic encephalopathy affecting mainly language, cognition and behaviour in children, independently whether the original spikes arises from the site of a brain lesion or are only functional as in BFEC.

Another peculiar phenomenon present in these patients is epileptic negative myoclonus (ENM) during wakefulness. ENM is a motor disorder characterized by a sudden, brief loss of postural tone, associated with a paroxysmal EEG abnormality (usually a spike) without any clinical or polygraphic evidence of an antecedent positive motor phenomenon in the agonist and antagonist muscles (Rubboli et al., 1995; Capovilla et al., 2000; Parmeggiani et al., 2004). ENM can be bilateral, in relation to diffuse paroxysmal activity (Tassinari et al., 1968); or focal associated with a spike in the central region of the contralateral hemisphere (Guerrini et al., 1993). Clinical manifestations of ENM vary in location and intensity and may be head-drops, brief atonia of hands causing the drop of objects, or falls due to ENM in lower limbs. In some cases these "inhibitory seizures" in lower limbs are subtle and may cause a difficulty in walking. Even episodes of faecal incontinence were reported in two children as manifestations of ENM in the pelvic floor muscles (Capovilla et al., 2000). An easy manœuvre to detect ENM in upper limbs is to ask the child to extend to the front both arms, and one can see very brief and partial drops of one arm. The diagnosis of ENM relies on the polygraphic demonstration of a brief interruption of the tonic EMG activity, time-locked to a cortical spike. Status epilepticus with repetitive asymmetrical atonia has been reported (Kanazawa et al., 1990). Unilateral brief focal atonia was found in association with rolandic spikes (Oguni et al., 1992, 1997). Regarding treatment of ENM, Ethosuximide has been reported to be effective in ENM occurring in partial epilepsies of childhood (Oguni et al., 1998, Capovilla et al., 1999), but we'll discuss it in more detail under treatment of all the variants of CSWSS.

The reasons why only a portion of patients with lesional or functional spikes develop SBS or CSWS are not clear, neither is clear why occasionally children may present ESES without clinical seizures or neuropsychologic impairments (Dalla Bernardina et al., 1978). Duration of ESES has been correlated with clinical features (Tassinari et al., 2000). The localization of interictal foci seem also to play a major role in influencing the degree of cognitive dysfunction, suggesting that ESES's clinical picture results from a localized disruption of EEG activity caused by focal epileptic activity during sleep (Tassinari & Rubboli, 2006). Probably, age of appearance of SBS is also relevant, as we'll see analysing the difference in time of onset of ABFEC, SEBCECTS, LKS and CSWSS when they appear in children having already BCECTS.

We have evidence of one factor that can elicit increases in SW discharges and SBS evolving into ESES: certain antiepileptic drugs (AED). This was demonstrated for the old AEDs such as Phenobarbital and Phenytoin (Guerrini *et al.*, 1995; Veggiotti *et al.*, 1999; Fejerman *et al.*, 2000; Hamano *et al.*, 2002), for Carbamazepine (Shields & Saslow, 1983; Lerman, 1986; Caraballo *et al.*, 1989; Namba & Maegaki, 1999; Corda *et al.*, 2001; Kochen *et al.*, 2002; Kikumoto *et al.*, 2006), and for Valproic Acid (Prats *et al.*, 1998). Of the new drugs, anecdotical evidence was reported for Oxcarbazepine (Hahn *et al.*, 2004; Grosso *et al.*, 2006), for Lamotrigine (Catania *et al.*, 1999; Cerminara *et al.*, 2004) and for Topiramate (Montenegro & Guerreiro, 2002).

We'll see under treatment which are the best steps to prevent the development of ESES and how to treat ESES once it has appeared, irrespective of the associated clinical manifestations. Nevertheless, independently from the different points of view regarding nosology of the four conditions which have in common SBS evolving into ESES, and whether they belong or not to the category of definite epileptic syndromes (Fejerman, 2003), we present their clinical features.

Atypical Benign Focal Epilepsy of Childhood

The initial report of ABFEC (Aicardi & Chevrie, 1982) included 7 patients with normal neuropsychological development and neurologic examination, who started after 2 years of age with partial seizures of the BCECTS type at night. Later, frequent partial or bilateral atonic and myoclonic seizures appeared leading to multiple daily falls. These atonic or inhibitory attacks appear in clusters of one of several weeks duration and are usually separated by seizure-free intervals of weeks or even months. Patients frequently stopped attending school several times during the year, but regain normal performance during the months of remission. EEGs in active epileptic periods show CSWS *(Fig. 1)* that are indistinguishable from the discharges seen in the typical CSWSS (Beaumanoir, 1995a; Fejerman *et al.*, 2000; Dalla Bernardina *et al.*, 2002, 2005). Diffuse paroxysmal activity during wakefulness is associated with the typical centrotemporal spikes of BCECTS *(Fig. 2)*. A benign outcome with spontaneous disappearance of seizures before adolescence was an important criterion for diagnosis, but the fact that misdiagnosis of Lennox-Gastaut syndrome in the first series of cases had been common, was emphasized (Aicardi & Chevrie, 1982). This cluster of electroclinical features was repeatedly recognized (Deonna *et al.*, 1986; Fejerman & Medina, 1986), and it was even given the synonymous of "pseudo-Lennox" syndrome (Doose *et al.*, 1996; Hahn, 2000; Hahn *et al.*, 2001).

In a review of the subject Aicardi (2000) presented a new series of 12 cases emphasizing the following findings: 1) the mean age at first atypical seizure was 50 months; 2) evolution in 2-6 bouts of 3-12 weeks in 11-12 patients; 3) seizure free and cognitive/behavioural recovery in the 12 cases; 4) regarding seizures, 9 patients had nocturnal partial seizures, 11 had atonic attacks, 12 had myoclonic jerks and 7 had other seizures; 5) the EEG findings included focal spikes and bursts of fast spike waves in wakefulness and CSWS in the 12 cases. In 2000 we reported 11 children with ABFEC showing that the worsening of electroclinical features occurred between 6 months and 2 years after onset of BCECTS in all cases. All the 11 children became seizure free

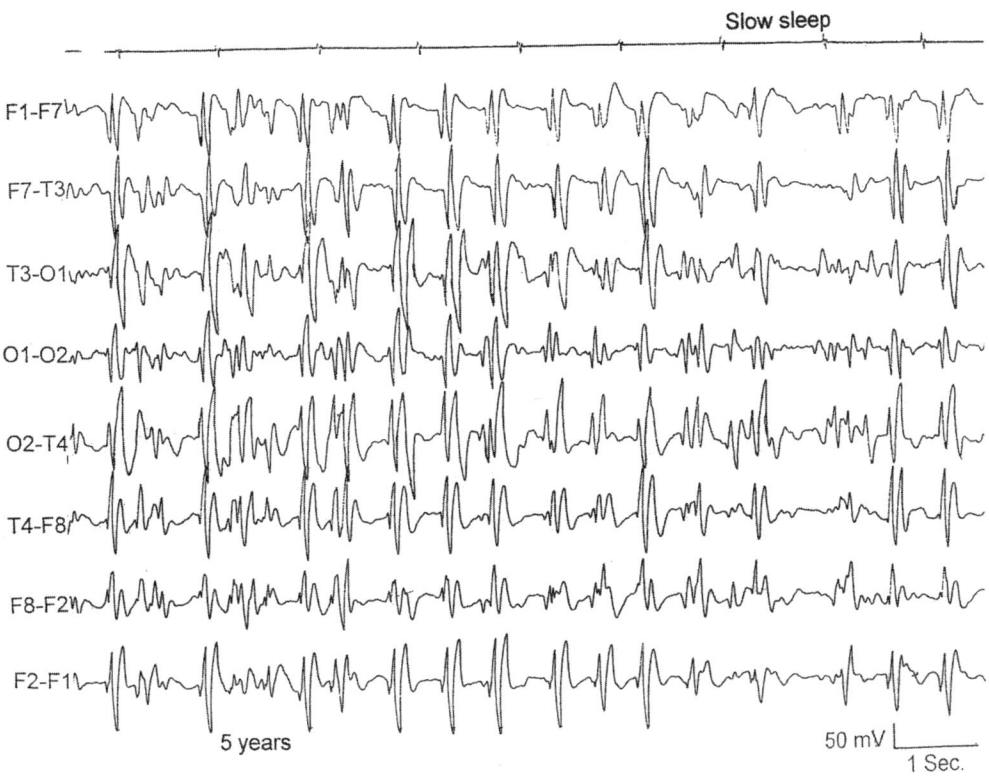

Figure 1. Five years old boy with clinical features of ABPEC. EEG shows continuous spike-and-wave activity in more than 85% of slow sleep.

and had no neuropsychological impairment by adolescence (Fejerman et al., 2000). ABFEC may also start in children who did not present previously clinical or EEG features of BCECTS, but this eventuality is rare. Obviously, in these cases there was no chance to use AED before the appearance of ABFEC.

In chapter 11 we present our series of 59 children with unilateral polymicrogyria including a few patients with clastic unilateral brain lesions probably associated with polymicrogyria who presented the same clinical and EEG features, and even the same responses to changes in treatment as the idiopathic cases with ABFEC (Caraballo et al., 1999a).

Since some authors use the term "pseudo-Lennox", the Lennox-Gastaut syndrome (LGS) is the first differential diagnosis. Similarities are the epileptic falls and the absences, but the EEG patterns are different and the presence of clinical and/or EEG evidence of tonic seizures is only seen in LGS. Epilepsy with myoclonic-astatic seizures is discarded as soon as a period of transitory improvement arrives and centrotemporal spikes are clearly seen in the EEG.

In *Table I* we include data about our present series of 16 patients with ABFEC.

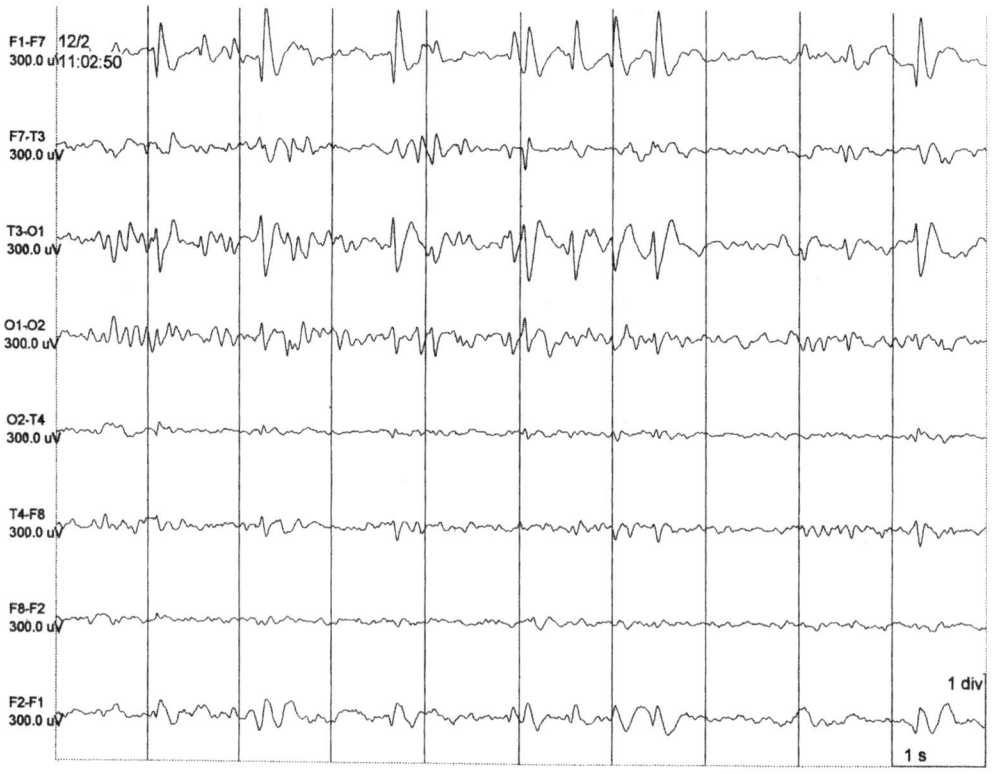

Figure 2. EEG while awake in the same patient of Fig. 1 shows centrotemporal spikes with higher amplitude in left side.

Table I. Follow-up of 16 children with ABFEC*

Patient No.	Age at onset of BCECTS (years)	Age at worsening (years)	Age at last seizure (years)	Age at normal EEG (years)	Age when AED treatment stopped (years)	Present age (years)
1	5	7	10	10.5	12	21
2	3.5	5	9	12	12	24
3	6	7.5	12	12.5	14.5	22
4	5	5.5	13	13	16	23.5
5	4.5	6	12	15	15	24
6	7.5	8.5	11	11.5	14	19.5
7	5.5	7.5	9	13	12	23.5
8	6.5	8	14	17	17.5	28.5

9	2	2.5	7	7	10	19
10	4	6	8	10	12	23
11	4	5.5	7	10	12	19
12	5	8	10	11	-	12
13	6	7.5	11	12	12	13
14	4	6	9	-	-	10
15	7	8.5	-	-	-	11
16	7.5	9	-	-	-	10

ABFEC: Atypical benign focal epilepsy of childhood; BCECTS: Benign childhood epilepsy with centrotemporal spikes; AED: antiepileptic drug
* Three patients not included in this table presented features of ABFEC at onset.

Status of benign childhood epilepsy with centrotemporal spikes

In 1987 Fejerman and Di Blasi reported the first two cases of status epilepticus of BCECTS (SEBCECTS). These children had not only electrical status during sleep but also persistent focal seizure status while awake and during sleep. Seizures with facial localization, speech arrest and sialorrhea were resistant to AED for 5 weeks in one case and for 10 days in the other; Only the administration of steroids stopped the electroclinical status. Again, as seen in *figures 3 & 4*, the ictal waking EEG in one case showed continuous paroxysmal activity with higher amplitude in Rolandic areas, and the ictal sleep EEG in the other case showed continuous spikes and waves with higher amplitude on the hemisphere which previously showed the centrotemporal spikes. Since 1987, other cases of SEBCECTS have been reported with slight clinical differences or a better response to AEDs (Roulet *et al.*, 1989; Boulloche *et al.*, 1990; Colamaria *et al.*, 1991; Septien *et al.*, 1992; Deonna *et al.*, 1993; Shafir & Prensky, 1995; Salas-Puig *et al.*, 2002; Gregory *et al.*, 2002).

In one case, persistent drooling, dysarthria and dysphagia was interpreted as an oromotor deficit "indirectly correlated to the abundance and the bilateral topography of interictal discharges recorded during sleep" (de Saint Martin *et al.*, 1999). Incidentally, the same symptomatology was interpreted in once child as a reversible anterior opercular syndrome which persisted for 2 weeks and was associated with continuous bilateral epileptic discharges with right predominance (Christen *et al.*, 2000). We agree with the latter interpretation.

In 2000 we presented 7 children with SEBCECTS and in this condition the median time elapsed between onset of BCECTS and the appearance of electroclinical status was 4 years, which is significantly higher than in the cases of ABPEC. Again, all the cases recovered completely with normalization of EEGs and free of seizures before 12 years of age (Fejerman *et al.*, 2000). *Figure 5* shows one more example of EEG during status of BCECTS.

In *Table II* we include data about our present series of cases with SEBCECTS.

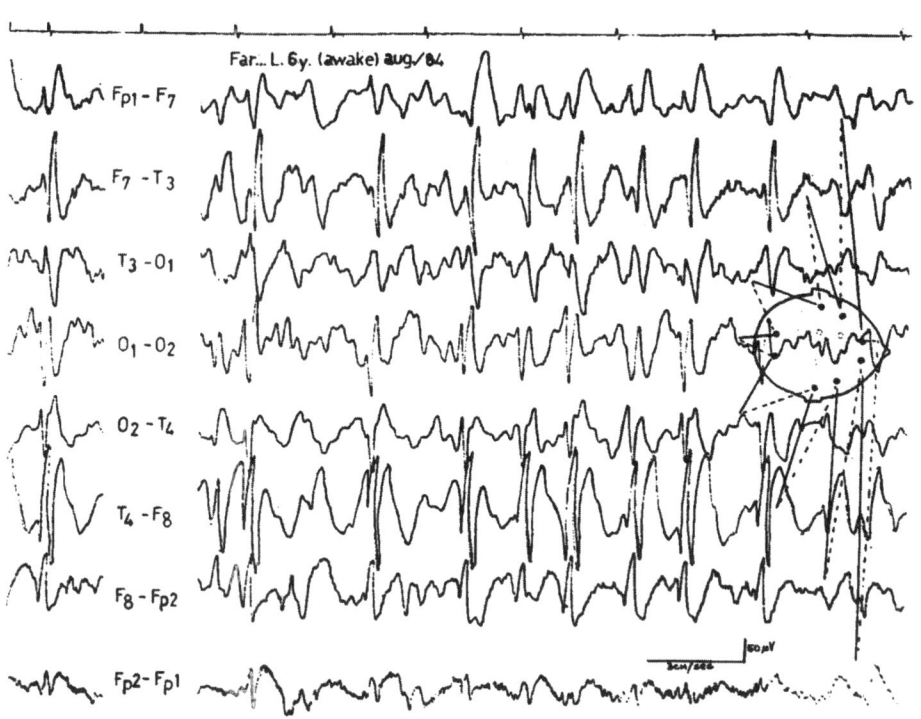

Figure 3. Six years old boy. Awake ictal EEG showing continuous paroxysmal activity of generalized spikes. Amplitude is higher in centrotemporal areas. (Reproduced with permission from *Epilepsia* 1987; 28 (4): 351-5).

Table II. Follow-up of 10 children with Status of BCECTS*

Patient No.	Age at onset of BCECTS (years)	Age at worsening (years)	Age at last seizure (years)	Age at normal EEG (years)	Age when AED treatment stopped (years)	Present age (years)
1	3	8	10	12	12	25
2	3	8	10	10	12	19
3	7.5	9	11.5	14	14	19
4	3	6	8	10	10	27
5	3	7	8.5	9	11	26
6	6	7	8	9	10	19
7	3	8	9	10	11	19
8	4	6	9	11	13	14
9	5	7.5	11	–	12	13
10	3	6	11	–	–	12

BCECTS: Benign childhood epilepsy with centrotemporal spikes; AED: antiepileptic drug
* One patient not included in this table presented status at onset of BCECTS.

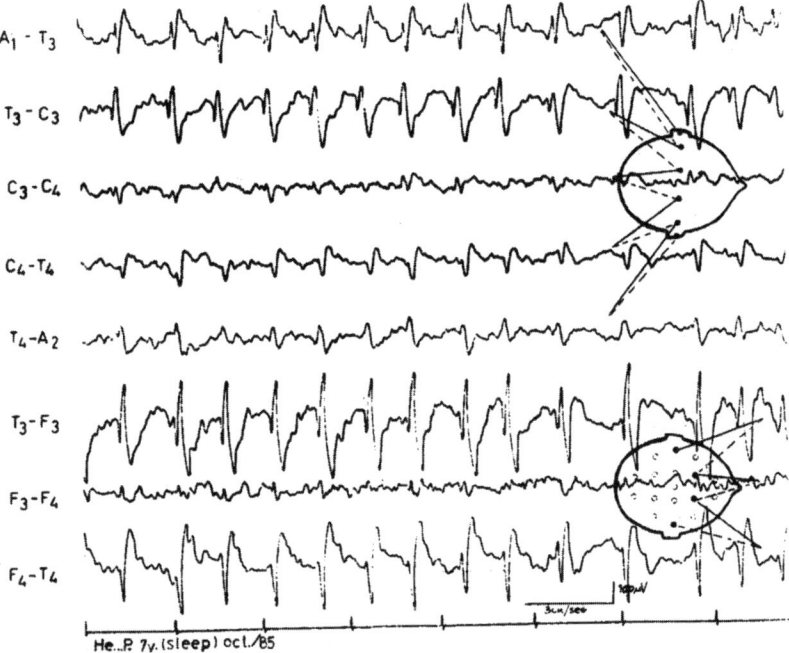

Figure 4. Seven years old boy. Sleep EEG with continuous bilateral spike discharges. Amplitude is higher on left side. Partial motor status epilepticus was present during the entire EEG tracing. (Reproduced with permission from *Epilepsia* 1987; 28 (4): 351-5).

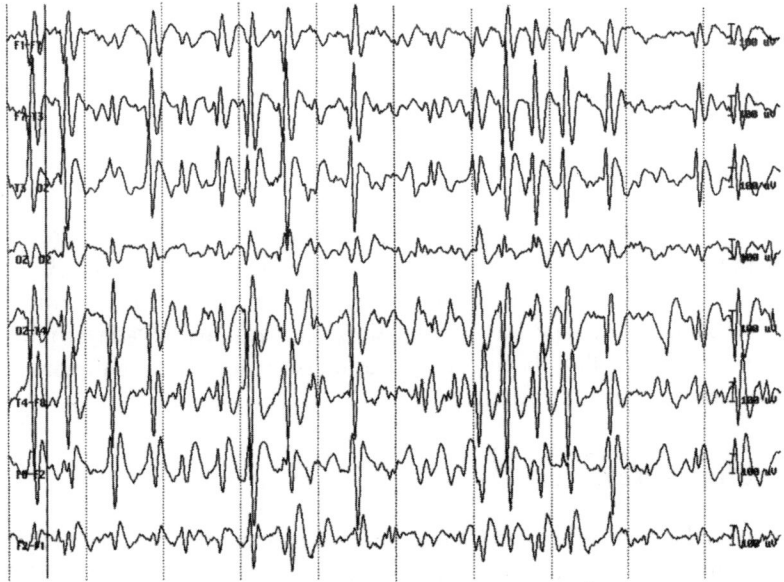

Figure 5. Seven years old girl with status of BCECTS which lasted 2 days. Ictal EEG while awake shows rhythmic bilateral spike activity with higher amplitude in centrotemporal areas.

Landau Kleffner syndrome

In 1957 Landau and Kleffner described 6 children with a "syndrome of acquired aphasia with convulsive disorder" (Landau & Kleffner, 1957). The language disorder was later recognized as being different from typical childhood aphasia, which is usually expressive. Instead, the aphasia of the Landau-Kleffner syndrome is an auditory verbal agnosia (Rapin *et al.*, 1977). The language disorder was initially considered to be a seizure manifestation because epileptiform activity from one or both temporal lobes is generally present on EEG recordings. Seizures are not a constant feature, and when present, they may precede or follow the onset of the language disorder.

Mantovani and Landau (1980) followed the 6 original cases plus 4 others and found that the outcome was variable: 5 of the children had recovered good language function as adults. Their hypothesis that outcome correlated with seizure frequency was not substantiated by subsequent reports (Deonna *et al.*, 1977; Holmes *et al.*, 1981).

In 1989 the International League Against Epilepsy placed this syndrome under the classification of "epilepsies and syndromes undetermined as to whether they are focal or generalized" (Commission on Classification..., 1989). In the same category, the syndrome of continuous spikes-and-waves during slow sleep was included as a definite entity. However, in recent years many common features between these two syndromes have been recognized, and there are questions as to whether they are two distinct entities or subclasses of a single syndrome (Deonna & Roulet, 1995; Hirsch *et al.*, 1995; De Negri, 1997; Smith, 1998; Rossi *et al.*, 1999; Tassinari *et al.*, 2000, 2002; Smith & Hoeppner, 2003). Furthermore, the mechanism of bilateral secondary synchronies after an initial functional spike focus seems to be the basis of language impairment and represent both for Landau-Kleffner syndrome and continuous spikes-and-waves during slow sleep syndrome an explanation for the inclusion of these syndromes among the epileptic encephalopathies as proposed by ILAE's Task Force on Classification (Engel, 2001).

Epidemiology

The incidence of Landau-Kleffner syndrome is unknown. At least 198 cases were reported by 1992 (Beaumanoir, 1992). In 1994 we presented 12 cases with a long follow-up (Soprano *et al.*, 1994). Even when Landau-Kleffner syndrome shares many clinical and EEG features with the syndrome of Continuous spikes-and-waves during slow sleep, acquired aphasia is a more frequent finding than the psychiatric disturbances described in association with continuous spike-wave activity in slow sleep.

Clinical features

Acquired aphasia is the more prominent feature, since seizures are present in only 70% to 80% of the patients and may appear before or after onset of aphasia (Beaumanoir, 1985, 1992; Deonna *et al.*, 1997). Age of onset ranges from 3 to 8 years, and boys are more frequently affected than girls (Beaumanoir, 1985; Panayiotopoulos, 2005). The onset of aphasia is often insidious and progressive with spontaneous improvements and aggravations in its course. The most common feature is verbal auditory agnosia, which is the reason why in many cases the first diagnosis is hearing loss (Rapin et al., 1977). Agnosia may extend to familiar noises. In some cases onset may be abrupt, and different types of aphasia may occur (Soprano et al., 1994). Variable time may elapse between the loss of the ability to understand language and the expressive aphasia. In general, it is stated that patients previously had been normal in both psychomotor and language development. However, detailed history of language characteristics show that 9 of 12 patients have had previous features of developmental dysphasia (Soprano et al., 1994). Rarely, stuttering may be the presenting feature (Tutuncuoglu et al., 2002), although it is difficult to differentiate pure stuttering from the repetitive nature of the impaired speech in early stages of acquired aphasia.

Neuropsychological and behavioural disturbances have been reported, and there are cases in which the overlapping between Landau-Kleffner syndrome and the syndrome of continuous spikes-and-waves during slow sleep is more prominent on clinical grounds. Alternating courses with behavioural disturbances and acquired aphasia has been described in children within the mentioned spectrum (Fejerman et al., 2000). Nevertheless, the most frequent findings are hyperkinesia and excitability. In fact, it is striking that children with such a severe handicap in understanding language only present psychotic or autistic features when aphasia appears in early ages (Deonna et al., 1982; Fejerman & Medina, 1986; Deonna 1991; Klein et al., 2000). In the context of a more global autistic regression, some young children show language regression with epileptiform EEGs, but it is controversial to state that these children are part of an extended Landau-Kleffner spectrum (McVicar & Shinnar, 2004, Baird et al., 2006). A recent investigation using sleep EEGs in 64 children with autism without history of epilepsy disclosed that there was no significant difference in epileptic discharges comparing those patients that showed regression with those which did not. No child presented electrical status epilepticus in slow sleep. These results are against the suggestion that subclinical epilepsy may be causative of regression in autism (Baird et al., 2006).

The most common types of seizures are: eyelid myoclonia, eye blinking, atypical absences, head drops and atonic fits in upper limbs, automatisms, and occasionally, partial motor seizures with secondary generalization.

Aetiology

Isolated cases of Landau-Kleffner syndrome were apparently associated with overt cerebral pathology (*e.g.*, acute inflammatory disease, arteritis, cysticercosis, tumours, and arachnoid cyst) (Cole et al., 1988; Otero et al., 1989; Pascual-Castroviejo et al., 1992; Nass et al., 1993; Perniola et al., 1993; De Volder et al., 1994). Pathological study in a surgical series of 14 patients with Landau-Kleffner syndrome yielded a variety of abnormalities (Smith et al., 1992). Perisylvian polymichrogyria has been reported in one case (Huppke et al., 2005). A new aetiology has recently been reported in a 5 year old girl with typical Landau Kleffner syndrome associated with mitochondrial respiratory chain-complex I deficiency (Kang et al., 2006). Nevertheless, the language symptomatology is interpreted as a dysfunctional disorder associated with the bilateral EEG discharges and deafferentation of temporal cortex (Landau & Kleffner, 1957; Gordon, 1990, 1997; Beaumanoir, 1992).

Cases of BCECTS evolving into LKS: Several authors have pointed to a relationship between the epileptic abnormalities of Landau-Kleffner syndrome and the benign epilepsies of childhood (Dulac *et al.*, 1983; Cole *et al.*, 1988; Deonna & Roulet, 1995). Moreover, some patients were reported with a history of typical benign childhood epilepsy with centrotemporal spikes previous to the onset of Landau-Kleffner syndrome (Fejerman & Medina, 1986; Cole *et al.*, 1988; Deonna *et al.*, 1993; Fejerman *et al.*, 2000; Smith & Hoeppner, 2003). In 2000 we reported 3 cases that started with typical BCECTS and after 3 to 5 years presented the clinico-EEG features of LKS (Fejerman *et al.*, 2000). In *Table III* data about our new series of patients with LKS are given. Even when the prevalence of this phenomenon is rare, the mentioned findings show numbers that are more than anecdotical. Discussion about its nosological significance is, however, yet open. One might say that the 4 cases represent a clear atypical evolution of BCECTS, and that there is enough evidence to explain the course into an epileptic encephalopathy as the LKS. Other hypothesis might be that the appearance of the acquired epileptic aphasia was determined previously and that the centrotemporal spikes with the rolandic seizures were its first manifestation, or that BCECTS and LKS represent in these cases a continuum of one condition with variable phenotypes.

EEG and other neurophysiological studies

Waking EEG usually shows brief bursts of temporal or temporo-occipital spike and wave discharges, either symmetrical or asymmetrical. In fact, the most typical EEG findings appear during slow sleep as continuous 1.5 Hz to 5 Hz spike and wave discharges, which may be seen in approximately 85% of the record (Beaumanoir, 1992; Deonna & Roulet, 1995; De Negri, 1997; Smith, 1998). In *figure 6* we present the sleep EEG of a seven years old girl at the time she had a clear acquired epileptic aphasia. This patient had started at 5 years of age with typical electroclinical features of BCECTS. It has been stated that most of the cases have a unilateral primary epileptogenic region (Morrell *et al.*, 1995). Therefore, the presence of bilateral continuous spike-wave discharges is interpreted as a mechanism of secondary bilateral synchronies (Tassinari *et al.*, 2000; Fejerman *et al.*, 2000).

Table III. Follow-up of 4 children with LKS*

Patient No.	Age at onset of BCECTS (years)	Age at worsening (years)	Age at last seizure (years)	Age at normal EEG (years)	Age when AED treatment stopped (years)	Present age (years)
1	3	8	9	11	11	19.5
2	5	8	10.5	14	14	26
3	3	7	3	11.5	12	29
4	4	8	9	10.5	11.5	12

LKS: Landau-Kleffner syndrome; BCECTS: Benign childhood epilepsy with centrotemporal spikes; AED: antiepileptic drug.
* These patients are not part of our series of 17 cases with LKS.

The correlation between the frequency and severity of EEG abnormalities and the degree of language disturbances has been questioned, although in active periods of aphasia, epileptiform activities in the EEG are more prominent. Again, at present, all patients with Landau-Kleffner syndrome show, at some time during its course, the sleep-EEG pattern of continuous spike and wave discharges (Tassinari *et al.*, 2002). In long-term follow-up of series of patients with Landau-Kleffner syndrome, a strict correlation between length of continuous spike and wave discharges and persistence of language impairment was found (Robinson *et al.*, 2001; Veggiotti *et al.*, 2002). Finally, epileptiform activities in EEG were also seen in a percentage of patients with developmental dysphasia, adding difficulties to the interpretation of physiopathogenic mechanisms in Landau-Kleffner syndrome (Maccario *et al.*, 1982; Echenne *et al.*, 1992; Picard *et al.*, 1998).

Magnetoencephalography was used to localize the source of epileptiform activity in children with Landau-Kleffner syndrome. A thorough study of 4 right-handed Landau-Kleffner syndrome patients including video-EEG and magnetoencephalography was performed as presurgical evaluation 3 to 6 years after the first language deterioration. Conclusion was that the intrasylvian cortex is a likely pacemaker of epileptic discharges in Landau-Kleffner syndrome and that magnetoencephalography provides useful presurgical information of the cortical spike dynamics (Paetau *et al.*, 1999). Magnetoencephalography was also performed in 19 patients with suspected

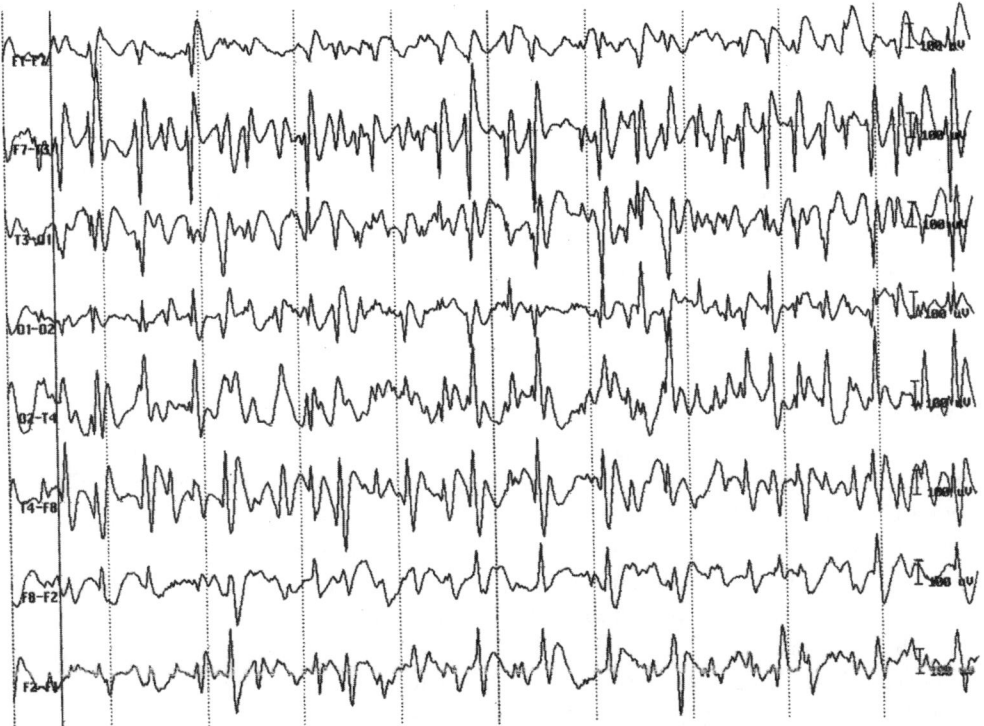

Figure 6. Seven years old girl with LKS. Sleep EEG shows diffuse continuous spike and waves discharges, with higher amplitude in centrotemporal areas.

diagnosis of Landau-Kleffner syndrome. Thirteen of the 19 children had perisylvian magnetoencephalography spikes, which were bilateral in 10 and unilateral in 3 of the children. These results suggest that magnetoencephalography might help to obviate the need for invasive video-EEG recordings when surgery is being considered for patients with this condition (Sobel et al., 2000).

Abnormal auditory evoked potentials have been reported in several patients with Landau-Kleffner syndrome. Some authors found normal brainstem auditory evoked potentials and clearly abnormal long latency evoked potentials, specifically the P300 (Fejerman & Medina, 1986; Caraballo et al., 1999b). Others reported abnormal brainstem auditory evoked potentials and middle-latency evoked potentials (Isnard et al., 1995). Five children having recovered from Landau-Kleffner syndrome were compared to controls using early, middle latency, and late auditory evoked potentials. Unilateral voltage reduction of late auditory evoked potentials over the temporal areas previously involved by epileptic discharges was found, suggesting a permanent dysfunction in the associative auditory cortex (Wioland et al., 2001). All studies support the hypothesis of a deficit in the activation of the auditory cortical areas.

Pathophysiology

It has been suggested that the EEG discharges and seizures are manifestations of underlying abnormalities of the cortex in the speech areas, rather than the cause of the aphasia (Holmes et al., 1981). A specific hypothesis has been proposed for pathophysiology of Landau-Kleffner syndrome: a persistent paroxysmal activity during the age-dependent period of synaptogenesis might strengthen synaptic contacts that should have degenerated to allow neuronal aggregates mediate normal behaviour. This reinforcement of inappropriate contacts in the developing temporoparietal cortex produces a permanent language dysfunction when paroxysmal activities are bilateral (Morrell et al., 1995; Smith, 1998). Therefore, early treatment would be the only way to prevent persistent aphasia. This mechanism also explains why eventual normalization of the EEG is not necessarily paralleled with improvement of aphasia.

A new pathogenetic interpretation was provided studying 4 children with Landau-Kleffner syndrome compared to 4 controls. MRI volumetric analysis was performed focusing on various neocortical regions and emphasizing the auditory association cortex. Age of onset of the Landau-Kleffner syndrome in the patients ranged between 3 and 4.5 years, whereas the MRI volumetry was done at ages 5 to 6.5 years. Greater than 25% volume reduction in both superior temporal areas was demonstrated only after comparison with controls, and it was worse in the side with more epileptiform activity in 2 of the children. The authors were not able to determine if volume changes existed before language regression and, thus, could not distinguish tissue loss from decreased growth or dysgenesis. Besides, 2 patients received steroid treatment before the MRI study (Takeoka et al., 2004). The main question arising is whether the reduction of temporal cortical volume is cause or effect of the Landau-Kleffner syndrome. Incidentally, one of the two authors who described originally the syndrome commented the just mentioned findings and envisioned the following sequence of events:
1) Early on temporal lobe epileptiform activity produces the positive symptom of clinical seizures and the negative symptom of language dysfunction;
2) Excitotoxicity of unrelieved epileptic activity causes focal cortical atrophy;

3) Cortical atrophy prevents language recovery despite disappearance of epileptiform activity (Bourgeois & Landau, 2004).

If the findings of volume reduction are ratified, longitudinal volumetric analysis might become a useful tool to evaluate evolution and treatment effects in patients with Landau Kleffner syndrome.

Differential diagnosis

Progressive degenerative neurologic disorders usually affect language as part of the neuropsychological deterioration. Structural lesions in the dominant hemisphere of children less than 5 years of age do not impair language development because that function is served by the non-dominant hemisphere. Hence, receptive or expressive aphasia is unusual in young children unless they have a bitemporal lobe dysfunction. Therefore, acute or subacute aphasia in children aged 2 to 8 years, without unilateral acquired paresis or encephalitic symptoms, is most probably due to Landau-Kleffner syndrome (Fejerman & Engel, 2006).

The boundaries between Landau-Kleffner syndrome and the syndrome of epilepsy with continuous spikes-and-waves during slow wave sleep have been widely discussed (Hirsch et al., 1990, 1995; Tassinari, 1995; Smith, 1998; Tassinari et al., 2002). This type of EEG has also been found in several children with benign childhood epilepsy with centrotemporal spikes, particularly in the reported cases with clinical and EEG status lasting weeks (Fejerman & Di Blasi, 1987; Roulet et al., 1989; Fejerman, 1996, 2000). Intermediate cases between status of benign childhood epilepsy with centrotemporal spikes and Landau-Kleffner syndrome are also occasionally seen (Shafrir & Prensky, 1995; Fejerman, 1996).

In early-onset cases of Landau-Kleffner syndrome, differential diagnosis with developmental dysphasia associated with EEG discharges could be difficult. The same applies to children with autistic features, regression, and epileptiform EEGs (Tuchman & Rapin, 1997; Tuchman, 2006). We already quoted the study of Baird et al. (2006) demonstrating that regression in 39 out of 64 children with autism was not related to EEG subclinical epileptiform activity. Elective mutism can be readily discarded on clinical grounds and with EEG. Nevertheless, many cases of Landau-Kleffner syndrome are initially diagnosed as psychosis or severe emotional disturbance on account of their recent inability to understand spoken language, their hyperkinesia, and their anxiety. In a significant number of cases, diagnosis is delayed because an extensive workup for deafness is undertaken.

Diagnostic work-up

Neurologic examination is normal, and special care should be given to recognition of aphasia, mainly at onset, as auditory verbal agnosia. Neuropsychological evaluation is fundamental to determine the nature of the language disorder and level of intelligence (Deonna, 1997). In many cases children keep their ability to write and to communicate through nonverbal means (Gordon, 1990; Soprano et al., 1994).

EEG shows a pattern of bilateral symmetrical or asymmetrical multifocal spikes and spike-waves most frequently located in the temporal and parieto-occipital regions. Sleep enhances the EEG paroxysms up to the level of exhibiting spike-wave discharges in more than 85% of slow wave sleep (Beaumanoir, 1985; Paquier *et al.*, 1992). It is therefore necessary to perform at least a 1-2 hours sleep EEG in all cases to make sure that enough slow sleep is recorded.

When available, magnetoencephalography might be useful as part of presurgical evaluation in refractory cases.

Except in occasional cases associated with cerebral structural pathologies, MRI is normal. There is no doubt that high resolution MRI is mandatory in every child with features of LKS. As mentioned before, MRI volumetric analysis of superior temporal areas may yield clues to understand pathogenesis and evaluate evolution.

Functional imaging with PET and SPECT has repeatedly revealed unilateral or bilateral disturbances involving the temporal lobe (Maquet *et al.*, 1990; Mouridsen *et al.*, 1993; Guerreiro *et al.*, 1996; Da Silva *et al.*, 1997). A 4 year old boy with repeated episodes of receptive aphasia was studied with PET. Glucose metabolism PET scan during aphasia showed intense hypermetabolism in the left temporal neocortex, while a repeated PET scan during remission showed hypometabolism in the same region (Luat *et al.*, 2005). A child with LKS presenting episodic receptive aphasia was recently studied with PET showing dynamic changes of glucose metabolism in the temporal lobe during episodes of aphasia and remission (Luat *et al.*, 2006). It is clear that SPECT and PET are not essential for diagnosis of LKS, but may be useful to localize hemispheric metabolic asymmetries.

Treatment

We are detailing in one section of this chapter the treatment alternatives of the 4 conditions associated with the appearance of ESES, namely ABPEC, SEBCECTS, LKS and CSWSS. However, since epilepsy surgery treatment was only reported for children with LKS, we comment on it here.

Multiple subpial transection of the cortex to abolish epileptic discharges was used in a series of 14 children with acquired epileptic aphasia who had been unable to use language to communicate for at least 2 years; sustained improvement was obtained in 11 of them. According to the authors, success depends on selection of cases having severe EEG abnormality that can be demonstrated to be unilateral in origin despite a bilateral manifestation (Morrell *et al.*, 1992, 1995). In another small series, 5 children with Landau-Kleffner syndrome aged 5.5 to 10 years underwent multiple subpial transection, and behaviour and seizure frequency improved dramatically. Improvement in language also occurred in all children, although none of them reached an age-appropriate level of language even when their electrical status epilepticus during sleep was eliminated by the procedure (Irwin *et al.*, 2001).

More recently, six children with Landau-Kleffner syndrome were implanted with the vagal nerve stimulation device and three of them apparently showed improvement in quality of life (Park, 2003).

Prognosis and long term follow-up

The outcome of Landau-Kleffner syndrome varies. The seizures are usually controlled with antiepileptic drugs, and EEG abnormalities disappear after a few years.

The language disorder, however, may never resolve in almost half of the patients (Mantovani & Landau, 1980). Both improvement and aggravation of aphasia have been reported (Deonna, 1991). In many cases, correlation was found between increase in EEG discharges and aphasia, or even between abnormalities in the P300 wave during evoked potential studies and aphasia (Fejerman & Medina, 1986). The presence or absence of seizures, as well as their frequency, has no correlation with the outcome of language deficiency (Gordon, 1990). A residual impairment in verbal short-term memory is frequent. Brain activation during immediate serial recall of lists of 4 words, compared to single word repetition, using positron emission tomography were measured in three Landau-Kleffner syndrome patients after recovery and in 14 healthy controls. The patients had shown abnormally increased or decreased glucose metabolism in left or right superior temporal gyrus at different stages during the active phase of the disease. At the time of the study, the patients were 6 years to 10 years from the active phase of the disease. Results showed that two patients had impaired performance in verbal short-term memory. The data suggest that impaired verbal short-term memory at late outcome of Landau-Kleffner syndrome might be related to a persistent decrease of activity in the areas involved in the epileptic focus during the active phase (Majerus et al., 2003).

Out of 10 children with electrical status epilepticus during sleep and global or specific deterioration with long-term follow-up, 3 had Landau-Kleffner syndrome and showed that electrical status epilepticus during sleep persisted for 1 to 5 years and language impairment was not modified by treatment with Valproic acid or Benzodiazepines (Scholtes et al., 2005). In a retrospective review of EEGs with ESES and clinical information of 90 patients, 18 cases were diagnosed as LKS. The authors stated that prognosis of LKS was substantially better than CSWSS (Van Hirtum-Das et al., 2006).

Outcome at adulthood has been reported in seven young adults, five who had continuous spike-and-wave during slow-sleep syndrome and two with Landau-Kleffner syndrome in childhood. The intellectual functions of the two patients with Landau-Kleffner syndrome were normal, but their everyday lives were disrupted by severe, disabling language disturbances. The authors emphasized the role of location of interictal EEG focus and age of onset as prognostic factors (Praline et al., 2003). Another long-term follow-up was reported in five children with CSWS, of which 4 met criteria for diagnosis of Landau Kleffner syndrome. Again, age of onset and location of interictal EEG focus were considered as the main prognostic factors (Veggiotti et al., 2002). Dementia, or more precisely, long-term deterioration of intellectual functions, is uncommon in Landau-Kleffner syndrome (Dugas et al., 1995). However, in early onset cases, neuropsychological impairment is more severe (Deonna et al., 1982; Bishop, 1985).

Continuous spike and wave during slow wave sleep syndrome (CSWSS)

Electrical status epilepticus during sleep in children was first reported in 1971 (Patry *et al.*, 1971), describing 6 patients with the particular EEG pattern characterized by apparently subclinical spike and waves occurring almost continuously during sleep. Five of the 6 children had epileptic seizures, while the other one had no language, and 5 of the 6 children were mentally retarded. Tassinari, one of the three authors of the first report, introduced a few years later the terms "electrical status epilepticus during slow sleep" (ESES) and "encephalopathy related to ESES" (Tassinari *et al.*, 1977a, 1977b). Questioning about the term of status without detectable simultaneous clinical signs, and the finding of ESES in non-epileptic children, prompted the use of the term "epilepsy with continuous spikes and waves during slow sleep" (Tassinari *et al.*, 1985, 1992). Under this term was accepted in the 1989 classification of ILAE (Commission..., 1989). In 1995, a book was devoted to the subject and in a chapter on CSWSS or ESES it was stated that "ESES" is not a particular epileptic condition (Tassinari, 1995). Later on, the boundaries between CSWSS and LKS were considered less defined and the text "including acquired epileptic aphasia (Landau-Kleffner syndrome)" was added to the title "ESES or CSWSS" in the third edition of the same book (Tassinari *et al.*, 2002) and in a comprehensive textbook on epilepsy (Smith, 1998). In the last edition of the "blue book" on Epileptic syndromes in infancy, childhood, and adolescence, the encephalopathy with CSWSS was defined as an age-related and self-limited disorder, characterized by the following features (Tassinari *et al.*, 2005): 1) Epilepsy with different types of seizures including focal or generalized clonic or tonic-clonic seizures, absences, myoclonic or atonic seizures, etc.; 2) Neuropsychological impairment with global or selective regression of cognitive functions; 3) Transient motor impairment with ataxia, dyspraxia dystonia or unilateral deficits; 4) Typical EEG findings with diffuse or more or less unilateral ESES occurring in up to 85% of slow sleep. CSWSS syndrome, as defined above is a rare disorder, although several hundred of cases had already been reported (Galanopoulou *et al.*, 2000). In a study of 12,854 children with epilepsy the incidence of CSWSS syndrome was of 0.5% (Morikawa *et al.*, 1989). A slight preponderance in males is reported (Tassinari *et al.*, 2005).

Clinical features

Neuropsychological development: normal neuropsychological development was registered in the literature in only 60 to 75% of the cases (Dalla Bernardina *et al.*, 1989; Morikawa *et al.*, 1989, 1995; Tassinari *et al.*, 1992). A rapid neuropsychological impairment takes place after the appearance of ESES with deterioration of IQ, language, cognitive functions and behaviour. The latter include hyperkinesis, aggressiveness, bizarre or psychotic behaviours. Mental and behavioural deterioration evoking a frontal lobe syndrome has been described in children with spikes or spike-waves discharges in frontal lobe (Roulet-Perez *et al.*, 1993).

Motor impairment: is never permanent in functional cases and the most disabling motor disturbances are gate difficulties due to negative myoclonus in lower limbs. Orofacial dysfunction with dysarthria and dyspraxia (associated with persisting sialorrhea) has been reported in relation with ESES arising from Rolandic spikes (Fejerman & Di Blasi, 1987; Colamaria *et al.*, 1991). In a particularly symptomatic case of CSWSS which appeared years after a West syndrome, unilateral ESES was associated with a transitory "motor neglect" of one arm lasting during the morning hours and disappearing during evenings (Veggiotti *et al.*, 2005).

Seizures: it has been stated that a significant number of cases have seizures before the stage of ESES, and that in the majority of the cases these seizures were motor and focal, and occurred during sleep (Bureau, 1995, Tassinari *et al.*, 2005). Once the ESES is developed, the children present absence seizures, seizures with falls (usually due to negative myoclonus) or even status of absences or motor seizures. In one series of cases, epilepsy was severe in 93% of cases with numerous seizures per day (Bureau, 1995). Based on seizure patterns, three groups were proposed: 1) Patients with rare and nocturnal motor seizures (11%); 2) Patients with unilateral and/or generalized motor seizures occurring during sleep and also absences during wakefulness (44.5%); 3) Patients with rare nocturnal motor seizures and frequent atonic seizures leading to falls while awake (Tassinari *et al.*, 2002, 2005). Interestingly, tonic seizures are not registered in children with this syndrome, neither while awake, nor during sleep (Bureau, 1995; Tassinari *et al.*, 2005).

EEG features

Before the appearance of ESES waking EEGs show frequent focal spikes and associated diffuse SW discharges. During sleep there is an increase of these abnormalities *(Fig. 7)*. As we'll discuss later, in symptomatic cases with unilateral or predominantly unilateral involvement, a background asymmetry can be seen.

Once entering the ESES stage, the waking EEGs show diffuse bursts of 2-3 Hz discharges. As soon as the patients fall asleep, continuous diffuse SW, mainly at 1.5-2.5 Hz, appear *(Fig. 8)*. A quantitative measure of the EEG abnormalities is the spike-wave index (SWI), which represents the sum of all the minutes with SW discharges multiplied by 100 and divided by the total NREM recorded minutes (Galanopoulou *et al.*, 2000). Persistence of ESES during 85% to 100% of slow sleep was initially considered and essential criterion for diagnosis (Patri *et al.*, 1971; Tassinari *et al.*, 1985), but it was accepted later that CSWSS syndrome can be diagnosed in cases with a SWI less than 85% (Billard *et al.*, 1982; Yasuhara *et al.*, 1991; Beaumanoir, 1995b). During REM sleep the SWI decreases and focal spike discharges may become more prominent.

Aetiology

The syndrome of CSWSS appears in a significant number of children with pre-existing encephalopathies [up to 40% in one series (Bureau, 1995)]. The fact that the same clinico-EEG features are shared by previously normal children, does not point to a precise aetiology, but to the physiopathogenic mechanisms involved in the genesis of ESES. A family history of epilepsy is not markedly increased (Jayakar & Seshia, 1991; Bureau, 1995).

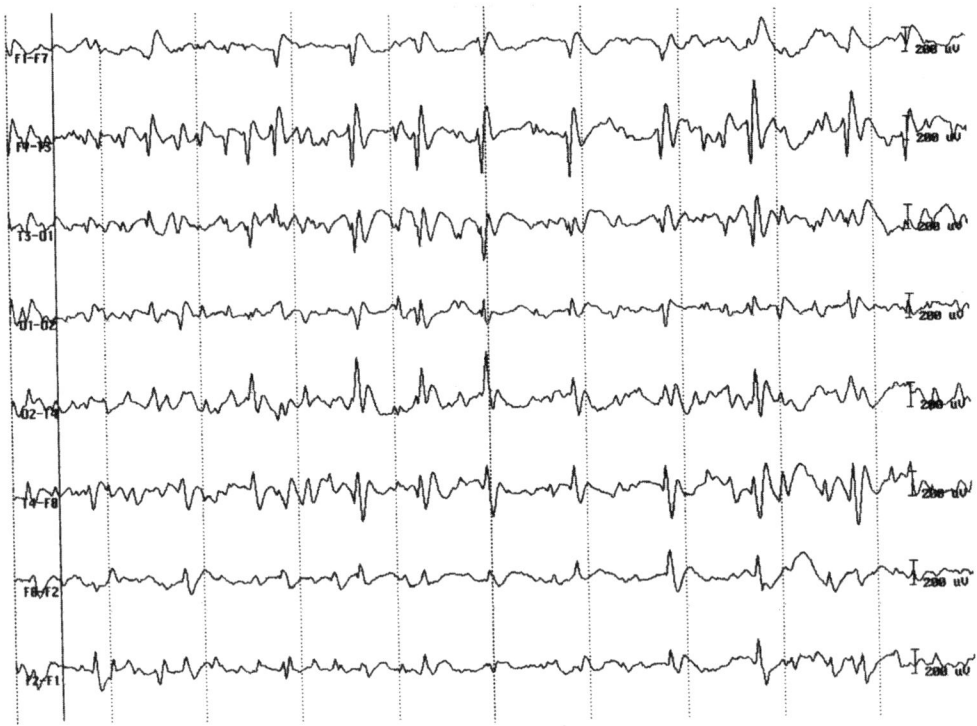

Figure 7. Eight years old girl with history of Rolandic seizures at 6 years of age. At 8 years she started with learning difficulties and some behaviour problems. Sleep EEG shows frequent bilateral spikes dominant in centrotemporal regions.

Differential Diagnosis

Diagnosis rest on recognition of clinical features and the demonstration of ESES in the EEG. This can be done with brief sleep recordings, but all-night sleep studies are recommended. Imaging studies will show focal or bilateral abnormalities according to the proportion of symptomatic cases. Abnormal neuroradiological signs were found in about 1/3 of the cases (Bureau, 1995).

Differential diagnosis is first due with the three related syndromes (ABPEC, SEBCECTS and LKS). However, the main responsibility lies in ruling out the Lennox-Gastaut syndrome (LGS). They have in common the presence of atypical absences, epileptic falls due to atonic or myoclonic-atonic seizures, and clonic or tonic-clonic seizures either focal or generalized, associated with neuropsychologic deterioration. EEG patterns are different and the main distinguishing feature is that tonic seizures occur almost always in LGS and never in CSWSS. Another epileptic syndrome to think about is epilepsy with myoclonic-astatic seizures (EMAS), but again, the EEG patterns are different and the neuropsychologic impairment which may be seen in around 1/3 of the patients with EMAS takes much more time to become evident than in CSWSS (Fejerman et al., 2005).

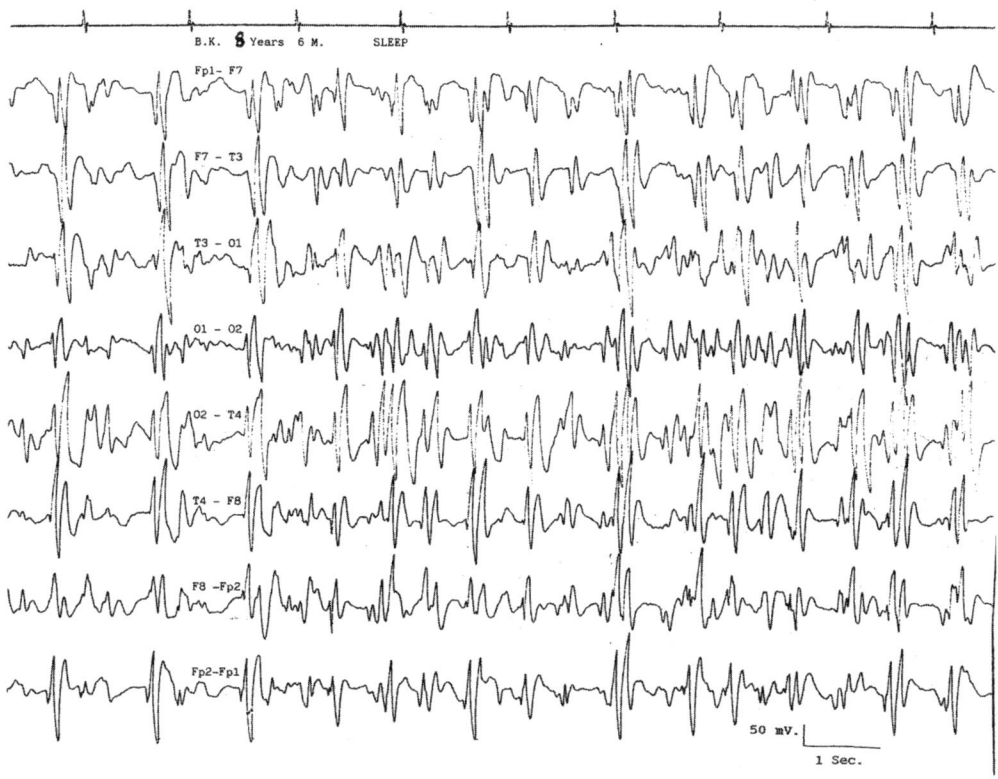

Figure 8. The same girl described in Fig. 7 after presenting clear bizarre behaviours. Sleep EEG shows now continuous spike and wave activities in more than 85% of the record.

Treatment

As stated before, we'll consider later in this chapter treatment for the 4 conditions which have ESES as a common group.

Prognosis and long-term evolution

It was generally stated that prognosis of CSWSS in terms of epilepsy was that seizures disappeared in all cases, whether they were lesional or non-lesional and whether epilepsy had been severe or not (Morikawa *et al.*, 1995; Dalla Bernardina *et al.*, 1989; Bureau, 1999; Tassinari *et al.*, 2005). In series with large follow up, the duration of epilepsy ranged from 4 years to 14 years and in 44% of the cases seizures disappeared before the end of ESES (Bureau, 1999; Tassinari *et al.*, 2005). ESES also disappears in all cases, with an average persistence until 11 years of age (Tassinari *et al.*, 2000). Focal abnormalities instead, may persist for a long time after the disappearance of ESES (Bureau, 1995). Despite the disappearance of seizures and the normalization of the EEG, the persistence of neuropsychological impairments obliges to be cautious regarding prognosis, even when certain degree of improvement in cognition and behaviour is seen in most of the patients. In a long follow up of 25 patients, low IQ scores and behavioural disturbances persisted in 50% of the cases (Tassinari et al., 2005). The poor prognosis is not related to the age of discovery of ESES or to the severity of epilepsy, but it may be related to the duration of ESES. A comprehensive and long-term follow up of one case showed details about evaluation of the boy's behaviour, language and cognitive functions suggesting a dysexecutive syndrome (Hommet et al., 2000). During the follow up of 4 cases for more than 8 years, no case of CSWSS evolving into another epileptic syndrome was encountered (Morikawa et al., 1995). In a 8 years old boy with occipito-temporal CSWS followed up during 2 years, major deficits in visual perception with normal verbal intelligence were found (Eriksson et al., 2003). Moreover, persistence of ESES during 17 months without behavioural changes was also reported (Gokyigit et al., 1986).

In *Table IV* data about our present series of 5 cases with CSWSS are shown.

Discussion

Epilepsy with CSWSS was defined in the ILAE's 1989 classification as the association of various types of seizures with an EEG pattern of continuous diffuse spike-waves during slow sleep which lasts years and causes the appearance of neuropsychologic impairments (Commission, 1989). The wide range of clinical manifestations associated with CSWSS has been repeatedly mentioned, especially regarding the points in common between LKS a CSWSS syndrome (Tassinari et al., 2005; Beaumanoir et al., 1995a, 1995b; Smith, 1998). The concept of different clinical syndromes with ESES was discussed (De Negri 1997). We are including here a new variant of clinical expressions in children with ESES appearing as an atypical evolution of BCECTS (see later in this Chapter). The finding of CSWS in ≥ 85% of the slow wave sleep was the inclusion criterion in a study performed on 32 patients observed in three centers in Italy (Veggiotti et al., 1999). Based on aetiology, a group of 13 cryptogenic cases and a group of 19 symptomatic cases were disclosed. The first group comprised 5 patients matching with the definitions of CSWSS syndrome,

Table IV. Follow-up of 5 children with CSWSS

Patient No.	Age at onset of BCECTS (years)	Age at worsening (years)	Age at last seizure (years)	Age at normal EEG (years)	Age when AED treatment stopped (years)	Present age (years)
1	3	6	6.5	7	14	19
2	4	7	9.5	12	14	22
3	3.5	6	8	10	12	24
4	3	6.5	9	11	13	13.5
5	5	7.5	-	-	-	10

CSWSS: Continuous spike-and-wave during slow sleep syndrome; BCECTS: Benign childhood epilepsy with centrotemporal spikes; AED: antiepileptic drug.

5 patients with typical clinic-EEG features of LKS, and 3 patients with status of BCECTS. The second group was composed by children with important pre-existing CNS lesions including hydrocephalus, prenatal clastic lesions and neuronal migration disorders as most common. In total, only 34% of the patients had the typical syndrome of CSWSS. The authors concluded that the ESES pattern itself should not define the syndrome.

We proposed, instead, that either idiopathic or symptomatic cases with ESES can present the clinical features of ABFEC, SEBCECTS, LKS or the syndrome of CSWSS. Physiopathogenic interpretation of the relation between location of initial spikes and symptomatology during ESES pointed to propagation of spike discharges into parasagital regions with frontal predominance for ABFEC (Aicardi 2000, Hahn 2000), into lower Rolandic areas in SEBCECTS (Fejerman & Di Blasi, 1987; Colamaria et al., 1991), propagation to posterior Sylvian areas in LKS (Morrell et al., 1995), and to frontal and perhaps limbic areas in the typical CSWSS syndrome (Fejerman et al., 2000). We also intended to demonstrate that 26 children with typical clinico-EEG features of idiopathic BCECTS evolved into ABFEC, SEBCECTS, LKS, and CSWSS (Fejerman et al., 2000). The most interesting point was that even when all the cases were idiopathic, the long term prognosis varied according to the final syndromes: children evolving into ABFEC and SEBCECTS had an ultimate good prognosis, while cases evolving into LKS and CSWSS syndrome had a guarded prognosis in terms of language or cognitive and behavioural impairments.

The feature in common of all these four atypical evolutions or syndromes related to BCECTS was the early onset of Rolandic seizures and CTS (e.g. between 3 and 5 years of age). This early onset in idiopathic partial epilepsies with evolution into ESES spectrum disorders was also registered in an interesting comparative study between 16 children with this evolution and 25 patients with idiopathic partial epilepsies without complications serving as controls (Saltik et al., 2005). Two families associating BCECTS and Epileptic syndrome with CSWS in first degree relatives were recently reported (De Tiege et al., 2006). The authors stated that their data suggested the existence of a common genetic basis between BCECTS and cryptogenic epilepsies with CSWSS, and that "these epileptic syndromes constitute edges of a continuum". However, the histories of the two probands show that they started at 4 and 2.5 years of age with clinic-EEG features of BCECTS, and around one year later, "despite of treatment with Valproate", developed CSWSS with clinical evidence of the typical syndrome of CSWSS in the first case and of ABPEC in the second. Both probands had antecedents of BCECTS in their respective fathers and grandparents. Interestingly, one of the cases had developmental delay before onset of BCECTS, which gives us the opportunity to recognize that the coexistence of BCECTS and CSWSS may be seen in idiopathic and in probably symptomatic cases. The fact that the second proband had to be implanted with a vagal stimulator points to a failure of all AEDs and perhaps the mixture of familial genetic factors plus some added personal non-genetic influence. How do we interpret then this coexistence: are both syndromes part of a continuum or just atypical evolutions of BCECTS?

We also want to call attention to the fact that a number of patients with BCECTS evolve into a different kind of CSWSS which we termed "mixed forms of atypical evolutions" because the patients presented ESES associated with clinical features of ABFEC, SEBCECTS, LKS and typical CSWSS (Fejerman et al., 2000). That is to say that the same children present ESES with alternating periods of inhibitory seizures, plus absences, plus myoclonia, with learning disorders but without language or behavioural problems (ABFEC), periods of status of Rolandic seizures during wakefulness and sleep (SEBCECTS), periods of acquired epileptic aphasia (LKS), and periods of bizarre behaviour with or without seizures (CSWSS) *(Fig. 9)*.

In *Table V* we show data of our new series of 4 patients with mixed forms of atypical evolution of BCECTS.

In *Table VI* we show data on follow-up of 39 patients with atypical evolution of BCECTS. *Tables I to VI* refer to patients followed at the J.P. Garrahan Hospital in Buenos Aires. In *Table VII* features on atypical evolution of BCECTS in 25 patients followed-up at the unit of child Neuropsychiatry in Verona are shown.

Regarding the cases of idiopathic occipital epilepsies (CEOP) showing also evolution into the ESES spectrum disorders, the general experience is more limited. Our first case with the Gastaut type of CEOP evolving into CSWSS presented a severe neuropsychologic deterioration *(Fig. 10)*, and our cases with this complication in the course of Panayiotopoulos syndrome also showed mixed symptoms of language, cognition, and behavioural impairments *(Fig. 11)*. One of the two reported cases in the literature with initial Gastaut type and one of the three with initial Panayiotopoulos syndrome remained with residual neuropsychiatric abnormalities (Fejerman *et al.*, 1991, 1998; Tenembaum *et al.*, 1997; Caraballo *et al.*, 2001; Ferrie *et al.*, 2002).

In *Tables VIII & IX* we present data about our 6 cases of PS who showed atypical clinical evolutions within the ESES spectrum in the EEG. Four of them had frequent inhibitory seizures associated with the ESES without significant neurosychological impairment. One patient presented typical electroclinical features of CSWSS and another patient showed a mixed form of atypical evolution. This last patient is now seizure free but with some residual language impairment, significant cognitive deficit and moderate mental retardation. By definition these 6 cases were idiopathic. Incidentally, one of the 4 children who evolved into ABFEC with inhibitory seizures, had at onset and at the same time clinical and EEG features of PS and BCECTS.

Finally, in *figure 12* we present a synthesis of concepts exposed in this chapter regarding the different pathways by which benign focal epilepsies in childhood, either BCECTS, Panayiotopoulos syndrome (PS) or the Gastaut type of COE, may arrive to the clinical spectrum associated

Table V. Follow-up of 4 children with mixed forms of atypical evolutions

Patient No.	Age at onset of BCECTS (years)	Age at worsening (years)	Age at last seizure (years)	Age at normal EEG (years)	Age when AED treatment stopped (years)	Present age (years)
1	3	6	7	7	12	14
2	3.5	4	6	13	-	14
3	3	4	6	-	-	10.5
4	4	5	6	-	-	12.5

BCECTS: Benign childhood epilepsy with centrotemporal spikes; AED: antiepileptic drug.

Table VI. Neuropsychological data on follow-up of 39 patients with atypical evolutions of BCECTS

Types of atypical evolutions	Number of Patients	Residual language impairment (N of patients)	Residual cognitive deficits (N of patients)	Residual behaviour abnormalities (N of patients)	Mental retardation (N of patients)
ABFEC	16	–	–	–	–
Status of BCECTS	10	–	1 mild learning disorder	–	–
LKS	4	2	2*	–	2 mild*
CSWSS	5	3	3*	2 patients*	2 moderate* 1 mild*
Mixed forms of atypical evolutions	4	2	1 moderate* 1 mild*	1 moderate* 1 mild*	1 moderate* 1 mild*

ABFEC: Atypical benign focal epilepsy of childhood; BCECTS: Benign childhood epilepsy with centrotemporal spikes; LKS: Landau Kleffner syndrome; CSWSS: Continuous spike-and-waves during slow sleep syndrome.
*The same as with language impairment.

Table VII. Atypical evolutions in 25 patients with BCECTS followed-up at the Unit of child neuropsychiatry, University of Verona*

Clinical features	N of patients
Absences	16
Absence status	9 of the 16 with absences
Inhibitory seizures	13
Language disturbances	9
Aphasia	3 of the 9 with language disturbances
Total duration of episodes with atypical features throughout evolution	
Less than 1 month	8
2 to 3 months	4
4 to 6 months	2
7 to 12 months	5
13 to 18 months	4
24 to 26 months	2

* Atypical features stopped between 8 and 13 years of age. EEG with electrical status epilepticus during sleep was present in 24 patients.

with ESES. In rare instances, children with BCECTS or with idiopathic occipital epilepsies present at onset the features of ABFEC, status of BCECTS or CSWSS. Obviously, according to common criteria, in the majority of patients with LKS and CSWSS there is no clearly evidence of precedent benign focal epilepsies of childhood.

Table VIII. Follow-up of 6 children with atypical evolutions of PS*

Patient No.	Age at onset of PS (years)	Age at worsening (years)	Age at last seizure (years)	Age at normal EEG (years)	Age when AED treatment stopped (years)	Age (years)
1	2.5	3.5	5	8	12	14
2	4	7	9	9	11	15
3	6	7	-	-	-	8
4	5	6.5	8	9	10	12
5	3	5	-	-	-	7
6	6	8	10	12	12	13

PS: Panayiotopoulos syndrome; AED: antiepileptic drug.
* Patient No. 6 was not included in our series of 192 cases with PS.

Table IX. Neuropsychological data on follow-up of 6 patients with atypical evolutions of PS*

Types of atypical evolutions	Number of Patients	Residual language impairment (N of patients)	Residual cognitive deficits (N of patients)	Residual behaviour abnormalities (N of patients)	Mental retardation (N of patients)
ABFEC	4	-	1 mild	-	-
CSWSS	1**	1 mild	1 mild	-	1 mild
Mixed forms of atypical evolutions	1	1 mild	1 moderate	-	1 moderate

PS: Panayiotopoulos syndrome; ABFEC: Atypical benign focal epilepsy of childhood; CSWSS: Continuous spike-and-waves during slow sleep syndrome.
* Status epilepticus, either motor or autonomic, is frequent in PS but it is not considered as part of an atypical evolution. No patient evolved into Landau Kleffner syndrome.
** This is a new patient with only 2 years of follow-up.

Treatment

In chapters 7 and 8 we already commented on all therapeutic alternatives for BCECTS and ICOE. We also quoted and presented data showing evidence of AED inducing aggravation of EEG and clinical symptoms in patients. Specific reports on this effect of Carbamazepine in patients with BCECTS (Caraballo et al., 1989; Guerrini et al., 1993, 1995; Prats et al., 1998; Fejerman et al., 2000; Kochen et al., 2002) were published. In the 2 cases of Caraballo et al. (1989) negative myoclonus induced by carbamazepine was documented through polygraphic recording, and in one of them the ESES disappeared after discontinuation of carbamazepine and reappeared on reintroduction of that AED. A quite recent report showed the same effect on one child with PS (Kikumoto et al., 2006). Data were given on more anecdotal cases treated with Phenobarbital and

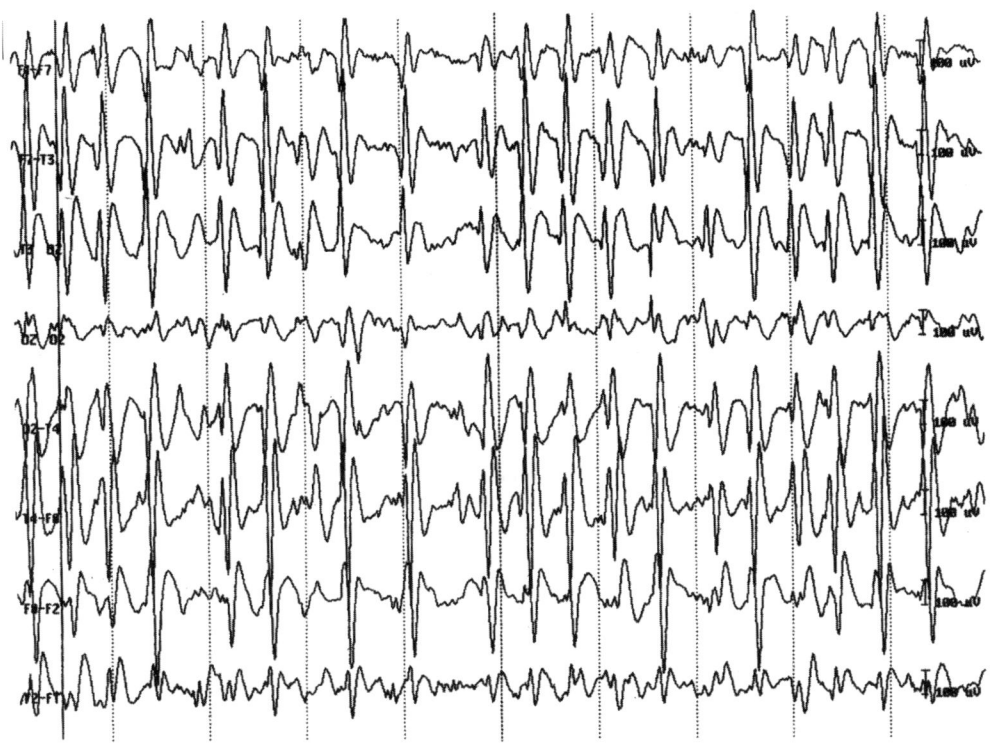

Figure 9. Six years old boy who started with BCECTS at age 4. Six months after medication with Carbamazepine he presented a "mixed form of atypical evolution". Slow sleep EEG shows diffuse continuous spike and wave activity.

Phenytoin (Guerrini *et al.*, 1995, 1998; Fejerman *et al.*, 2000; Saltik *et al.*, 2005). Valproate has been recommended for LKS (Marescaux *et al.*, 1990), although this drug has also been shown to induce continuous spike-wave discharges and worsening of clinical seizures in patients with BFEC (Prats *et al.*, 1998; Fejerman *et al.*, 2000; Prats Viñas, 2002).

There are consistent references about the preference of Benzodiazepines or Sulthiame to treat BFEC because they seem to cause a reduction in EEG discharges (De Negri *et al.*, 1993, 1997; Mitsudome *et al.*, 1997; Rating *et al.*, 2000; Engler, 2003, Chahine & Mikati, 2006). Incidentally, the power of Benzodiazepines to reduce rapidly the EEG discharges was recently considered misleading for diagnosis of distinct syndromes within the ESES spectrum. Clonazepam controlled spike-wave activities in two children with ESES but had no effect on cognitive and motor disorders, preventing a proper diagnosis (Bahi-Buisson *et al.*, 2006).

Sulthiame seems to be the oldest drug of choice according to several reports (Lerman & Lerman-Sagie, 1995; Gross-Selbeck, 1995; Wakai *et al.*, 1997; Doose *et al.*, 1998; Fejerman *et al.*, 2000; Huppke *et al.*, 2005).

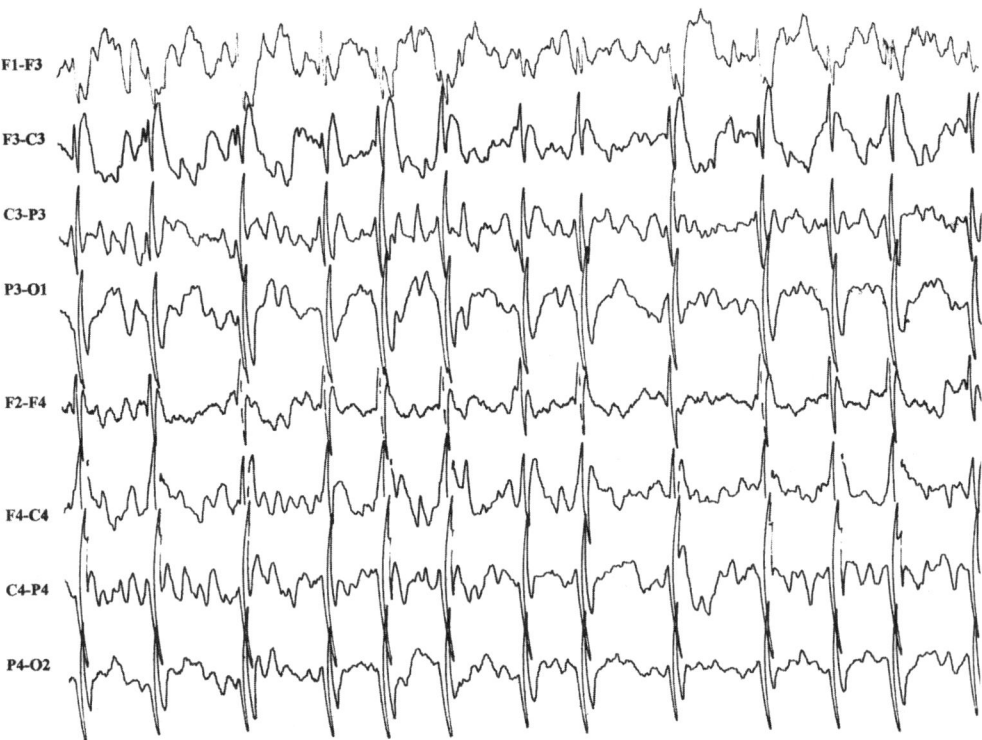

Figure 10. Sixteen years old boy who started at 8 years with frequent visual seizures and EEG with occipital spike wave paroxysms. Frequent visual and motor seizures, severe behavioural disturbances and learning impairment appeared. Sleep EEG shows continuous spike and waves during slow sleep.

Among the new AED, Lamotrigine was involved in inducing ESES in a couple of cases (Catania *et al.*, 1999; Cerminara *et al.*, 2004). There is one report stating that Gabapentin (GBP) was effective in controlling seizures in children with BCECTS, but the duration of the trial was not long enough to know about atypical evolutions in those cases (Burgeois *et al.*, 1998). A study with Oxcarbacepine with a follow up of 18 months considered it effective in preventing seizures, normalizing EEGs, and even in preserving cognitive functions and behavioural abilities (Tziridou *et al.*, 2005). Oxcarbazepine induced epileptic negative myoclonus in a child with symptomatic focal epilepsy (Hahn *et al.*, 2004), and more recently, was considered responsible of atypical evolution in three patients with BCECTS who already had some atypical features (Grosso *et al.*, 2006). We also saw two patients with Oxcarbazepine who developed ABFEC. Regarding to Topiramate, it was involved in one report (Montenegro & Guerreiro, 2002) and we also had one patient with BCECTS evolving into CSWSS after introduction of Topiramate, but we did not reintroduce the drugs to verify if it was associated with the reappearance of ESES. One case of LKS was treated with Levetiracetam (LVT) with control of seizures and language improvement (Kossoff *et al.*, 2003). LEV was tried in 12 children with CSWSS syndrome including cryptogenic

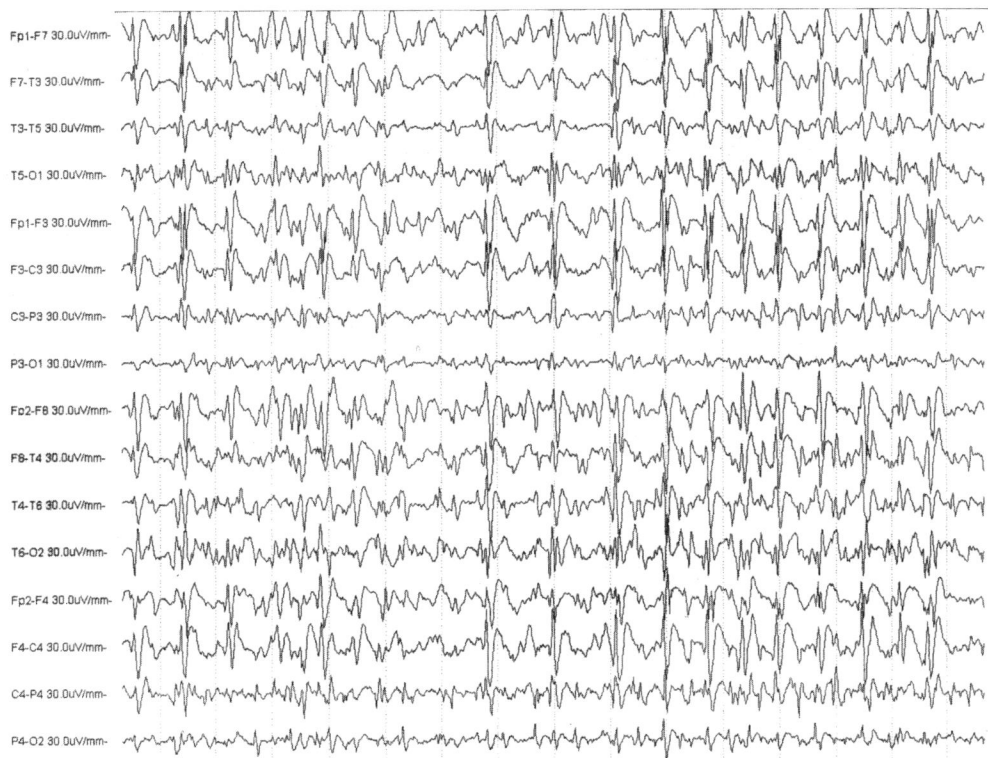

Figure 11. Six years old boy who started with Panayiotopoulos syndrome at 3 years of age. At 5.5 years of age absences and bizarre behaviours appeared. Sleep EEG shows almost continuous spike and waves activities.

and symptomatic cases (Aebi *et al.*, 2005). The study was retrospective and four patients showed retention of the drug after one year of treatment. The authors recognized that additional studies are needed in order to asses the place of LVT in the treatment of these epileptic conditions.

Treatment with high-dose corticosteroids was reported to yield the best results, and prolonged chronic or intermittent therapy may be necessary (Marescaux *et al.*, 1990; Lerman *et al.*, 1991; Caraballo *et al.*, 1999b; Tsuru *et al.*, 2000). In a series of 8 patients with Landau-Kleffner syndrome and 2 with the syndrome of continuous spike-and-waves during slow sleep treated with Prednisone 1 mg/kg/day for at least 6 months, all but 1 showed significant improvement in language, cognition, and behaviour (Sinclair and Snyder 2005). A multicenter control study to compare the efficacy of early versus delayed corticosteroid treatment in patients with typical Landau-Kleffner syndrome was recently recommended (Hirsch *et al.*, 2006). In 15 patients with electrical status epilepticus during slow-sleep, including one case with Landau-Kleffner syndrome, a strategy with a sequential order of different treatments was presented: 1) High-dose valproate (VPA); 2) A combination of VPA and Ethosuximide (ESM); 3) Short cycles of high-dose diazepam (DZP) for 7 days; 4) Intramuscular synthetic ACTH-Z therapy for 11-43 days. A remission of CSWS in the EEG was achieved by high-dose VPA in 7 of 15 trials, by VPA + ESM in 3/7 trials, by short cycles of high-dose DZP in 2/4 trials and by ACTH-Z therapy in 2/5 trials. A permanent remission

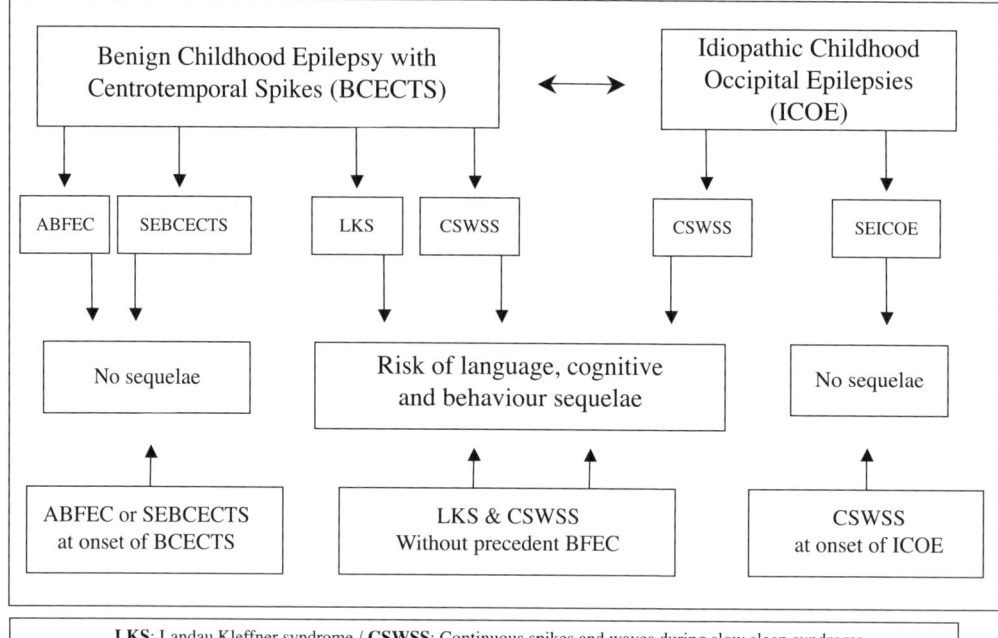

Figure 12. Benign focal epilepsies of childhood and disorders related with ESES.

of ESES syndrome was only achieved with high-dose VPA and/or combination of VPA + ESM in 10 patients (Inutsuka *et al.*, 2006). In isolated cases, the use of intravenous immunoglobulins was successful (Fayad *et al.*, 1997; Lagae *et al.*, 1998). In one report, 2 of 5 children with Landau-Kleffner syndrome receiving 2 g/kg of intravenous gamma-globulin over 4 days showed excellent response; in both children the severe language and EEG abnormalities completely resolved (Mikati *et al.*, 2002).

Proposed scheme of treatment

Now we center our interest in two questions: 1) Is it possible to prevent the evolution of Benign focal epilepsies of childhood BFEC) into ABPEC, SEBCECTS, status epilepticus in idiopathic childhood occipital epilepsies (SEICOE), LKS or CSWSS syndrome?; 2) What is the treatment of choice once one of these conditions is installed?

1) *How to prevent the atypical evolutions of BFEC*

According to present evidence, the risk of atypical evolutions of BFEC due to AEDs commonly used to treat BFEC is low (Corda *et al.*, 2001). Nevertheless, we should try to recognize factors of risk on clinical grounds and on EEGs in order to take steps to prevent complications. A main item is early onset of BCECTS (Fejerman *et al.*, 2000; Kramer *et al.*, 2002; Saltik *et al.*, 2005). The other salient factor of risk is constituted by several interictal EEG findings: multiple asynchronous spike-wave foci, long spike-wave clusters, generalized "absence-like spike-wave discharges, and, in general, an abundance of abnormalities during wakefulness and sleep (Massa et al., 2001).

The recommendations to prevent atypical evolutions may then be:
a) Avoid the use of classic AEDs (PB, PH, CMZ, VA) and some of the new AEDs (LTG, OXC, GBP) in patients with BFEC presenting atypical clinical features and/or excessive EEG abnormalities;
b) When these risks are evident, start treatment with Sulthiame or Benzodiazepines;
c) In patients with BFEC with clear generalized spike-wave discharges, VA may be a good chance. It is also the first choice in patients with the Gastaut type of CEOP;
d) In patients without the mentioned risks and presenting seizures only during night sleep, we recommend single doses of Clobazam at night;
e) Finally, a good alternative to discuss with parents in these patients without risks, is not to use medication.

2) *Treatment strategies in children with any of the epileptic encephalopathies with ESES, including the symptomatic cases*

a) Start discontinuation of the AED that the patient is taking and introduce Benzodiazepines, Ethosuximide (ETS), or Sulthiame. (SLT). A combination of two of these may also be used. One alternative is to admit the patient, stop the AEDs supposedly involved in the aggravation of the disease, or at least having showed no benefit, and administrate high oral doses of Diazepam (DZ) for one or two weeks. Thereafter the patient may be followed with ambulatory controls with DZ, or switched to Clobazam (CLZ), or lowering progressively the doses of DZ and adding Ethosuximide or Sulthiame (SLT). In our experience, we had good results with SLT in doses up to 20 mg/kg/day. If the case does not merit a hospital admission, or if there are difficulties or resistance to do it, the switch should be done more cautiously either adding CLZ, ETS, or SLT with a slow titration while the previous AEDs are being discontinued.
b) If no significant improvement is seen, the following indication is steroids in high doses. In our first two cases with SEBCECTS steroids were clearly effective to stop status and after a couple of weeks they were discontinued. In LKS steroids have to be maintained for several months at least, and sometimes improvement starts to be seen after two months (Caraballo et al., 1999b).
c) We reported on one case of status of the Gastaut type of CEOP who only responded to intravenous immunoglobulins (Fejerman et al., 1991; Tenembaum et al., 1997), and several cases with successful use of immunoglobulins in cases of LKS were also reported (Fayad et al., 1997; Lagae et al., 1998; Mikati et al., 2002).
d) We have already commented on the reported cases of LKS who underwent successful subpial transections (Morrell et al., 1992, 1995; Irwin et al., 2001) and Vagal nerve stimulation (Park, 2003).

References

• Aebi A, Poznanski N, Verheulpen D, *et al*. Levetiracetam efficacy in epileptic syndromes with continuous spikes and waves during slow sleep: experience in 12 cases. *Epilepsia* 2005; 46 (12): 1937-42.

• Aicardi J, Chevrie JJ. Atypical benign partial epilepsy of childhood. *Dev Med Child Neurol* 1982; 24: 281-92.

• Aicardi J. Atypical semiology of Rolandic epilepsy in some related syndromes. *Epileptic Disorders* 2000; 2 (Suppl 1): S5-S10.

• Bahi-Buisson N, Savini R, Eisermann M, *et al*. Misleading effects of clonazepam in symptomatic electrical status epilepticus during sleep syndrome. *Pediatr Neurol* 2006; 34 (2): 146-50.

• Baird G, Robinson RO, Boyd S, Charman T. Sleep electroencephalograms in young children with autism with and without regression. *Dev Med Child Neurol* 2006; 48 (7): 604-8.

• Beaumanoir A. The Landau-Kleffner syndrome. In: Roger J, Dravet C, Bureau M, *et al*. (Eds). *Epileptic syndromes in infancy, childhood and adolescence*. London: John Libbey, 1985: 181-91.

• Beaumanoir A. The Landau-Kleffner syndrome. In: Roger J, Dravet C, Bureau M, *et al*. (Eds). *Epileptic syndromes in infancy, childhood and adolescence* (2nd ed.). London: John Libbey, 1992: 231-44.

• Beaumanoir A. (1995a) About continuous or subcontinuous spike-wave activity during wakefulness: electroclinical correlations. In: Beaumanoir A, Bureau M, Deonna T, *et al*. (Eds). *Continuous spikes and waves during slow sleep: acquired epileptic aphasia and related conditions*. London: John Libbey, 1995: 115-8.

• Beaumanoir A. (1995b) EEG Data. In: Beaumanoir A, Bureau M, Deonna T, *et al*. (Eds). *Continuous spikes and waves during slow sleep: acquired epileptic aphasia and related conditions*. London: John Libbey, 1995: 217-23.

• Billard C, Autret A, Laffont F, *et al*. Electrical status epilepticus during sleep in children: a reappraisal from eight new cases. In: Sterman MB, Shouse MN, Passouant P (Eds). *Sleep and epilepsy*. London & New York: Academic Press, 1982: 481-91.

• Bishop DV. Age of onset and outcome in acquired aphasia with convulsive disorders (Landau-Kleffner syndrome). *Dev Med Child Neurol* 1985; 27: 705-12.

• Boulloche J, Husson A, Le Luyer B, Le Roux P. Dysphagie, troubles du langage et pointes-ondes centro-temporales. *Arch Franc Pediatr* 1990; 47: 115-7.

• Bourgeois B, Brown W, Pellock JM, *et al*. Gabapentin (Neurontin) monotherapy in children with Benign childhood epilepsy with centrotemporal spikes (BECTS): a 36-week, double blind, placebo-controlled study. *Epilepsia* 1998; 39 (6): 163 (Abstract).

• Bourgeois BF, Landau WM. Landau-Kleffner syndrome and temporal cortical volume reduction: cause or effect? *Neurology* 2004; 63 (7): 1152-3.

• Bureau M. Continuous spikes and waves during slow sleep (CSWS): definition of the syndrome. In: Beaumanoir A, Bureau M, Deonna T, *et al*. (Eds). *Continuous spikes and waves during slow sleep: acquired epileptic aphasia and related conditions*. London: John Libbey, 1995: 17-26.

• Bureau M. Electroclinical aspects and evolution of the syndrome of epilepsy with continuous spikes and waves during slow sleep (CSWS). *Epilepsi* (Turkey) 1999; 3: 102-10.

• Capovilla G, Beccaria F, Veggiotti P, *et al*. Ethosuximide is effective in the treatment of epileptic negative myoclonus in childhood partial epilepsy. *J Child Neurol* 1999; 14 (6): 395-400.

• Capovilla G, Rubboli G, Beccaria F, *et al*. Intermittent falls and fecal incontinence as a manifestation of epileptic negative myoclonus in idiopathic partial epilepsy of childhood. *Neuropediatrics* 2000; 31: 273-5.

• Caraballo R, Fontana E, Michelizza B, *et al*. CBZ inducing atypical absences, drop-spells and continuous spike and waves during slow sleep (CSWS). *Boll Lega It Epil* 1989; 66/67: 379-81.

- Caraballo R, Cersosimo R, Fejerman N. (1999a) A particular type of epilepsy in children with congenital hemiparesis associated with unilateral polymichrogyria. *Epilepsia* 1999; 40 (7): 865-7.

- Caraballo R, Yepez AL, Cersosismo R, Medina C, Fejerman N. (1999b) Afasia epiléptica adquirida. *Rev Neurol* 1999; 29 (10): 899-907.

- Caraballo RH, Astorino F, Cersosimo R, Soprano AM, Fejerman N. Atypical evolution in childhood epilepsy with occipital paroxysms (Panayiotopoulos type). *Epileptic Disord* 2001; 3 (3): 157-62.

- Catania S, Cross H, de Sousa C, Boyd S. Paradoxic reaction to lamotrigine in a child with benign focal epilepsy of childhood with centrotemporal spikes. *Epilepsia* 1999; 40 (11): 1657-60.

- Cerminara C, Montanaro ML, Curatolo P, Seri S. Lamotrigine-induced seizure aggravation and negative myoclonus in idiopathic rolandic epilepsy. *Neurology* 2004, 63 (2): 373-5.

- Chahine LM, Mikati MA. Benign pediatric localization-related epilepsies. *Epileptic Disord* 2006; 8 (4): 243-58.

- Christen HJ, Hanefeld F, Kruse E, *et al*. Foix-Chavany-Marie (anterior operculum) syndrome in childhood: a reappraisal of Worster-Drought syndrome. *Dev Med Child Neurol* 2000; 42 (2): 122-32.

- Colamaria V, Sgro V, Caraballo R, *et al*. Status epileptics in benign rolandic epilepsy manifesting as anterior operculum syndrome. *Epilepsia* 1991; 32: 329-34.

- Cole AJ, Andermann F, Taylor L, *et al*. The Landau-Kleffner syndrome of acquired epileptic aphasia: unusual clinical outcome, surgical experience, and absence of encephalitis. *Neurology* 1988; 38: 31-8.

- Commission on Classification and Terminology of the International League Against Epilepsy. Proposal for revised classification of epilepsies and epileptic syndromes. *Epilepsia* 1989; 30 (4): 389-99.

- Corda D, Gelisse P, Genton P, *et al*. Incidence of drug-induced aggravation in benign epilepsy with centrotemporal spikes. *Epilepsia* 2001; 42 (6): 754-9.

- Croona C, Kihlgren M, Lundberg S, *et al*. Neuropsychological findings in children with benign childhood epilepsy with centrotemporal spikes. *Dev Med Child Neurol* 1999; 41: 813-8.

- Da Silva EA, Chugani DC, Muzik O, Chugani HT. Landau-Kleffner syndrome: metabolic abnormalities in temporal lobe are a common feature. *J Child Neurol* 1997; 12: 489-95.

- Dalla Bernardina B, Tassinari CA, Dravet C, *et al*. Épilepsie partielle bénigne et état de mal électroencéphalique pendant le sommeil. *Rev Electroencephalogr Neurophysiol Clin* 1978; 8 (3): 350-3.

- Dalla Bernardina B, Fontana E, Michelizza B, *et al*. Partial epilepsies of childhood, bilateral synchronization, continuous spike-waves during slow sleep. In: Manelis S, Bental E, Loeber JN, *et al*. (Eds). *Advances in epileptology*. New York: Raven Press, 1989: 295-302.

- Dalla Bernardina B, Sgró V, Fejerman N. Epilepsy with centrotemporal spikes and related syndromes. In: Roger J, Bureau M, Dravet CH, *et al*. (Eds). *Epileptic syndromes in infancy, childhood and adolescence* (3rd ed.). Eastleigh: John Libbey, 2002: 181-202.

- Dalla Bernardina B, Sgró V, Fejerman N. Epilepsy with centrotemporal spikes and related syndromes. In: Roger J., Bureau M., Dravet CH, *et al*. (Eds). *Epileptic syndromes in infancy, childhood and adolescence* (4th ed.). Montrouge: John Libbey Eurotext, 2005: 203-25.

- De Negri M, Baglietto MG, Biancheri R, *et al*. Electrical status epilepticus in childhood: treatment with short cycles of high dosage benzodiazepine. *Brain Dev* 1993; 15 (4): 311-2.

- De Negri M. Electrical status epilepticus during sleep (ESES). Different clinical syndromes: towards a unifying view? *Brain Dev* 1997; 19: 447-51.

- De Negri M, Baglietto MG, Gaggero R. Benzodiazepine (BDZ) treatment of benign childhood epilepsy with centrotemporal spikes. *Brain Dev* 1997; 19 (7): 506.

- De Saint-Martin A, Petiau C, Massa R, *et al*. Idiopathic Rolandic epilepsy with "interictal" facial myoclonia and oromotor deficit: a longitudinal EEG and PET study. *Epilepsia* 1999; 40: 614-20.

- De Tiege X, Goldman S, Verheulpen D, *et al*. Coexistence of idiopathic rolandic epilepsy and CSWS in two families. *Epilepsia* 2006; 47 (10): 1723-7.

- De Volder AG, Michel C, Thauvoy C, *et al*. Brain glucose utilization in acquired childhood aphasia associated with a sylvian arachnoid cyst: recovery after shunting as demonstrated by PET. *J Neurol Neurosurg Psychiatry* 1994; 57: 296-300.

- Deonna T, Beaumanoir A, Gaillard F, Assal G. Acquired aphasia in childhood with seizure disorder: a heterogeneous syndrome. *Neuropediatrie* 1977; 8: 263-73.

- Deonna T, Fletcher P, Voumard C. Temporary regression during language acquisition: a linguistic analysis of a 21/2 year old child with epileptic aphasia. *Dev Med Child Neurol* 1982; 24: 156-63.

- Deonna T, Ziegler AL, Despland PA. Combined myoclonic-astatic and "benign" focal epilepsy of childhood ("atypical benign partial epilepsy of childhood"). A separate syndrome? *Neuropediatrics* 1986; 17 (3): 144-51.

- Deonna T. Acquired epileptiform aphasia in children (Landau-Kleffner syndrome). *J Clin Neurophysiol* 1991; 8: 288-98.

- Deonna T, Roulet E, Fontan D, Marcoz JP. Speech and oromotor deficits of epileptic origin in benign partial epilepsy of childhood with rolandic spikes (BPERS). Relationship to the acquired aphasia-epilepsy syndrome. *Neuropediatrics* 1993; 24 (2): 83-7.

- Deonna T, Roulet E. Acquired epileptic aphasia (AEA): definition of the syndrome and current problems. In Beaumanoir A, Bureau M, Deonna T, *et al*. (Eds). *Continuous spikes and waves during slow sleep. Electrical status epilepticus during slow sleep. Acquired epileptic aphasia and related conditions*. London: John Libbey, 1995: 37-45.

- Deonna T. Trastornos del lenguaje y epilepsia. In: Narbona J, Chevrie-Muller C (Eds). *El lenguaje del niño*. Barcelona: Masson, 1997: 387-400.

- Doose H, Neubauer B, Carlsson G. Children with benign focal sharp waves in the EEG-developmental disorders and epilepsy. *Neuropediatrics* 1996; 27 (5): 227-41.

- Doose AH, Baier WK, Ernst JP. Benign partial epilepsy: treatment with sulthiame. *Dev Med Child Neurol* 1998; 30: 683-4.

- Dugas M, Franc S, Loic GC, Lecendreux M. Evolution of acquired epileptic aphasia with or without continuous spikes and waves during slow sleep. In: Beaumanoir A, Bureau M, Deonna T, *et al*. (Eds). *Continuous spikes and waves during slow sleep. Electrical status epilepticus during slow sleep. Acquired epileptic aphasia and related conditions*. London: John Libbey, 1995: 47-55.

- Dulac O, Billard C, Arthuis M. Aspects électro-cliniques et évolutifs dans le syndrome aphasie-épilepsie. *Arch Fr Pediatr* 1983; 40: 299-308.

- Echenne B, Cheminal R, Rivier F, *et al*. Epileptic encephalopathic abnormalities and developmental dysphasias: study of 32 patients. *Brain Dev* 1992; 14: 216-25.

- Engel J Jr; International League Against Epilepsy (ILAE). A proposed diagnostic scheme for people with epileptic seizures and with epilepsy: report of the ILAE Task Force on Classification and Terminology. *Epilepsia* 2001; 42 (6): 796-803.

- Engler F, Maeder-Ingvar M, Roulet E, Deonna T. Treatment with sulthiame (Ospolot) in benign partial epilepsy of childhood and related syndromes: an open clinical and EEG study. *Neuropediatrics* 2003; 34 (2): 105-9.

- Eriksson K, Kylliainen A, Hirvonen K, *et al*. Visual agnosia in a child with non-lesional occipito-temporal CSWS. *Brain Dev* 2003; 25 (4): 262-7.

- Fayad MN, Choueiri R, Mikati M. Landau-Kleffner syndrome: consistent response to repeated intravenous gamma-globulin doses: a case report. *Epilepsia* 1997; 38: 489-94.

- Fejerman N, Medina CS. *Convulsiones en la infancia* (2nd ed.). Buenos Aires: El Ateneo, 1986.

- Fejerman N, Di Blasi AM. Status epilepticus of benign partial epilepsies in children: report of two cases. *Epilepsia* 1987; 28 (4): 351-5.

- Fejerman N, Tenembaum S, Medina CS, *et al*. Continuous spike-waves during slow-wave sleep and awake in a case of childhood epilepsy with occipital paroxysms: clinical correlations. *Epilepsia* 1991; 32 (Suppl 1): 16.

- Fejerman N. Atypical evolutions of benign partial epilepsies in children. *Int Pediatr* 1996; 11: 351-6.

- Fejerman N, Caraballo R, Tenembaum S. Epilepsias parciais idiopaticas. In: Costa da Costa J, Palmini A, Yacubian EMT, Cavalheiro EA (Eds). *Fundamentos Neurobiológicos das Epilepsias*. Sao Paulo: Lemos, 1998.

- Fejerman N, Caraballo R, Tenembaum S. Atypical evolutions of benign localization-related epilepsies in children: Are they predictable? *Epilepsia* 2000; 41 (4): 380-90.

- Fejerman N. Epileptic syndromes and diseases. In: Aminoff M, Daroff rB (Eds). *Encyclopedia of the Neurological Sciences*. San Diego: Academic Press, 2003: 264-88.

- Fejerman N, Caraballo R, Cersosimo R. Ketogenic diet in patients with Dravet syndrome and myoclonic epilepsies in infancy and early childhood. In: Delgado-Escueta AV, Guerrini R, Medina MT, *et al*. (Eds). *Myoclonic Epilepsies, Advances in Neurology Series*. Lippincott Williams & Wilkins, 2005: 299-305.

- Fejerman N, Engel J. Landau Kleffner syndrome. In: Engel J, Fejerman N (Eds). MedLink Neurology (Section of Epilepsy). San Diego: MedLink Corporation, 2006. Available at www.medlink.com.

- Fejerman N. Benign childhood epilepsy with centrotemporal spikes. In: Engel J, Pedley TA (Eds). *Epilepsy: a comprehensive textbook*. Philadelphia: Lippincott Williams & Wilkins, 2007: In Press.

- Ferrie CD, Koutroumanidis M, Rowlinson S, Sanders S, Panayiotopoulos CP. Atypical evolution of Panayiotopoulos syndrome: a case report. *Epileptic Disord* 2002; 4 (1): 35-42.

- Galanopoulou A, Bojko A, Lado F, Moshe SL. The spectrum of neuropsychiatric abnormalities associated with electrical status epilepticus in sleep. *Brain Dev* 2000; 22: 279-95.

- Gokyigit A, Apak S, Caliskan A. Electrical status epilepticus lasting for 17 months without behavioural changes. *Electroencephalogr Clin Neurophysiol* 1986; 63: 32-34.

- Gordon N. Acquired aphasia in childhood: the Landau-Kleffner syndrome. *Dev Med Child Neurol* 1990; 32: 267-74.

- Gordon N. The Landau-Kleffner syndrome: increase understanding. *Brain Dev* 1997; 19: 311-6.

- Gregory DL, Farrell K, Wong PK. Partial status epilepticus in benign childhood epilepsy with centrotemporal spikes: are independent right and left seizures a risk factor? *Epilepsia* 2002; 43 (8): 936-40.

- Grosso S, Balestri M, Di Bartolo RM, *et al*. Oxcarbazepine and atypical evolution of benign idiopathic focal epilepsy of childhood. *Eur J Neurol* 2003; 13 (10): 1142-5.

- Gross-Selbeck G. Treatment of "benign" partial epilepsies of childhood, including atypical forms. *Neuropediatrics* 1995; 26 (1): 45-50.

- Guerreiro MM, Camargo EE, Kato M, *et al*. Brain single photon emission computed tomography imaging in Landau-Kleffner syndrome. *Epilepsia* 1996; 37: 60-7.

- Guerrini R, Dravet C, Genton P, *et al*. Epileptic negative myoclonus. *Neurology* 1993; 43: 1078-83.

- Guerrini R, Belmonte A, Strumia S, Hirsch E. Exacerbation of epileptic negative myoclonus by carbamazepine or phenobarbital in children with atypical benign rolandic epilepsy. *Epilepsia* 1995; 36 (Suppl 3): S65.

- Guerrini R, Belmonte A, Genton P. Antiepileptic drug-induced worsening of seizures in children. *Epilepsia* 1998; 39 (Suppl 3); S2-S10.

- Guzzetta E, Battaglia D, Veredice C, *et al.* Early thalamic injury associated with epilepsy and continuous spike-wave during slow sleep. *Epilepsia* 2005; 46 (6): 889-900.

- Hahn A. Atypical benign partial epilepsy/pseudo-Lennox syndrome. *Epileptic Disord* 2000; 2 (Suppl 1): S11-S17.

- Hahn A, Pistohl J, Neubauer BA, Stephani U. Atypical "benign" partial epilepsy or pseudo-Lennox syndrome. Part I: symptomatology and long-term prognosis. *Neuropediatrics* 2001; 32 (1): 1-8.

- Hahn A, Fischenbeck A, Stephani U. Induction of epileptic negative myoclonus by oxcarbazepine in symptomatic epilepsy. *Epileptic Disord* 2004; 6 (4): 271-4.

- Hamano S, Mochizuki M, Morikawa T. Phenobarbital-induced atypical absence seizure in benign childhood epilepsy with centrotemporal spikes. *Seizure* 2002; 11 (3): 201-4.

- Hirsch E, Marescaux C, Maquet P, *et al.* Landau-Kleffner syndrome: a clinical an EEG study of five cases. *Epilepsia* 1990; 31: 756-67.

- Hirsch E, Maquet P, Metz-Lutz MN, *et al.* The eponym "Landau-Kleffner syndrome" should not be restricted to childhood-acquired aphasia with epilepsy. In: Beaumanoir A, Bureau M, Deonna T, *et al.* (Eds). *Continuous spikes and waves during slow sleep. Electrical status epilepticus during slow sleep. Acquired epileptic aphasia and related conditions.* London: John Libbey, 1995: 57-62.

- Hirsch E, Valenti MP, Rudolf G, *et al.* Landau-Kleffner syndrome is not an eponymic badge of ignorance. *Epilepsy Res* 2006; 70 (2-3 Suppl): 239-47.

- Holmes GL, McKeever M, Saunders Z. Epileptiform activity in aphasia of childhood: an epiphenomenon? *Epilepsia* 1981; 22: 631-9.

- Hommet C, Billard C, Barthez MA, *et al.* Continuous spikes and waves during slow sleep (CSWS): outcome in adulthood. *Epileptic Disorders* 2000; 2 (2): 107-12.

- Huppke P, Kallenberg K, Gartner J. Perisylvian polymichrogyria in Landau-Kleffner syndrome. *Neurology* 2005; 64 (9): 1660.

- Inutsuka M, Kobayashi K, Oka M, *et al.* Treatment of epilepsy with electrical status epilepticus during slow sleep and its related disorders. *Brain Dev* 2006; 28 (5): 281-6.

- Irwin K, Birch V, Lees J, *et al.* Multiple subpial transection in Landau-Kleffner syndrome. *Dev Med Child Neurol* 2001; 43 (4): 248-52.

- Isnard J, Fischer C, Bastuji H, *et al.* Auditory early (BAEP) and middle-latency (MLAEP) evoked potentials in patients with CSWS and Landau-Kleffner syndrome. In: Beaumanoir A, Bureau M, Deonna T, *et al.* (Eds). *Continuous spikes and waves during slow sleep. Electrical status epilepticus during slow sleep. Acquired epileptic aphasia and related conditions.* London: John Libbey, 1995: 99-103.

- Jayakar PB, Seshia SS. Electrical status epilepticus during slow-wave sleep: a review. *J Clin Neurophysiol* 1991; 8 (3): 299-311.

- Kanazawa O, Kawai I. Status epilepticus characterized by repetitive asymmetrical atonia: two cases accompanied by partial seizures. *Epilepsia* 1990; 31 (5): 536-43.

- Kang HC, Kim HD, Lee YM, Han SH. Landau-Kleffner syndrome with mitochondrial respiratory chain-complex I deficiency. *Pediatr Neurol* 2006; 35 (2): 158-61.

- Kikumoto K, Yoshinaga H, Oka M, *et al.* EEG and seizure exacerbation induced by carbamazepine in Panayiotopoulos syndrome. *Epileptic Disord* 2006; 8 (1): 53-6.

- Klein SK, Tuchman RF, Rapin I. The influence of premorbid language skills and behaviour on language recovery in children with verbal auditory agnosia. *J Child Neurol* 2000; 15 (1): 36-43.

- Kobayashi K, Nishibayashi N, Ohtsuka Y, *et al*. Epilepsy with electrical status epilepticus during slow sleep and secondary bilateral synchrony. *Epilepsia* 1994; 35 (5): 1097-103.

- Kochen S, Giagante B, Oddo S. Spike-and-wave complexes and seizure exacerbation caused by carbamazepine. *Eur J Neurol* 2002; 9: 41-7.

- Kossoff EH, Boatman D, Freeman JM. Landau-Kleffner syndrome responsive to levetiracetam. *Epilepsy Behav* 2003; 4 (5): 571-5.

- Kramer U, Zelnik N, Lerman-Sagie T, Shahar E. Benign childhood epilepsy with centrotemporal spikes: clinical characteristics and identification of patients at risk of multiple seizures. *J Child Neurol* 2002; 17 (1): 17-9.

- Lagae LG, Silberstein J, Gillis PL, Casaer PJ. Successful use of intravenous immunoglobulins in Landau-Kleffner syndrome. *Pediatr Neurol* 1998; 18: 165-8.

- Landau WM, Kleffner FR. Syndrome of acquired aphasia with convulsive disorder in childhood. *Neurology* 1957; 7: 523-30.

- Lerman P. Seizures induced or aggravated by anticonvulsants. *Epilepsia* 1986; 27 (6): 706-10.

- Lerman P, Lerman-Sagie T, Kivity S. Effect of early corticosteroid therapy for Landau-Kleffner syndrome. *Dev Med Child Neurol* 1991; 33: 257-60.

- Lerman P, Lerman-Sagie T. Sulthiame revisited. *J Child Neurol* 1995; 10 (3): 241-2.

- Lombroso CT, Erba G. Primary and secondary bilateral synchrony in epilepsy. *Arch Neurol* 1970; 22: 321-34.

- Luat AF, Asano E, Juhasz C, *et al*. Relationship between brain glucose metabolism positron emission tomography (PET) and electroencephalography (EEG) in children with continuous spike-and-wave activity during slow-wave sleep. *J Child Neurol* 2005; 20 (8): 682-90.

- Luat AF, Chugani HT, Asano E, *et al*. Episodic receptive aphasia in a child with Landau-Kleffner Syndrome: PET correlates. *Brain Dev* 2006; 28 (9): 592-6.

- Maccario M, Hefferen SJ, Keblusek SJ, Lipinski KA. Developmental dysphasia and electroencephalographic abnormalities. *Dev Med Child Neurol* 1982; 24: 141-55.

- Majerus S, Laureys S, Collette F, *et al*. Phonological short-term memory networks following recovery from Landau and Kleffner syndrome. *Hum Brain Mapp* 2003; 19 (3): 133-44.

- Mantovani JF, Landau WF. Acquired aphasia with convulsive disorder: course and prognosis. *Neurology* 1980; 30: 524-9.

- Maquet P, Hirsch E, Dive D, *et al*. Cerebral glucose utilization during sleep in Landau-Kleffner syndrome: a PET study. *Epilepsia* 1990; 31: 778-83.

- Marescaux C, Hirsch E, Finck S, *et al*. Landau-Kleffner syndrome: a pharmacologic study of five cases. *Epilepsia* 1990; 31: 768-77.

- Massa R, de Saint-Martin A, Carcangiu R, *et al*. EEG criteria predictive of complicated evolution in idiopathic Rolandic epilepsy. *Neurology* 2001; 57: 1071-9.

- McVicar KA, Shinnar S. Landau-Kleffner syndrome, electrical status epilepticus in slow wave sleep, and language regression in children. *Ment Retard Dev Disabil Res Rev* 2004; 10 (2): 144-9.

- Mikati MA, Saab R, Fayad MN, Choueiri RN. Efficacy of intravenous immunoglobulin in Landau-Kleffner syndrome. *Pediatr Neurol* 2002; 26 (4): 298-300.

• Mitsudome A, Ohfu M, Yasumoto S, et al. The effectiveness of clonazepam on the rolandic discharges. *Brain Dev* 1997; 19 (4): 274-8.

• Montenegro MA, Guerreiro MM. Electrical status epilepticus of sleep in association with Topiramate. *Epilepsia* 2002; 43 (11): 1436-40.

• Morikawa T, Seino M, Watanabe Y, et al. Clinical relevance of continuous spike-waves discharges during slow-wave sleep. In: Manelis S, Bental E, Loeber JN, Dreifuss FE (Eds). *Advances in epileptology*. New York: Raven Press, 1989: 359-63.

• Morikawa T, Seino M, Watanabe M. Long-term outcome of CSWS syndrome. In: Beaumanoir A, Bureau M, Deonna T, et al. (Eds). *Continuous spikes and waves during slow sleep: acquired epileptic aphasia and related conditions*. London: John Libbey, 1995: 27-36.

• Morrell F, Whisler WW, Smith MC, et al. Clinical outcome in Landau-Kleffner syndrome treated by multiple subpial transection. *Epilepsia* 1992; 33 (Suppl 3): 100.

• Morrell F, Whisler WW, Smith MC, et al. Landau-Kleffner syndrome: treatment with subpial intracortical transection. *Brain* 1995; 118: 1529-46.

• Mouridsen SE, Videbaek C, Sogaard H, Andersen AR. Regional blood-flow measured by HMPAO and SPECT on a 5-year-old boy with Landau-Kleffner syndrome. *Neuropediatrics* 1993; 24: 47-50.

• Nanba Y, Maegaki Y. Epileptic negative myoclonus induced by carbamazepine in a child with BECTS. Benign childhood epilepsy with centrotemporal spikes. *Pediatr Neurol* 1999; 21 (3): 664-7.

• Nass R, Heier L, Walker R. Landau-Kleffner syndrome: temporal lobe tumor resection results in good outcome. *Pediatr Neurol* 1993; 9: 303-5.

• Oguni H, Sato F, Hayashi K, Wang PJ, Fukuyama Y. A study of unilateral brief focal atonia in childhood partial epilepsy. *Epilepsia* 1992; 33 (1): 75-83.

• Oguni H, Uehara T, Imai K, Osawa M. Atonic epileptic drop attacks associated with generalized spike-and-slow wave complexes: video-polygraphic study in two patients. *Epilepsia* 1997; 38 (7): 813-8.

• Oguni H, Uehara T, Tanaka T, et al. Dramatic effect of ethosuximide on epileptic negative myoclonus: implications for the neurophysiological mechanism. *Neuropediatrics* 1998; 29 (1): 29-34.

• Otero E, Cordova S, Diaz F, et al. Acquired epileptic aphasia (the Landau-Kleffner syndrome) due to neurocysticercosis. *Epilepsia* 1989; 30 (5): 564-8.

• Paetau R, Granstrom ML, Blomstedt G, et al. Magnetoencephalography in presurgical evaluation of children with the Landau-Kleffner syndrome. *Epilepsia* 1999; 40 (3): 326-35.

• Panayiotopoulos CP. *The Epilepsies*. Oxfordshire: Bladon medical publishing, 2005.

• Paquier PF, Van Dongen HR, Loonen CB. The Landau-Kleffner syndrome or "acquired aphasia with convulsive disorder". Long-term follow up of six children and a review of the recent literature. *Arch Neurol* 1992; 49: 354-9.

• Park YD. The effects of vagus nerve stimulation therapy on patients with intractable seizures and either Landau-Kleffner syndrome or autism. *Epilepsy Behav* 2003; 4 (3): 286-90.

• Parmeggiani L, Seri S, Bonanni P, Guerrini R. Electrophysiological characterization of spontaneous and carbamazepine-induced epileptic negative myoclonus in benign childhood epilepsy with centrotemporal spikes. *Clin Neurophysiol* 2004; 115 (1): 50-8.

• Pascual-Castroviejo I, Lopez Martin V, Martinez Bermejo A, Perez Higueras A. Is cerebral arteritis the cause of the Landau-Kleffner syndrome? Four cases in childhood with angiographic study. *Can J Neurol Sci* 1992; 19: 46-52.

• Patry G, Lyagoubi S, Tassinari CA. Subclinical "electrical status epilepticus" induced by sleep in children. A clinical and electroencephalographic study of six cases. *Arch Neurol* 1971; 24 (3): 242-52.

- Perniola T, Margari L, Buttiglione M, *et al*. A case of Landau-Kleffner syndrome secondary to inflammatory demyelinating disease. *Epilepsia* 1993; 39: 551-6.

- Picard A, Cheliout Heraut F, Bouskraoui M, *et al*. Sleep EEG and developmental dysphasia. *Dev Med Child Neurol* 1998; 40: 595-9.

- Praline J, Hommet C, Barthez MA, *et al*. Outcome at adulthood of the continuous spike-waves during show sleep and Landau-Kleffner syndromes. *Epilepsia* 2003; 44 (11): 1434-40.

- Prats JM, Garaizar C, García-Nieto ML, Madoz P. Antiepileptic drugs and atypical evolution of idiopathic partial epilepsy. *Pediatr Neurol* 1998; 18: 402-6.

- Prats-Vinas JM. Complicated benign partial epilepsy. *Rev Neurol* 2002; 35 (1): 73-9.

- Rapin I, Mattis S, Rowan AJ, Golden GG. Verbal auditory agnosia in children. *Dev Med Child Neurol* 1977; 19: 192-207.

- Rating D, Wolf C, Bast T. Sulthiame as monotherapy in children with benign childhood epilepsy with centrotemporal spikes: a 6-month randomized, double-blind, placebo-controlled study. Sulthiame Study Group. *Epilepsia* 2000; 41 (10): 1284-8.

- Robinson RO, Baird G, Robinson G, Simonoff E. Landau-Kleffner syndrome: course and correlates with outcome. *Dev Med Child Neurol* 2001; 43 (4): 243-7.

- Rossi PG, Parmeggiani A, Posar A, *et al*. Landau-Kleffner syndrome (LKS): long-term follow-up and links with electrical status epilepticus during sleep (ESES). *Brain Dev* 1999; 21 (2): 90-8.

- Roulet E, Deonna T, Despland PA. Prolonged intermittent drooling and oromotor apraxia in benign childhood epilepsy with centrotemporal spikes. *Epilepsia* 1989; 30: 564-8.

- Roulet Perez E, Davidoff V, Despland PA, Deonna T. Mental and behavioural deterioration of children with epilepsy and CSWS: acquired epileptic frontal syndrome. *Dev Med Child Neurol* 1993; 35 (8): 661-74.

- Rubboli G, Parmeggiani L, Tassinari CA. Frontal inhibitory spike component associated with epileptic negative myoclonus. *Electroencephalography & clinical neurophysiology* 1995; 95: 201-5.

- Salas-Puig J, Perez-Jimenez A, Thomas P, *et al*. Opercular epilepsies with oromotora dysfunction. In: Guerrini R, Aicardi J, Andermann F, Hallet R (Eds). *Epilepsy and movement disorders*. London: Cambridge University Press, 2002: 251-68.

- Saltik S, Uluduz D, Cokar O, *et al*. A clinical EEG study on idiopathic partial epilepsies with evolution into ESES spectrum disorders. *Epilepsia* 2005; 46 (4): 524-33.

- Scholtes FB, Hendriks MP, Renier WO. Cognitive deterioration and electrical status epilepticus during slow sleep. *Epilepsy Behav* 2005; 6 (2): 167-73.

- Septien L, Gras P, Giroud M, Dumas R. Syndrome bi-operculaire antérieur aigu d'origine critique dans l'épilepsie à paroxysmes rolandiques. *Rev Neurol* 1992 ; 148: 712-5.

- Shafrir Y, Prensky AL. Acquired epileptiform opercular syndrome: a second case report, review of the literature, and comparison to the Landau-Kleffner syndrome. *Epilepsia* 1995; 36: 1050-7.

- Shields WD, Saslow E. Myoclonic, atonic, and absence seizures following institution of carbamazepine therapy in children. *Neurology* 1983; 33 (11): 1487-9.

- Sinclair DB, Snyder TJ. Corticosteroids for the treatment of Landau-Kleffner syndrome and continuous spike-wave discharge during sleep. *Pediatr Neurol* 2005; 32 (5): 300-6.

- Smith MC, Pierre-Louis SJ, Kanner AM, *et al*. Pathological spectrum of acquired epileptic aphasia of childhood. *Epilepsia* 1992; 33 (Suppl 3): 115.

- Smith MC. Landau-Kleffner syndrome and continuous spikes and waves during slow sleep. In: Engel J, Pedley TA (Eds). *Epilepsy: a comprehensive textbook*. Philadelphia/New York: Lippincott-Raven, 1998: 2367-77.

- Smith MC, Hoeppner TJ. Epileptic encephalopathy of late childhood: Landau-Kleffner syndrome and the syndrome of continuous spikes and waves during slow-wave sleep. *J Clin Neurophysiol* 2003; 20 (6): 462-72.

- Sobel DF, Aung M, Otsubo H, Smith MC. Magnetoencephalography in children with Landau-Kleffner syndrome and acquired epileptic aphasia. *Am J Neuroradiol* 2000; 21 (2): 301-7.

- Soprano AM, Garcia EF, Caraballo R, Fejerman N. Acquired epileptic aphasia: neuropsychologic follow-up of 12 patients. *Pediatr Neurol* 1994; 11 (3): 230-5.

- Takeoka M, Riviello JJ Jr, Duffy FH, *et al.* Bilateral volume reduction of the superior temporal areas in Landau-Kleffner syndrome. *Neurology* 2004; 63 (7): 1289-92.

- Tassinari CA, Regis H, Gastaut H. A particular form of muscular inhibition in epilepsy: the related epileptic silent period (R.E.S.P). *Proc Aust Ass Neurol* 1968; 5: 595-602.

- Tassinari CA, Terzano G, Capocci G, *et al.* (1977a) Epileptic seizures during sleep in children. In: Penry JK (Ed). *Epilepsy*. The 8th International Symposium. New York: Raven Press, 1977: 345-54.

- Tassinari CA, Dravet C, Roger J. (1977b) CSWS: encephalopathy related to electrical status epilepticus during slow sleep. *Electroencephalogr Clin Neurophysiol* 1977 ; 43: 529-30.

- Tassinari CA, Bureau M, Dravet C, *et al.* Epilepsy with continuous spike-waves during sleep. In: Roger J, Dravet C, Bureau M, *et al.* (Eds). *Epileptic syndromes in infancy, childhood and adolescence*. London: John Libbey, 1985: 194-204.

- Tassinari CA, Bureau M, Dravet C, *et al.* Epilepsy with continuous spikes and waves during slow sleep-otherwise described as ESES (Epilepsy with electrical status epilepticus during slow sleep). In: Roger J, Bureau M, Dravet C, *et al.* (Eds). *Epileptic syndromes in infancy, childhood and adolescence* (2nd Ed.). London: John Libbey, 1992: 245-56.

- Tassinari CA. The problems of continuous spikes and waves during slow sleep or electrical status epilepticus during slow sleep today. In: Beaumanoir A, Bureau M, Deonna T, *et al.* (Eds). *Continuous spikes and waves during slow sleep. Electrical status epilepticus during slow sleep. Acquired epileptic aphasia and related conditions*. London: John Libbey, 1995: 251-5.

- Tassinari CA, Rubboli G, Volpi L, *et al.* Encephalopathy with electrical status epilepticus during slow sleep or ESES syndrome including the acquired aphasia. *Clin Neurophysiol* 2000; 111 Suppl 2: S94-S102.

- Tassinari CA, Rubboli G, Volpi L, *et al.* Electrical status epilepticus during slow sleep (ESES or CSWS) including acquired epileptic aphasia (Landau-Kleffner syndrome). In: Roger J., Bureau M., Dravet CH, *et al.* (Eds). *Epileptic syndromes in infancy, childhood and adolescence* (3rd Ed.). Eastleigh: John Libbey, 2002: 265-83.

- Tassinari CA, Rubboli G, Volpi L, *et al.* Electrical status epilepticus during slow sleep (ESES or CSWS) including acquired epileptic aphasia (Landau-Kleffner syndrome). In: Roger J., Bureau M., Dravet CH, *et al.* (Eds). *Epileptic syndromes in infancy, childhood and adolescence* (4th Ed.). Montrouge: John Libbey Eurotext Ltd, 2005: 295-314.

- Tassinari CA, Rubboli G. Cognition and Paroxysmal EEG Activities: From a Single Spike to Electrical Status Epilepticus during Sleep. *Epilepsia* 2006; 47 Suppl 2: 40-3.

- Tenembaum SN, Deonna T, Fejerman N, *et al.* Continuous spike-waves and dementia in childhood epilepsy with occipital paroxysms. *J Epilepsy* 1997; 10: 139-45.

- Tsuru T, Mori M, Mizuguchi M. Effects of high-dose intravenous corticosteroid therapy in Landau-Kleffner syndrome. *Pediatr Neurol* 2000; 22 (2): 145-7.

- Tuchman RF, Rapin I. Regression in pervasive developmental disorders: seizures and epileptiform electroencephalogram correlates. *Pediatrics* 1997; 99: 560-6.

- Tuchman RF. Autism and Epilepsy: What Has Regression Got to Do with It? *Epilepsy currents* 2006; 6 (4): 107-11.

- Tutuncuoglu S, Serdaroglu G, Kadioglu B. Landau-Kleffner syndrome beginning with stuttering: case report. *J Child Neurol* 2002; 17 (10): 785-8.

- Tzitiridou M, Panou T, Ramantani G, *et al*. Oxcarbazepine monotherapy in benign childhood epilepsy with centrotemporal spikes: A clinical and cognitive evaluation. *Epilepsy Behav* 2005; 7 (3): 458-67.

- Van Hirtum-Das M, Licht EA, Koh S, *et al*. Children with ESES: variability in the syndrome. *Epilepsy Res* 2006; 70 Suppl 1: S248-S258.

- Van Lierde A. Therapeutic data. In: Beaumanoir A, Bureau M, Deonna T, *et al*. (Eds). *Continuous spikes and waves during slow sleep: acquired epileptic aphasia and related conditions*. London: John Libbey, 1995: 225-7.

- Veggiotti P, Beccaria F, Papalia G, *et al*. Continuous spikes and waves during sleep in children with shunted hydrocephalus. *Childs Nerv Syst* 1998; 14 (4-5): 188-94.

- Veggiotti P, Beccaria F, Guerrini R, *et al*. Continuous spike-and-wave activity during slow-wave sleep: syndrome or EEG pattern? *Epilepsia* 1999; 40 (11): 1593-601.

- Veggiotti P, Termine C, Granocchio E, *et al*. Long-term neuropsychological follow-up and nosological considerations in five patients with continuous spikes and waves during slow sleep. *Epileptic Disord* 2002; 4 (4): 243-9.

- Veggiotti P, Cardinali S, Granocchio E, *et al*. Motor impairment on awakening in a patient with an EEG pattern of "unilateral, continuous spikes and waves during slow sleep". *Epileptic Disord* 2005; 7 (2): 131-6.

- Verrotti A, Latini G, Trotta D, *et al*. Typical and atypical rolandic epilepsy in childhood: a follow-up study. *Pediatr Neurol* 2002; 26 (1): 26-9.

Wakai S, Ito N, Ueda D, Chiba S. Landau-Kleffner syndrome and sulthiame (letter). *Neuropediatrics* 1997; 28: 135-6.

- Weglage J, Demsky A, Pietsch M, Kurlemann G. Neuropsychological, intellectual, and behavioural findings in patients with centrotemporal spikes with and without seizures. *Dev Med Child Neurol* 1997; 39 (10): 646-51.

- Wioland N, Rudolf G, Metz-Lutz MN. Electrophysiological evidence of persisting unilateral auditory cortex dysfunction in the late outcome of Landau and Kleffner syndrome. *Clin Neurophysiol* 2001; 112 (2): 319-23.

- Wirrell EC, Camfield PR, Gordon KE, *et al*. Benign rolandic epilepsy: atypical features are very common. *J Child Neurol* 1995; 10 (6): 455-8.

- Yasuhara A, Yoshida H, Hatanaka T, *et al*. Epilepsy with continuous spike-waves during slow sleep and its treatment. *Epilepsia* 1991; 32: 59-62.

Symptomatic focal epilepsies imitating atypical evolutions of idiopathic focal epilepsies in childhood

Roberto H. Caraballo, Ricardo Cersósimo, Natalio Fejerman
Buenos Aires, Argentina

To our knowledge, children with congenital hemiparesis associated with unilateral polymicrogyria (PMG) represent a quite defined group who is prone to present an epileptic encephalopathic course imitating atypical evolutions of idiopathic focal epilepsies as described in Chapter 10.

A classification scheme for malformations of cortical development has been proposed based on genetics, embryology, imaging and pathology, disclosing abnormal neuronal and glial proliferation, abnormal neuronal migration and abnormal cortical organization as the main mechanisms (Barkovich, 1996; Palmini, 2000; Kuzniecky & Barkovich, 2001; Barkovich et al., 2002).

MRI technology has allowed recognition of different types of unilateral or bilateral cortical dysplasias. Nevertheless, it sometimes remains difficult to identify certain cortical malformations that are only diagnosed by special histological or histochemical techniques (Barkovich et al., 1992; Barkovich & Kjos, 1992).

Cortical dysplasias are being recognized with increasing frequency as a cause of epilepsies that are often refractory (Andermann, 1993). However, unilateral polymicrogyria (PMG) is associated with a particular type of epilepsy with a relatively benign course (Caraballo et al., 1992, 1997a, 1999; Guerrini et al., 1993, 1998).

Colamaria and co-workers (1989) reported a boy with congenital hemiparesis, unilateral pachygyria and epilepsy. The authors described an ictal asterixis as a particular type of seizures, an electroclinical phenomenon that, according to the polygraphic EEG recording, corresponds to negative myoclonus (Colamaria et al., 1989). Two years later, the same group published a series of nine cases with similar features (Colamaria et al., 1991). Later on, it became evident through pathological studies and higher resolution MRI that those images called pachygyria corresponded in fact to polymicrogyria.

In 1992 we presented our first three patients with congenital hemiparesis, unilateral PMG and a particular type of epilepsy (Caraballo et al., 1992). These patients started with motor focal seizures evolving into particular electroclinical features characterized by myoclonias, pseudoataxia, atonic seizures and absences. The interictal EEG showed bilateral, symmetrical and asymmetrical, continuous or subcontinuous spikes and spike-waves during slow sleep. Interestingly, these patients showed a much more benign course than the patients with epilepsy associated with cortical dysplasias (Caraballo et al., 1992; Guerrini et al. 1993). Subsequently, we published a more detailed electroclinical description of eleven children, and later with one more case, confirming the favourable evolution (Caraballo et al. 1997a, 1999). Similar electroclinical features and evolution have been described by Guerrini et al. (1998) in a series of patients with multi-lobar PMG.

Polymicrogyria is secondary to abnormal cortical organization. In PMG, the neurons reach the cortex but do not form normal cortical or intracortical connections and result in multiple small gyri. The classic form is four-layered polymicrogyric with a molecular layer, an organized intercellular layer, a cell-sparse layer and a slightly unorganized inner cellular layer. There is, however, a wide range of histological abnormalities including cases with an unlayered and completely unorganized cortex (Barkovich et al., 1996, 2001; Palmini, 2000; Kuzniecky & Barkovich, 2001). PMG may be generalized, focal or multifocal. Among the latter, there are bilateral symmetric anterior, perisylvian and posterior PMG (Barkovich et al., 1996). Unilateral PMG may affect the whole hemisphere or only part of it. Large malformations are associated with hypoplasia of the affected hemisphere. Multilobar forms are usually located in the perisylvian cortex. PMG often seems unilateral on the MRI, but may turn out to be bilateral and extensive on microscopic examination of the brain (Guerrini et al., 1996).

As the mechanism underlying schizencephaly (SCHZ) is probably very similar to the one that causes PMG, we compared cases with unilateral closed-lip SCHZ and unilateral PMG and demonstrated that the electroclinical features of patients with PMG were different from those with SCHZ (Caraballo et al., 2004a). Patients with closed-lip SCHZ had epilepsy characterized by motor focal seizures with or without secondarily generalized tonic-clonic seizures, but not showing the particular electroclinical features associated with secondary bilateral synchronies (SBS) as the patients with unilateral PMG do (Caraballo et al., 2004a).

On account that the patients we are presenting here show seizures, EEGs evolutions alike those of children with idiopathic focal epilepsies complicated by atypical evolutions, we decided to include this chapter in the book. We understand that the pathophysiological mechanisms underlying the phenomenon of electrical status epilepticus during sleep (ESES) are similar both in children with idiopathic epilepsies who present an atypical evolution and in children with PMG who develop the mentioned particular type of epilepsy, as we'll see later.

Epidemiology

The incidence and prevalence of epilepsy in large series of children with cerebral palsy have been reported (Aksu, 1990; Hadjipanayis et al., 1997). A review of patients with hemiparetic cerebral palsy showed that in 7% of the cases it was associated with unilateral cortical dysplasias (Wiklund et al., 1991). We had reported an incidence of epilepsy in 29% of 682 patients with cerebral palsy.

Cortical dysplasias were detected in 21.6% of the cases (Caraballo *et al.*, 1997b). Similar results were found by Pascual-Castroviejo *et al.* (2001). In a more selective analyisis, we studied 36 patients with unilateral PMG out of a series of 120 children with hemiparetic cerebral palsy (Caraballo *et al.*, 2004a; Cersósimo, 2005). Our findings were coincident with those of Barkovich, who showed that in his series of patients, PMG is the most common cause of congenital hemiplegia (Barkovich, 2002).

Clinical features

Clinical features in children with unilateral PMG have been thoroughly studied (Caraballo *et al.*, 2004a; Guerrini *et al.*, 1996). Currently, 59 cases are being followed by our group. The majority of these cases have mild spastic hemiparesis, which is less frequently moderate, and never severe. Conversely, spastic hemiparesis is severe when the PMG is associated with a porencephalic cyst. The majority of patients also have mild or moderate mental retardation.

Seventy eight percent of the patients have seizures. Onset of epilepsy occurs between the ages of 1 and 6 years (mean, 2 years) with motor focal seizures with or without secondary generalization. History of febrile seizures is found in 20% of the cases. Occasionally, the seizures are complex focal seizures. The epilepsy is always focal, with or without secondary generalization, but never generalized at onset.

Between ages 2 and 9 years (mean 6 years), an evident change in seizures and EEG occurs. Frequent negative myoclonus with gait instability, positive myoclonus, and atypical absences appear in 75% of the cases with epilepsy. Less frequently, the patients have focal motor seizures with or without secondary generalization in this period.

The patients with multi-lobar PMG have both focal motor and atypical absences, and both focal and generalized interictal discharges (Guerrini *et al.*, 1998). The age of seizure onset is similar to that of unilateral PMG, as is the particular electroclinical evolution due to secondary bilateral synchronies. We studied four cases with multi-lobar PMG with epilepsy. Three of them showed clinical manifestations associated with ESES.

EEG features

At the onset of epilepsy, the interictal EEG shows focal spikes in the region were the PMG is present *(Fig. 1)*. Some patients have electroencephalographic focal abnormalities before the seizures start and occasionally the spikes may show the morphology of BCECTS *(Fig. 2)*.

In some cases, the interictal abnormalities occur without concomitant clinical manifestations. These patients should be followed closely as they may present clinical manifestations in the future, and AEDs treatment may be considered.

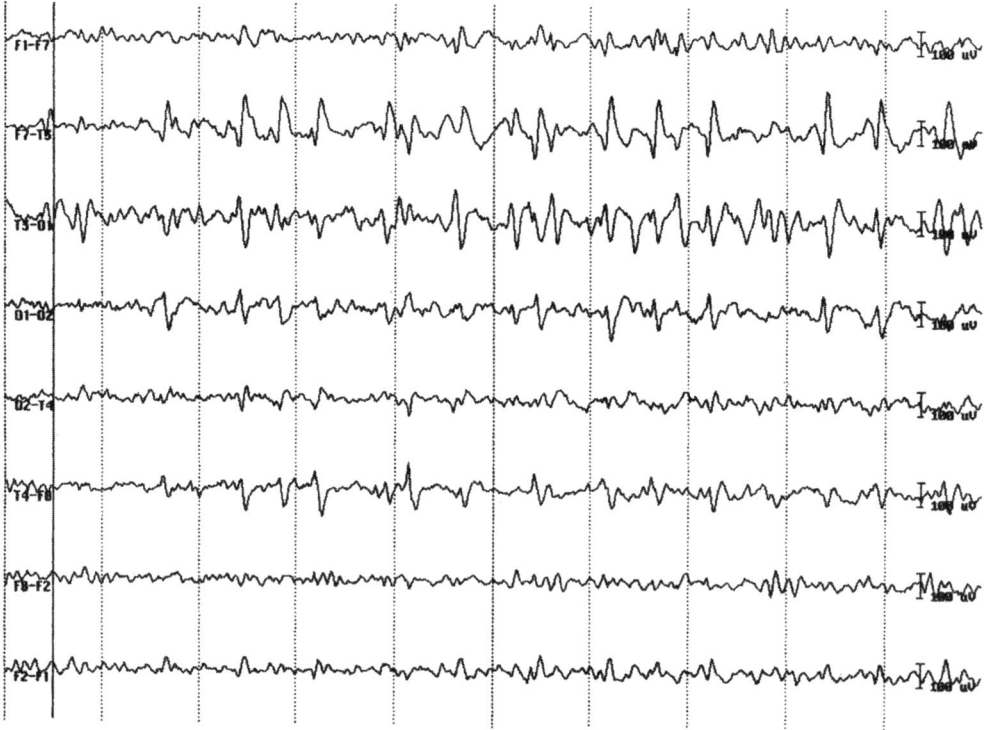

Figure 1. Eight years old boy with left PMG and recent history of right focal seizures. Interictal sleep EEG shows clear dominance of spikes in left hemisphere.

When the electroclinical picture changes, the interictal EEG shows asymmetric bilateral spikes while awake, and continuous symmetric or asymmetric spike-wave activity during slow-wave sleep constituting an ESES *(Fig. 3A, B)*. Other patients show bilateral high-frequency spike-wave discharges during slow-wave sleep but not frankly an ESES *(Fig. 4)* (Caraballo *et al.*, 1999; Dalla Bernardina *et al.*, 1996).

Aetiology

Most of the cases are sporadic (Caraballo *et al.*, 2004a). We found one familial case with affected mother and son (Caraballo *et al.*, 2000). It is interesting to note that only the son developed the particular type of epilepsy we are describing. This familial case 16-year-old boy was admitted at the age of 2 with a diagnosis of congenital hemiparesis while the rest of physical and neurological examination was normal. Right fronto-parietal cortical dysplasia with hemisphere atrophy was evident by computerized tomography scanning and magnetic resonance imaging. The latter, also disclosed abnormal thick cortex which was interpreted as PMG. He had a hemifacial motor seizure at the age of 7 years. At the age of 8, frequent atonic or negative myoclonus appeared.

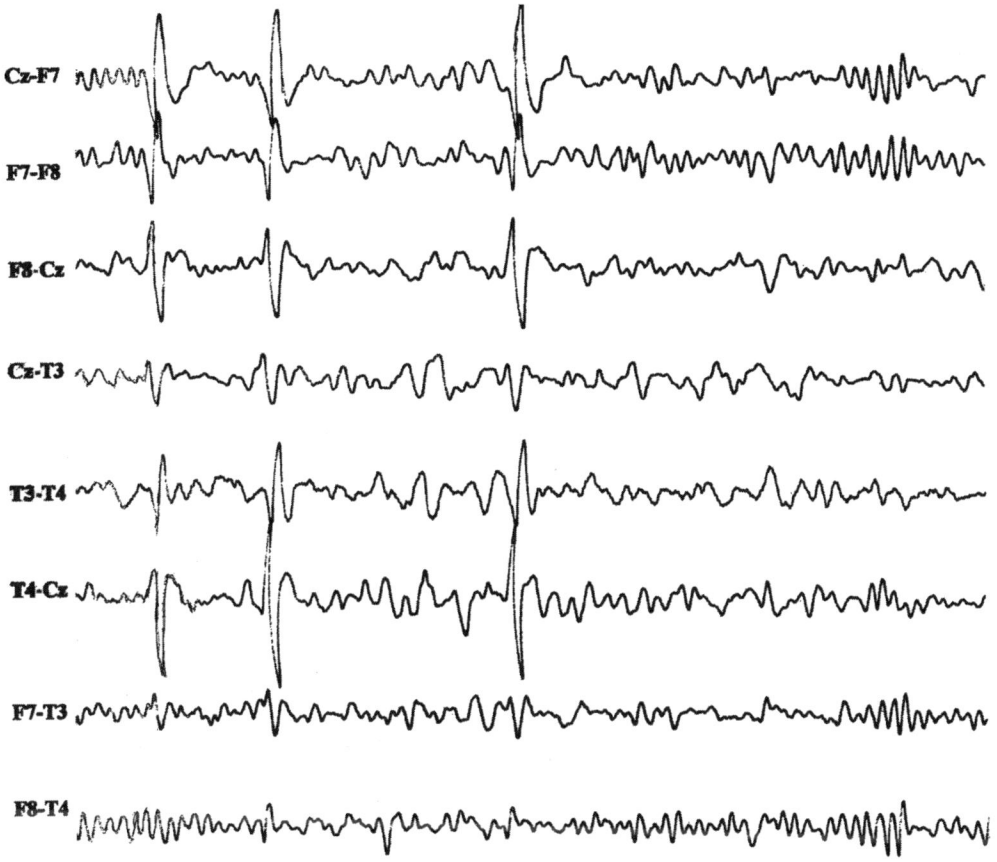

Figure 2. Four years old girl with right PMG. Routine EEG obtained before onset of seizures shows right fronto-temporal spikes.

Asymmetric bilateral spike discharges with a high voltage in the right hemisphere during the EEG recording were found. Seizures responded well to Clobazam and after two months the patient became seizure free and his EEG normalized up to the present time His cognitive functions were low normal and at 16 years his score in the Wechsler intelligence scale was 80. His mother, a 42-year-old woman (IQ 85) also had congenital hemiparesis. She never had seizures and her EEGs were normal. Magnetic resonance imaging showed right fronto-parietal cortical PMG with ipsilateral hemisphere atrophy *(Fig. 5A, B)*. In son and his mother the karyotype was normal. The presence of epilepsy only in the son shows a variable clinical phenotype.

Inheritance of PMG, including both parents and siblings, has been suggested in several reports (Ferrie *et al.*, 1995; Yoshimura *et al.*, 1998; Bartolomei *et al.*, 1999; Caraballo *et al.*, 2000), most commonly through X-linked transmission. Chang and co-workers (2006) identified four families in which unilateral right-sided PMG on MRI was present in more than one individual, with pathologic confirmation in one. These findings strongly suggest that unilateral PMG can have a

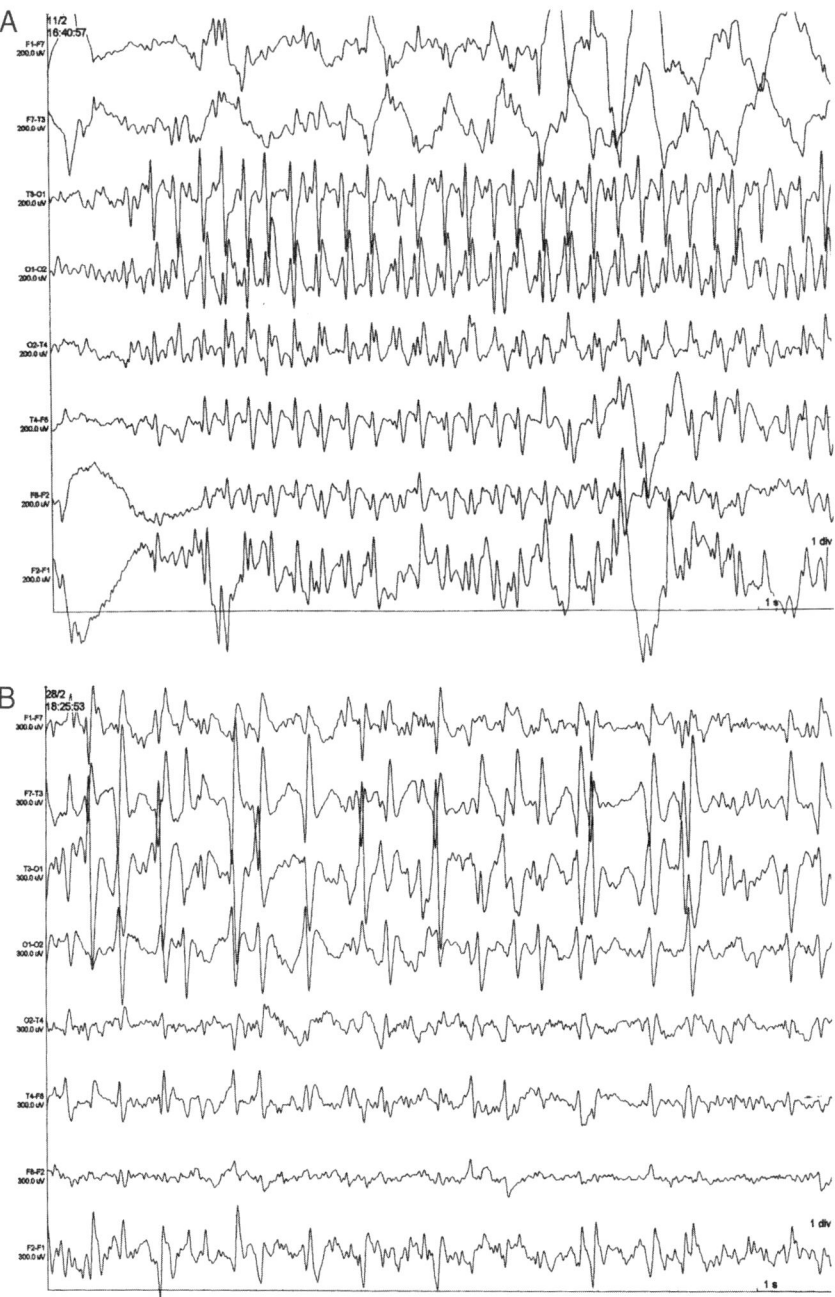

Figure 3. Six years old boy with left posterior PMG: who entered into the state of ESES. A: EEG while awake shows rhythmic bilateral spike-wave discharges with higher amplitude in left occipital region while having repetitive negative myoclonia. B: Sleep EEG shows bilateral continuous spike-wave activity clearly dominant on left hemisphere.

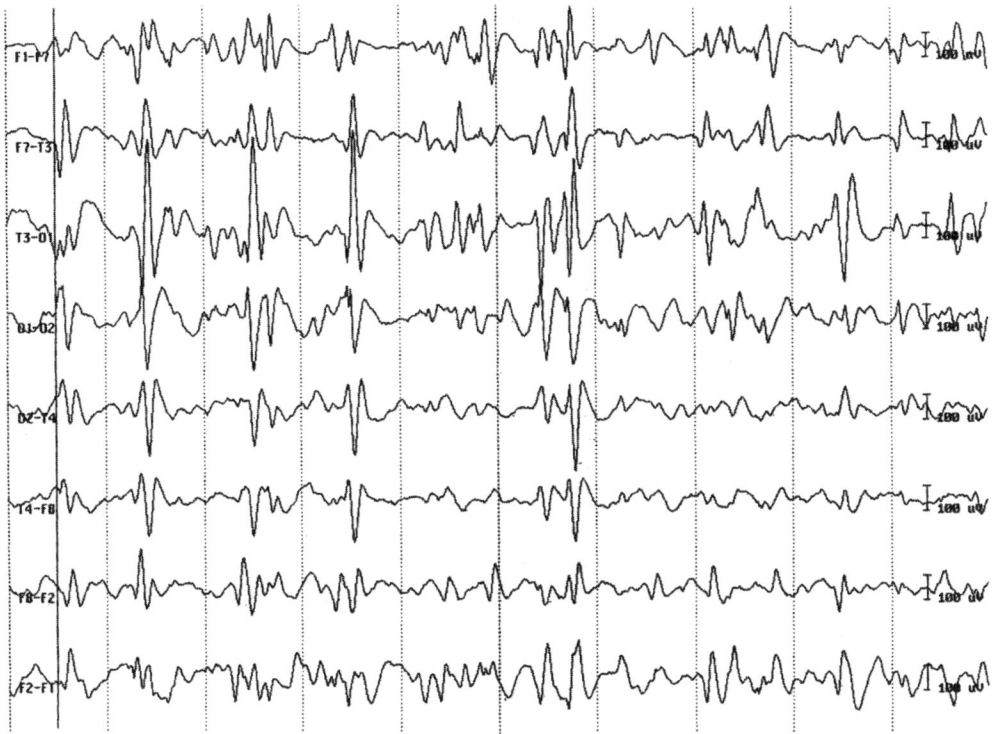

Figure 4. Eight years old boy with left PMG (the same patient as shown in Fig. 1). During the period of aggravation, his sleep EEG shows frequent spikes but not ESES.

germline genetic aetiology. However, there may be more than one causative locus, as the presence of multiple affected siblings with unaffected parents raises the possibility of autosomal recessive inheritance or dominant inheritance with germline mosaicism, while the mother-son pair suggests autosomal dominant or X-linked inheritance (Caraballo et al., 2000; Chang et al., 2006).

Unilateral PMG may be seen in patients with deletions at chromosome 22q11, the locus for DiGeorge syndrome and velocardiofacial syndrome, but it appears to be quite uncommon in these cases and is typically seen in association with other syndromic abnormalities (Bingham et al., 1998; Bird, Scambler, 2000; Sztriha et al., 2004). An unbalanced translocation resulting in 1q44qter monosomy and 12q13.3pter trisomy has been associated with unilateral right PMG, severe mental retardation, congenital hypotonia, dysmorphic facial features, and hypogenitalism (Zollino et al., 2003). One of the patients in our series also has Stickler syndrome. Stickler syndrome is a connective tissue disorder that can include ocular findings of myopia, cataract, and retinal detachment; hearing loss that is both conductive and sensorineural; midfacial underdevelopment and cleft palate; and mild spondyloepiphyseal dysplasia and/or precocious arthritis. This autosomal dominant syndrome can be extremely variable. To our knowledge, the finding of unilateral PMG in Stickler syndrome has not been described previously.

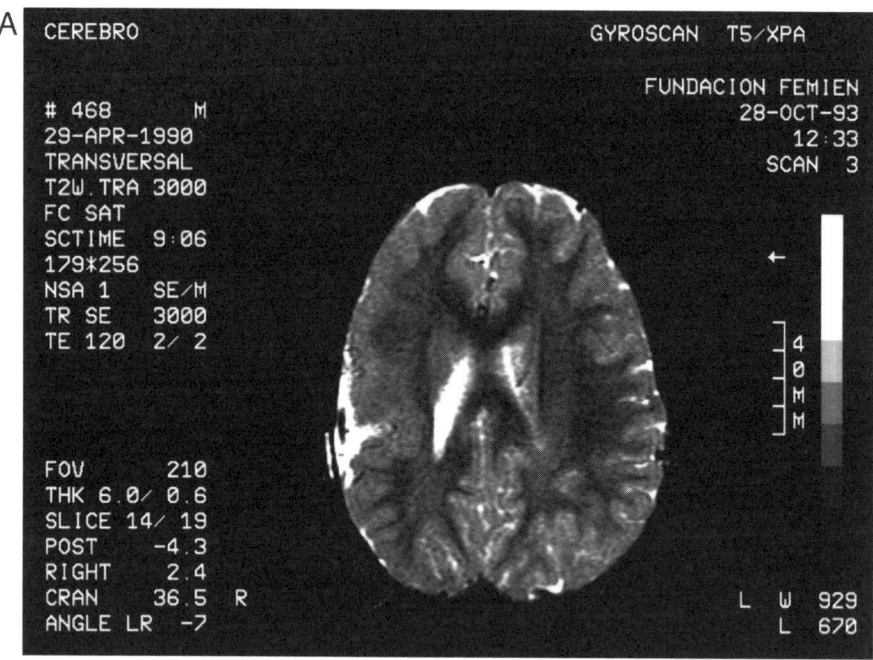

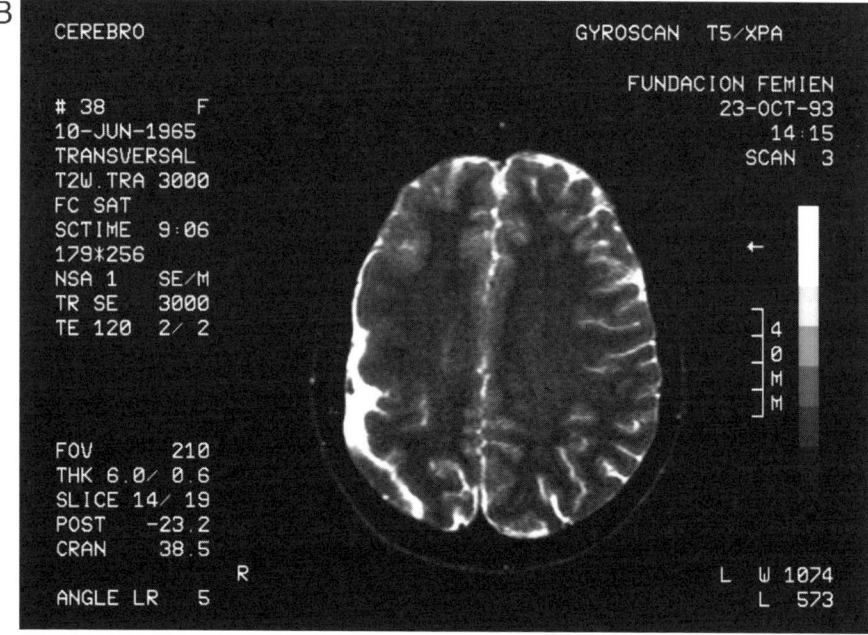

Figure 5. Mother and son. A: Ten years old boy. Axial T2-weighted brain MRI showing right fronto-parietal PMG with ipsilateral hemisphere atrophy. B: The brain MRI of his mother shows in the same sequence PMG with the same localization and associated also with ipsilateral hemisphere atrophy.

Inborn errors of metabolism may be aetiological factors. There are also cases secondary to cytomegalovirus infections during pregnancy. When an encephalomalacic lesion with or without the form of a porecenphalic cyst is associated with PMG, a vascular phenomenon should be suspected *(Fig. 6)*.

Pathophysiology

The mild spastic hemiparesis found in the majority of these patients may be explained by the cortical origin of the lesion, while it is common to find more spasticity in patients with clastic lesions.

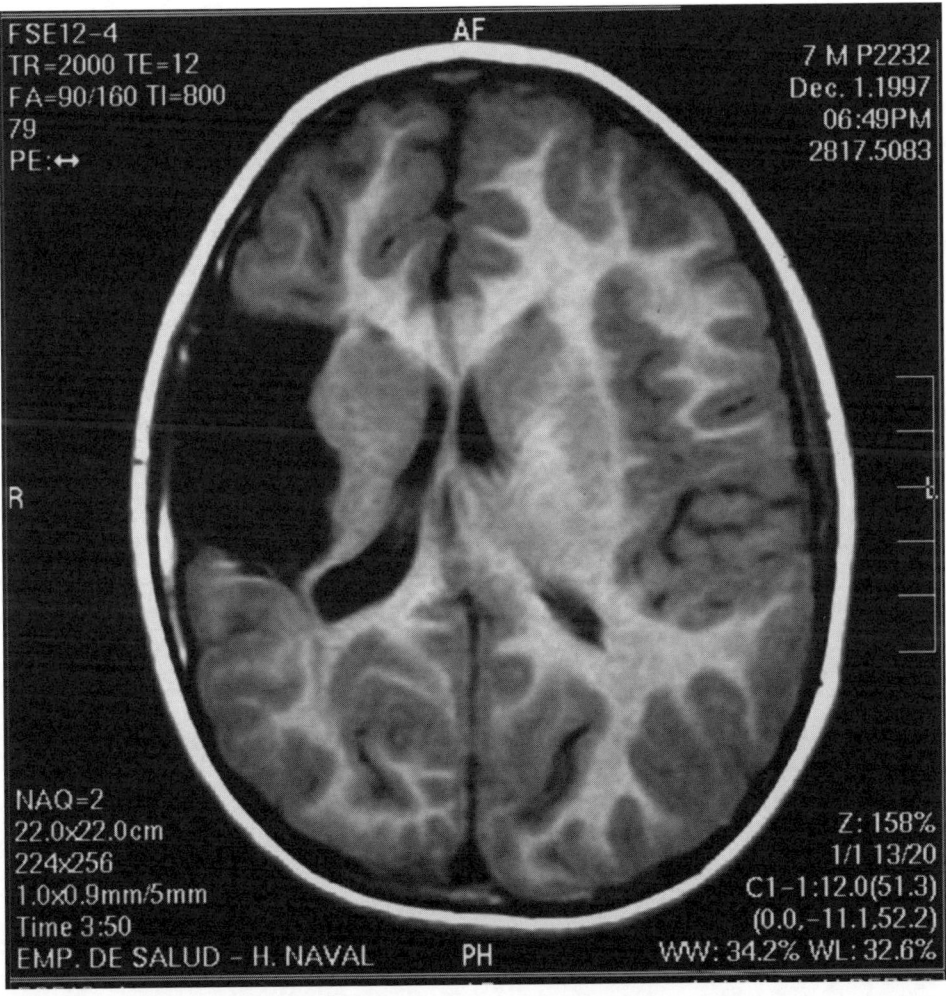

Figure 6. Eight years old boy. MRI: T1 sequence showing right fronto-parietal encephalomalacic lesion and PMG with ipsilateral hemisphere atrophy.

The EEG reveals unilateral synchronous spikes when awake that become diffuse and continuously synchronous during sleep. This may suggest that the epileptogenicity and propagation of electrical discharges between cortex and subcortex are different. Bilateral continuous or subcontinuous spike-wave discharges during slow-wave sleep with higher voltage over the dysplasic areas indicate a secondary bilateral synchrony (SBS) mechanism presumably correlating with atypical absences and epileptic negative myoclonus causing gait instability (Dalla Bernardina et al., 1990). The phenomenon of SBS in patients with other symptomatic or idiopathic focal epilepsies seems to be an age-dependent cause of the syndrome of continuous spike-wave activity during slow sleep, which usually disappears before adolescence (Dalla Bernardina et al., 1989; Tassinari et al., 1992). Kobayashi and co-workers (1992, 1994) suggested that SBS implies an initial diffusion of discharges through the corpus callosum, with or without intervention of centro-encephalic structures in their generalization. Spencer and co-workers (1985) also hypothesized about mesencephalic/diencephalic mechanisms for SBS.

Polymicrogyric abnormalities are often more widespread than can be shown by MRI and an extensive area of cortical abnormality may facilitate SBS. Enhanced excitation arising from the abnormal cortex in PMG and reduced inhibitory activity in the cortical surface surrounding PMG can trigger hypersynchronous neuronal discharges. It has been impossible to demonstrate whether the contralateral hemisphere is completely normal and how the contralateral hemisphere acts in the SBS mechanism.

In the majority of patients with unilateral PMG developing a status of epileptic negative myoclonus the location of cortical dysplasia is fronto-temporal, which may explain the phenomenon of SBS.

Right hemisphere is most frequently affected. There may be specific reasons for a differential hemispheric susceptibility to PMG. For example, the right cerebral hemisphere in the fetus demonstrates gyral complexity earlier than the left, particularly in the perisylvian region (Chang et al., 2006).

Finally, we want to emphasize again that this electroclinical picture seen in patients with unilateral PMG shares a similar pathopysiological mechanism to that described in children with idiopathic focal epilepsies who present atypical evolutions within the spectrum of ESES.

Diagnostic work-up

High resolution MRI is mandatory to identify the PMG in detail, and search for other types of lesion that may be associated in the same patients (Cersosimo, 2007). As stated before, unilateral PMG is most frequently located in the fronto-temporal regions and less frequently in the parieto-occipital regions *(Fig. 7A, B)*. The brain MRI may also show other types of cortical development malformation, such as schizencephaly (SCHZ) and nodular periventricular heterotopia. These neuroradiological findings could mean that this type of cortical malformation is due to abnormally late neuronal migration and affected cortical organization.

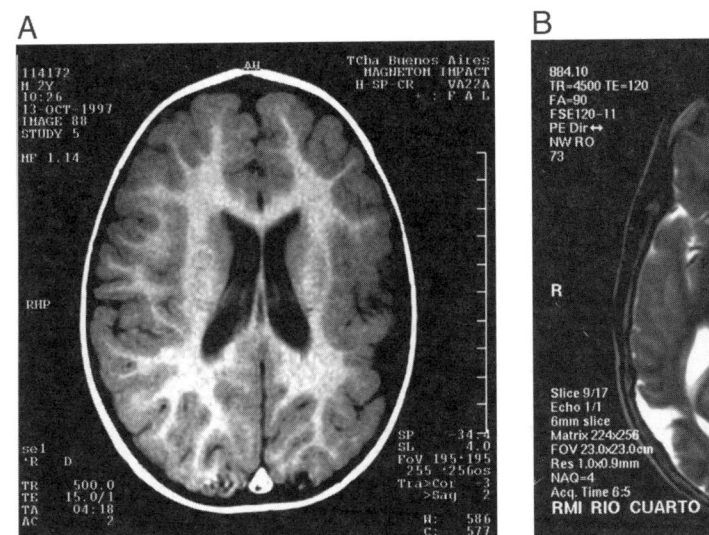
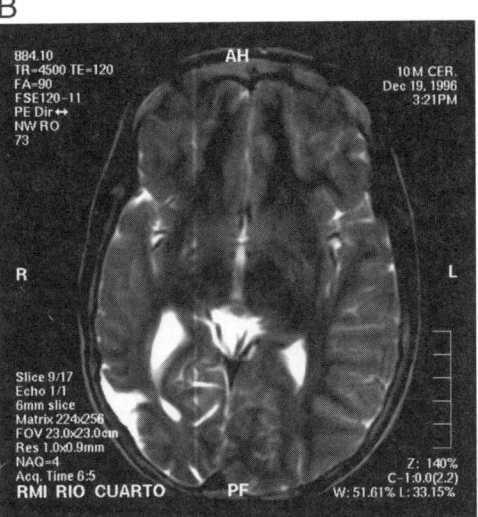

Figure 7. A: Nine years old boy. MRI with T1-weighted sequence showing left hemisphere atrophy with PMG on left frontal and perisylvian cortex; B: Ten years old boy. MRI T2 weighted sequence showing left posterior PMG.

In cases with microcephaly or suspicion of prenatal infections the CT scan may show periventricular calcifications associated with PMG. These findings may suggest an infection with cytomegalovirus.

Screening for prenatal infections and neurometabolic investigations should be indicated, and chromosome and FISH studies should also be performed.

EEG is fundamental and should be routinely performed in every child with congenital hemiparesis. If this child happens to have unilateral PMG, sleep EEGs should be repeated even before seizures appear. Obviously, if the patient not only presented isolated focal seizures but starts having frequent inhibitory seizures (negative myoclonus), or positive myoclonus, or absences, associated or not with neuropsychological and language deterioration, the presence of ESES should be suspected and a more prolonged sleep EEG obtained. Occurrence of ESES in patients with localized PMG does not seem to be rare at all (Caraballo *et al.*, 1997a, 1999, 2004a; Guerrini *et al.*, 1998).

Differential diagnosis

We are not entering in details neither about differential diagnosis of cerebral palsy in general nor about congenital hemiparesis in particular, because the aim in this chapter is to insist in recognizing this particular epileptic encephalopathy which occurs in children with unilateral PMG and which, curiously enough, shares pathophysiological mechanisms and almost similar evolutions with the reported in patients with idiopathic focal epilepsies in childhood. Therefore, early detection of PMG in a child with focal seizures is essential to start treatment and to attempt to avoid the development of ESES.

We published cases with a unilateral porencephalic cyst with a similar electroclinical picture. However, in these cases the cortical region surrounding the porencephalic lesion showed a polymicrogyric cortex explaining the electroclinical findings (Caraballo et al., 2004a).

This particular electroclinical pattern associated with unilateral PMG has not been described in other types of cortical development malformation. In addition, we compared the electroclinical features of patients with unilateral PMG and closed-lip SCHZ. Both conditions are secondary to abnormal cortical organization. Nevertheless, the patients with closed-lip SCHZ never developed electroclinical features due to SBS (Caraballo et al., 2004a). The fact that continuous or subcontinuous spike and waves during slow sleep due to SBS was found to be associated with unilateral PMG but not with cases with other cortical malformations may suggest that a unique anatomo-functional system is involved.

A series of 29 children with prenatal or perinatal unilateral thalamic injuries associated with symptomatic ESES or sleep SW overactivation was reported (Guzzetta et al., 2005). CSWS was detected in children with shunted hydrocephalus, suggesting involvement of thalamo-cortical circuitries (Veggiotti et al., 1998). The installation of ESES may also occur in patients with bilateral malformations of cortical development, which in general are not symmetrical and include polymicrogyric portions of cortex. In the cases with unilateral PMG without hemiparesis and mental retardation, the differentiation with cryptogenic or idiopathic focal epilepsy with SBS may be more difficult. However, the brain MRI findings will confirm the diagnosis.

We should be aware that patients with focal epilepsy, independently of the type of seizure and the epileptic syndrome (idiopathic, cryptogenic or symptomatic), may develop age-dependent SBS and its clinical manifestations (Dalla Bernardina et al., 1990). Of course, patients with hemiparesis associated with PMG may present only focal seizures not showing the mentioned evolution, or also common generalized seizures. Even a fortuitous association between focal neuronal migration disorders and typical BCECTS has been described (Ambrosetto, 1992; Sheth et al., 1997).

Within the spectrum of epileptic complications in children with congenital hemiparesis the main differential diagnosis is the appearance of reflex seizures causing frequent drops in children with central or parietal clastic lesions. These seizures are usually intractable to medication and constitute an indication for surgery (Oguni et al., 1998a; Caraballo et al., 2004b).

The final concept we want to introduce is that neuropediatricians should try to diagnose as early as possible the presence of these EEG abnormalities due to a particular neurophsyiological phenomenon in all children with structural cerebral pathology in order to avoid its clinical manifestations which increase the risk of neuropsychological impairment and hamper their quality of life.

Treatment

Care should be taken in the selection of AED treatment. A probable association between certain AEDs and the appearance of continuous spike-wave activity with negative myoclonus has repeatedly been reported in children with benign focal childhood epilepsy exposed to carbamazepine, phenobarbital, phenytoin and even valproate (Caraballo *et al.*, 1989; Prats *et al.*, 1998; Guerrini *et al.*, 1998; Fejerman *et al.*, 2000). This phenomenon has also been described in association with lamotrigine (Catania *et al.*, 1999; Cerminara *et al.*, 2004) and with topiramate (Montenegro & Guerreiro, 2002). The majority of our cases with unilateral PMG had been exposed to AEDs effective for focal seizures prior to the peculiar evolution of their epilepsy. In our experience, after the onset of continuous or subcontinuous electroclinical manifestations, the best results initially are obtained with benzodiazepines, sulthiame and ethosuximide, either in monotherapy or in combinations (Lerman, Lerman-Sagie, 1995; Oguni *et al.*, 1998b; Capovilla *et al.*, 1999; Fejerman *et al.*, 2000; Caraballo *et al.*, 2004a). For more details see Chapter 10.

In refractory cases, surgical treatment could be considered. In patients with CSWSS, surgery may be effective when a focal abnormality is demonstrated (Park *et al.*, 1994). Through motor and language fMRI study in 5 patients it was demonstrated that polymicrogyric cortex manteins functionality and that capability should be considered when surgery becomes absolutely necessary (Araujo *et al.*, 2006). Only one of our cases was operated on. He had extensive PMG on right hemisphere and his seizures were refractory to all medical treatments. He showed improvement in seizure frequency and quality of life. In *Figure 8 A & B* we show his pre and postsurgery EEGs. In hemiparetic children with extensive unilateral PMG and intractable seizures, total or subtotal hemispherectomy could be useful. Multiple subpial transections could represent a complement in severe cases, or an alternative in patients with absent or mild hemiparesis or incipient cognitive deterioration.

However, the main reason underlying our inclusion of this subject in a book on benign focal epilepsies in childhood is to emphasize that a significant proportion of children with mild hemiparesis, slight or moderate intellectual impairment and unilateral PMG may present an epilepsy with encephalopathic course similar to that seen in a minority of children with idiopathic focal epilepsies. This similarity is seen not only in the electrical and clinical features, but also in their evolution and their response to appropriate treatment, and therefore, surgical option should be deferred as much as possible.

Prognosis and long-term evolution

Providing careful selection of AEDs, a relatively benign course of epilepsy in patients with hemiparesis associated with unilateral PMG has repeatedly been reported (Caraballo *et al.*, 1992, 1997, 2004a; Aicardi, 1994; Guerrini *et al.*, 1996).

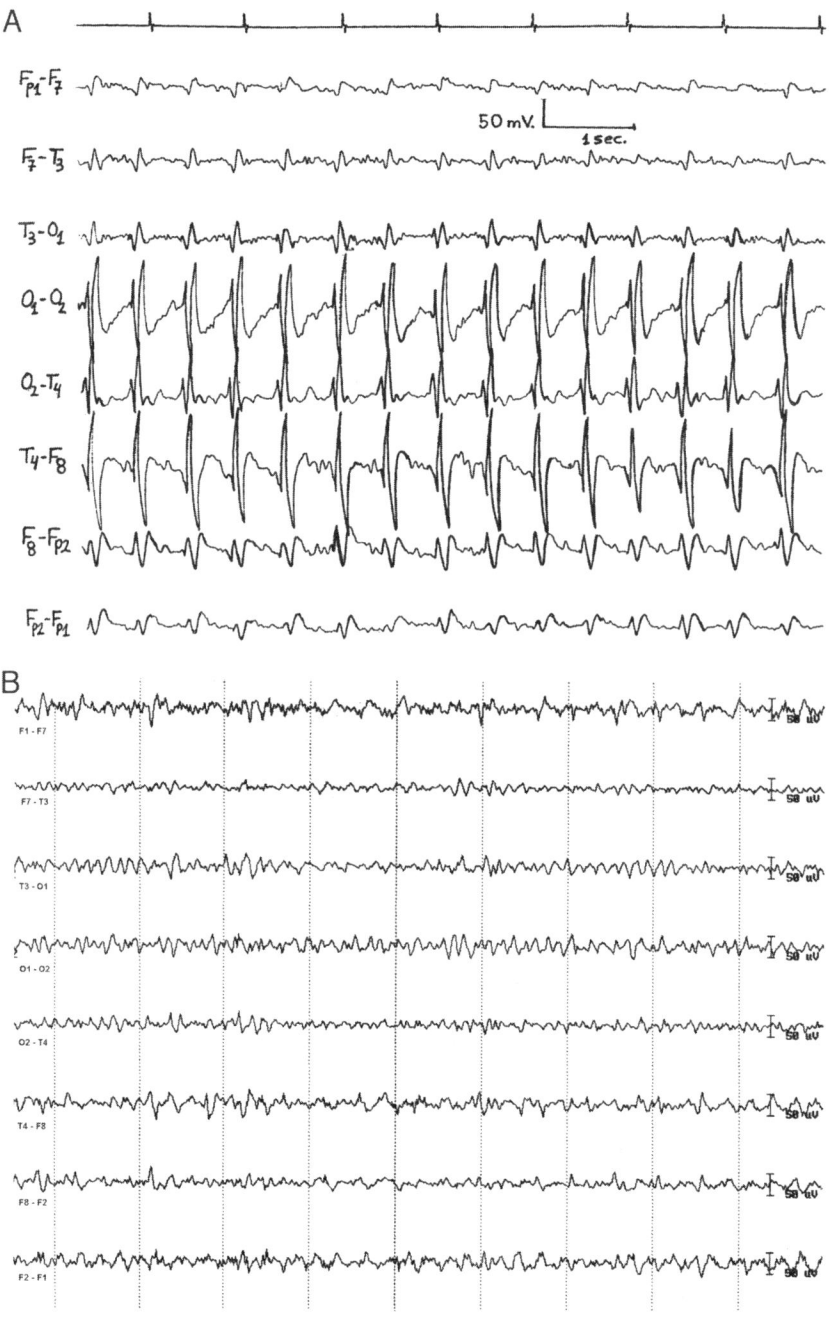

Figure 8. Eight years old boy. A: Slow sleep EEG shows asymmetric continuous spike-wave activity dominant in right hemisphere. B: Slow sleep EEG obtained in the last control after surgery shows right hemisphere slow-wave activity and isolated sharp waves in right fronto-temporal region.

Response to change of treatment is initially good in the majority of patients, but the evolution can vary. A significant number of patients may show one or more relapses of the same electro-clinical picture. The seizures usually remit completely before adolescence and few patients continue with sporadic seizures after this period of age.

Even though epilepsy in patients with cortical dysplasia is frequently refractory to AEDs, the majority of cases with unilateral PMG show a favourable outcome. However, 18% of patients in our series continued with seizures, so the prognosis of epilepsy in patients with PMG is not as benign as in idiopathic focal of epilepsy in childhood but, the outcome is more favourable when compared to patients with epilepsy secondary to other types of cortical dysplasia.

Present series of patients

Data about electroclinical features and neuroradiological findings in our series of 59 patients with unilateral PMG are described in *Table I*. Forty-four of them presented epileptic seizures. In *Table II* we detail about the 33 cases with unilateral PMG who presented the mentioned particular type of epilepsy. Finally in *Table III* we apply the scheme used in chapter 10 to recognize in children with unilateral PMG the same atypical evolutions as in children with idiopathic focal epilepsies.

In accordance with the different atypical evolutions recognized in patients with benign childhood epilepsies (Fejerman et al., 2000), we were able to disclose 19 patients with unilateral PMG having epilepsy with negative myoclonus, absences and focal motor seizures as seen in atypical

Table I. Initial electroclinical features in 59 patients with unilateral PMG

Sex	36 male; 23 female
Congenital hemiparesis (Mild spasticity) No hemiparesis	57 2
Localization of PMG	Fronto-temporal 39 Parieto-occipital 20
Mental retardation	Moderate 20 Mild 34 Normal IQ 5
Epilepsy	44/59 (78%)
Median age at onset of epilepsy	2 years (R: 4 months – 7 years)
Type of seizures at onset	Partial motor seizures with or without secondary generalization
Interictal EEG	Focal abnormalities

Table II. A particular type of epilepsy developing in 33 cases with unilateral PMG

Number and gender of cases	20 male; 13 female
Spasticity	Severe in 0 Mild in 33
Localization of unilateral PMG	Fronto-temporal 23 Parieto-occipital 10
Affected hemisphere	Right 19 Left 14
Median age at onset of seizures	22 months (R: 5 months – 6 years)
Median age at worsening of epilepsy	5.5 years (R: 3.5-9 years)
AED used before worsening of seizures	CBZ 13, PHB 7, PHT 5, OXC 5, VPA 3.

benign focal epilepsy of childhood (ABFEC), 7 patients with status epilepticus including oro-lingual seizures as in status of benign childhood epilepsy with centrotemporal spikes (SEBCECTS), 5 patients with focal motor seizures and mental disturbances including bizarre behaviours similar to those typical of CSWS syndrome, and 2 patients with what we called mixed forms of atypical evolutions including inhibitory seizures, absences, myoclonus, some language involvement and behavioural manifestations. In all these 33 patients the concomitantly EEG recording during slow-sleep showed continuous or subcontinuous, symmetrical or asymmetrical spike wave discharges. In this series of patients we didn't find any case with typical electroclinical features of Landau-Kleffner syndrome.

Follow-up ranged from 2 to 16 years (mean, 4.5 years). In the 33 patients the treatment with AEDs before developed the particular electroclinical pictures was: carbamazepine in 13, phenobarbital in 7, phenitoin in 5, oxcarbacepine in 5, and valproic acid in 3.

Fifteen patients had no relapses and have remained seizure free for more than 6 years, the other 18 patients had one or more relapses, but seven had no further seizures during the last 4 years. Ten children had their last relapse between 2 and 3 years ago but continue having seizures. One patient had five relapses of status epilepticus, and he was operated on as a case of refractory epilepsy. Pathologic examination of material from lesionectomy showed PMG. He has sporadic seizures after 10 years of follow-up.

Table III. Atypical evolutions in 33 cases with unilateral PMG and a particular type of epilepsy

Type of atypical evolution	ABFEC	SE	CSWSS	Mixed forms	LKS
Number of patients	19	7	5	2	0
Patients seizures-free at present	16	5	3	1	0

ABPEC: atypical benign focal epilepsy of childhood, SE: status epilepticus, CSWSS: continuous spike-waves during slow sleep syndrome, LKS: Landau-Kleffner syndrome.

References

- Aicardi J. Epilepsies Characterized by Simple Partial Seizures. In: Aicardi J (Ed). *Epilepsy in Children* (2nd ed.). New York: Raven Press, 1994: 130-64.

- Aksu F. Nature and prognosis of seizures in patents with cerebral palsy. *Dev Med Child Neurol* 1990; 32: 661-8.

- Ambrosetto G. Unilateral opercular macrogyria and benign childhood epilepsy with centrotemporal (rolandic) spikes: report of a case. *Epilepsia* 1992; 33: 499-503.

- Andermann F. Neuronal migration disorders and epilepsy: An overview. In: Fejerman N, Chamoles N (Eds). *New Trends in Pediatric Neurology*. Amsterdam: Elsevier Science Publishers, 1993: 81-5.

- Araujo D, de Araujo B, Pontes-Neto O, et al. Language and motor fMRI activation in Polymicrogyric cortex. *Epilepsia* 2006; 47 (3): 589-92.

- Barkovich AJ, Kjos B. Non-Lissencephaly cortical dysplasia: correlation of imaging findings with clinical deficits. *AJNR* 1992; 13: 85-94.

- Barkovich AJ, Gressens P, Evrard P. Formation, maturation and disorders of brain neocortex. *AJNR* 1992; 13: 423-46.

- Barkovich AJ, Kuzniecky R, Dobyns W, Jackson G, Becker L, Evrard P. A classification scheme for malformations of cortical development. *Neuropediatrics* 1996; 27: 59-63.

- Barkovich AJ. Magnetic Resonance Imaging of lissencephaly, polymicrogyria, schizencephaly, hemimegalencephaly and band heterotopia. In: Guerrini R., Canapicchi R, Zifkin B, Andermann F, Roger J, Pfanner P (Eds). *Dysplasias of Cerebral Cortex and Epilepsy*. Philadelphia: Lippincott-Raven Publishers, 1996: 115-29.

- Barkovich AJ, Kuzniecky R, Jackson G, Guerrini R, Dobyns W. A classification scheme for malformations of cortical development. Update. *Neurology* 2001; 57: 2168-78.

- Barkovich AJ. Magnetic resonance imaging: role in the understanding of cerebral malformations. *Brain Dev* 2002; 24: 2-12.

- Bartolomei F, Gavaret M, Dravet C, Guerrini R. Familial epilepsy with unilateral and bilateral malformations of cortical development. *Epilepsia* 1999; 40: 47-51.

- Bingham PM, Lynch D, McDonald-McGinn D, Zackai E. Polymicrogyria in chromosome 22 deletion syndrome. *Neurology* 1998; 51: 1500-2.

- Bird LM, Scambler P. Cortical dysgenesis in 2 patients with chromosome 22q11 deletion. *Clin Genet* 2000; 58: 64-8.

- Capovilla G, Beccaria F, Veggliotti P, et al. Ethosuximide is effective in the treatment of epileptic negative myoclonus in childhood partial epilepsy. *J Child Neurol* 1999; 14: 395-400.

- Caraballo R, Fontana E, Micheliza B, et al. Carbamazepina, assenze atipiche crisi atoniche e stato di PO continua del sonno (POCS). *Boll lega It Epil* 1989; 66/67: 379-81.

- Caraballo R, Kochen S, Cersósimo R, Fejerman N. Unilateral pachygyria with congenital hemiplegia and peculiar type of epilepsy (Abstract). *Pediatric Neurology* 1992; 8 (5): 398.

- Caraballo R, Cersósimo R, Fejerman N. (1997a) Un tipo particular de epilepsia en pacientes con hemiparesia congenita asociada a polimicrogiria o paquigiria unilateral. *Rev Neurol* (Barc) 1997; 25 (143): 1058-63.

- Caraballo R, Cersósimo R, Pociecha J, Galicchio S, Fejerman N. (1997b) Parálisis cerebral y epilepsia. (Abstract) *Rev Neurol* (Barc) 1997; 25: 773.

- Caraballo R, Cersósimo R, Fejerman N. A particular type of epilepsy in children with congenital hemiparesis associated with unilateral polymicrogyria. *Epilepsia* 1999; 40: 865-79.

• Caraballo R, Cersósimo R, Mazza E, Fejerman N. Focal polymicrogyria in mother and son. *Brain Dev* 2000; 22: 336-9.

• Caraballo R, Cersósimo R, Fejerman N. (2004a) Unilateral closed lip schizencephaly and epilepsy: a comparison with cases of unilateral polymicrogyria. *Brain & Development* 2004; 26: 151-7.

• Caraballo R, Semprino M, Cersósimo R, Sologuestua A, Arroyo H, Fejerman N (2004b). Parálisis cerebral hemiparética y epilepsia del sobresalto. *Rev Neurol* (Barc) 2004; 38: 123-7.

• Catania S, Cross H, de Sousa C, Boyd S. Paradoxic reaction to lamotrigine in a child with benign focal epilepsy of childhood with centrotemporal spikes. *Epilepsia* 1999; 40 (11): 1657-60.

• Cerminara C, Montanaro ML, Curatolo P, Seri S. Lamotrigine-induced seizure aggravation and negative myoclonus in idiopathic Rolandic epilepsy. *Neurology* 2004; 63 (2): 373-5.

• Cersósimo R. Hemiparesia congénita y epilepsia: estudio de 133 casos. *Medicina Infantil* 2005; XII: 164-74.

• Cersósimo R. Malformaciones del desarrollo cortical. In: Fejerman N, Fernandez-Alvarez E (Eds). *Neurología Pediatrica* (3rd ed.). Buenos Aires: Panamericana, 2007: 271-84.

• Chang BS, Apse K, Caraballo R, *et al*. A familial syndrome of unilateral polymicrogyria affecting the right hemisphere. *Neurology* 2006; 66: 133-5.

• Colamaria V, Grimau-Merino R, Sgró V, *et al*. Epilepsia focale con statu di punta-onda continua in sonno lento: asterixis critico in soggeto con emipachigiria. *Bol Lega It Epil* 1989; 66/67: 233-5.

• Colamaria V, Franco A, Zamponi N, *et al*. Emiplegia congenita, alterazioni corticale ed epilepssia. *Bol Lega It Epil* 1991; 74: 169-70.

• Dalla Bernardina B, Fontana E, Michelizza B, Colamaría V, Capovilla G, Tassinari C. Partial Epilepsies in Childhood Bilateral Synchronization, Continuous Spike-Waves During Slow Sleep. In: Manellis J, Bental E, Loeber N, Dreiffus F (Eds). *Advances in Epileptology: XVIIth Epilepsy International Symposium*. New York: Raven Press, 1989: 295-302.

• Dalla Bernardina B, Fontana E, Sgró V, *et al*. Generalized or partial atonic seizures – inhibitory seizures – in children with partial epilepsies (Abstract). *EEG Clin Neurophysiol* 1990; 75: 531.

• Dalla Bernardina B, Pérez-Jiménez A, Fontana E, *et al*. Electroencephalographic Findings Associated with Cortical Dysplasias. In: Guerrini R, Canapicchi R, Zifkin B, Andermann F, Roger J, Pfanner P (Eds). *Dysplasias of Cerebral Cortex and Epilepsy*. Philadelphia: Lippincott-Raven Publishers, 1996: 235-45.

• Ferrie C, Jackson G, Giannakodimos S, Panayiotopoulos C. Posterior agyria-pachygyria with polymicrogyria: Evidence for an inherited neuronal migration disorder. *Neurology* 1995; 45: 150-3.

• Fejerman N, Caraballo R, Tenembaum S. Atypical evolutions of benign localization-related epilepsies in children: Are they predictable. *Epilepsia* 2000. 41: 380-90.

• Guerrini R, Dravet C, Raybaud C, *et al*. Epilepsy and focal gyral anomalies detected by MRI: Electroclinic, morphological correlations and follow-up. *Dev Med Child Neurol* 1993; 34: 706-8.

• Guerrini R, Pammeggiani M, Bureau M, *et al*. Localized Cortical Dysplasia: Good Seizure Outcome After Sleep-Related Electrical Status Epilepticus. In: Guerrini R, Canapicchi R, Zifkin B, Andermann F, Roger J, Pfanner P (Eds). *Dysplasias of Cerebral Cortex and Epilepsy*. Philadelphia: Lippincott-Raven Publishers, 1996: 329-36.

• Guerrini R, Genton P, Bureau M, *et al*. Multilobar polymicrogyria, intractable drop attack seizures, and sleep-related electrical status epilepticus. *Neurology* 1998; 51: 504-12.

• Guzzetta E, Battaglia D, Veredice C, *et al*. Early thalamic injury associated with epilepsy and continuous spike-wave during slow sleep. *Epilepsia* 2005; 46 (6): 889-900.

- Hadjipanayis A, Hadjichristoulou C, Youroukos S. Epilepsy in patients with cerebral palsy. *Dev Med Child Neurol* 1997; 39: 659-63.

- Kobayashi K, Ohtsuka Y, Oka E, Ohtahara S. Primary and secondary bilateral synchrony in Epilepsy: Differentiation by stimulation of interhemispheric small time differences during short spike-wave activity. *Electroencephalogr Clin Neurophysiol* 1992; 83: 93-103.

- Kobayashi K, Nishibayashi N, Ohtsuka Y, Oka E, Ohtahara S. Epilepsy with electrical status epilepticus during slow sleep and secondary bilateral synchrony. *Epilepsia* 1994; 35: 1097-103.

- Kuzniecky R, Barkovich J. Malformations of cortical development and epilepsy. *Brain Dev* 2001; 23: 2-11.

- Lerman P, Lerman-Sagie T. Sulthiame revisted. *J Child Neurol* 1995; 10: 241-2.

- Montenegro MA, Guerreiro MM. Electrical status epilepticus of sleep in association with topiramate. *Epilepsia* 2002; 43 (11): 1436-40.

- Oguni H, Hayashi K, Usui N, *et al*. (1998a). Startle epilepsy with infantile hemiplegia: report of two cases improved by surgery. *Epilepsia* 1998; 39: 93-8.

- Oguni H, Uehara T, Tanaka T, Sunahara M, Hara M, Osawa M. (1998b) Dramatic effect of ethosuximide on epileptic negative myoclonus: implications for the neurophysiological mechanism. *Neuropediatrics* 1998; 29: 29-34.

- Palmini A. Disorders of cortical development. *Curr Opin Neurol* 2000; 13 (2): 183-92.

- Park YD, Hoffman JM, Radtke RA, DeLong GR. Focal cerebral metabolic abnormality in patients with continuous spikes-waves during slow-wave sleep. *J Child Neurol* 1994; 9: 139-43.

- Pascual-Castroviejo I, Pascual-Pascual SI, Viano J, Martinez V, Palencia R. Unilateral polymicrogyria: a common cause of hemiplegia of prenatal origin. *Brain Dev* 2001; 23: 216-22.

- Pratz JM, Garaizar C, García-Nieto ML, Madoz P. Antiepileptic drugs and atypical evolution of idiopathic partial epilepsy. *Pediatr Neurol* 1998, 18: 402-6.

- Sheth RD, Gutierrez AR, Riggs JE. Rolandic epilepsy and cortical dysplasia: MRI correlation of epileptiform discharges. *Pediatr Neurol* 1997; 17 (2): 177-9.

- Spencer SS, Spencer DD, Williamson PD, Mattson RH. Effects of corpus callosum sections on secondary bilateraly synchronous interictal EEG discharges. *Neurology* 1985; 35: 1689-94.

- Sztriha L, Guerrini R, Harding B, Stewart F, Chelloug N, Johansen JG. Clinical, MRI, and pathological features of polymicrogyria in chromosome 22q11 deletion syndrome. *Am J Med Genet* 2004; 127A: 313-7.

- Tassinari C, Bureau M, Dravet C, Dalla Bernardina B, Roger J. Epilepsy with continuous spike-wave during slow sleep otherwise described as ESES (Epilepsy with Electrical Status Epilepticus during Slow Sleep). In: Roger J., Bureau M, Dravet C, Dreiffus F, Perret A, Wolf P (Eds). *Epileptic Syndromes in Infancy, Childhood and Adolescence* (2nd ed.). London: John Libbey, 1992: 245-56.

- Veggiotti P, Cardinali S, Granocchio E, *et al*. Motor impairment on awakening in a patient with an EEG pattern of "Unilateral continuous spikes and waves during slow sleep". *Epileptic Disord* 2005; 7 (2): 131-6.

- Yoshimura K, Hamada F, Tomoda T, Wakiguchi H, Kurashige T. Focal pachy-polymicrogyria in three siblings. *Pediatr Neurol* 1998; 18: 435-8.

- Wiklund L., Uvebrant P, Flodniar K. Computed tomography as an adjunct in etiological analysis of hemiplegic cerebral palsy: children born at term. *Neuropediatrics* 1991; 22: 121-8.

- Zollino M, Colosimo C, Zuffardi O, *et al*. Cryptic t (1; 12Xq44; p13.3) translocation in a previously described syndrome with polymicrogyria, segregating as an apparently X-linked trait. *Am J Med Genet* 2003; 117A: 65-71.

Part IV
Idiopathic focal epilepsies in adolescence

Benign focal seizures of adolescence

Roberto H. Caraballo*, Ricardo Cersósimo*, Giuseppe Capovilla**, Natalio Fejerman*
*Buenos Aires, Argentina
**Mantova, Italy

The recognition of idiopathic focal epileptic syndromes in childhood took many years to be generally accepted because it was against the logical rule that focal seizures arise from focal epileptogenic areas which most probably have as substratum a focal cortical lesion (see Chapter 6).

Idiopathic focal epilepsies in infancy had been described in the late eighties and started to be accepted after the report of a series of familial cases with benign evolution (see Chapter 3).

As a logical sequence there were no reasons to deny the possibility that similar conditions might have their onset in adolescents. The first report of this event took place in 1972, in the French literature with the report of 14 patients with unprovoked isolated focal seizures in adolescents who were followed up for 4-12 years (Loiseau et al., 1972). However, this report was first acknowledged after the same group presented 83 adolescents with the same features and published the series of patients in Lancet under the title of "An unrecognized syndrome of benign focal epileptic seizures in teenagers" (Loiseau & Orgogozo, 1978). In 1992 Loiseau and Louiset updated their series and reported on 108 patients followed-up for 5 years or more. The authors still thought that it was a syndrome, although they preferred the term "Benign partial epileptic seizures of adolescents" because the patients usually did not present chronically recurrent seizures.

Thereafter, several series of patients have been reported from different centers (Mauri et al., 1996; King et al., 1998, 1999; Capovilla et al., 2001; Panayiotopoulos, 2005; Caraballo et al.,1999, 2004). The 10 cases of Mauri et al. were presented only as an abstract. The 8 cases of King et al. were part of an important first seizure study of 300 consecutive patients over 5 years of age. Ninety-two patients between 10 and 20 years of age were enrolled and 37 of them had partial epilepsies. Of these, 8 complied with more strict criteria for diagnosis of benign partial seizures of adolescents, but other 6 (classified as "unclassified") also were apparently idiopathic cases and had a benign course. Capovilla et al. presented 37 cases but a normal EEG was found in only 17 of the patients. The authors hypothesized that other forms of idiopathic focal epilepsies might be seen in adolescents. Nevertheless they suggested that even presenting spikes in the interictal EEGs, these patients should not be medicated.

The influence of ILAE's 1989 Classification (Commission..., 1989) including at the end of the table under "Special syndromes" a category of "Isolated seizures or isolated status epilepticus" moved the first author of the mentioned reports to place this condition as "Isolated partial seizures of adolescents" (Loiseau et al., 2002). Panayiotopoulos mentioned about 120 personal cases in a chapter on a book (2005). Caraballo et al. (2004) reported on 15 cases followed-up during 6 years on the first prospective study apart from the initial reports.

Finally, we are presenting here a large series of 44 patients including the 29 previously presented by our group.

Whether the patients described with BFSA represent an epileptic syndrome or only had a single seizure event with normal interictal EEG should be discussed. On behalf of the benefit to the neuropediatricians' practices achieved since the recognition of epileptic syndromes, we believe that BFSA should be considered as a benign, age-related, autolimited epileptic syndrome appearing during the second decade of life. It is a transitory condition, predominantly occurring in males, and with a peak of onset between 13 and 14 years of age. BFSA is characterized by simple focal motor and somatosensory seizures with secondary generalization occurring isolated or in a cluster in the first 24-48 hours after onset. The seizures occur predominantly when awake, and have a benign course. The interictal EEG, neurological examination and neuroradiological images are normal and a family history of epilepsy is rare (Loiseau & Louiset, 1992).

Epidemiology

According to Loiseau and Louiset (1992), a quarter of focal seizures (single or in a cluster of up to five seizures during 36 hours, never to occur again) with an onset between 12 and 18 years of age, have a benign course. BFSA may account for between 7.5% and 22% of patients having simple focal seizures in the second decade of life (Panayiotopoulos, 1996, 2005; King et al., 1999). However, to date no population-based study documents these figures. Around 200 cases have been described (Mauri et al., 1996; Panayiotopoulos, 1996; King et al., 1999; Capovilla et al., 2001; Loiseau et al., 2002; Caraballo et al., 1999, 2004).

In a 6-year period, we registered 15 adolescent patients with BFSA and within the same time, 17 teenagers were diagnosed as late-onset benign focal epilepsy of childhood, 8 patients with probably symptomatic focal epilepsy and 38 youngsters with symptomatic focal epilepsy. Now we expand the period to 10 years and we are reporting on 44 adolescents (11 to 18 years of age with BFSA) (Caraballo et al., 2004).

We believe that this entity is more frequent than reported in the literature. The reason may be the fact that BFSA is characterized by a single seizure or cluster of seizures, short-lived and transient that probably do not get to be controlled by an epileptologist. On the other hand, it is important that this type of patients be documented to know the exact prevalence in primary and other levels of care.

Clinical features

The age at onset of the seizures ranges from 11 to 18 years, with a mean age of 13.5 and a median age of 14 years. There is a 70% male preponderance. Physical examination and mental status of the patients are normal.

Simple focal seizures are the most frequent type of seizures, characterized by eye and/or head deviation, facial tonic or clonic focal seizures and visual symptoms followed by upper extremity clonic focal seizures. Seizures are followed by tonic-clonic seizures with secondary generalization in 50% of the cases. The motor seizures do not follow a Jacksonian march. In some cases a sensorymotor Jacksonian march was reported (Loiseau & Orgogozo, 1978) and this was a criterion selected for inclusion in the 8 cases presented by King et al. (1999). Rarely, the seizures are complex focal and characterized by motion arrest and oral automatisms, followed or not by secondarily generalized tonic-clonic seizures. Within the series of Capovilla et al. (2001), a subgroup of patients presented versive seizures. The duration of the seizures is around 2 minutes, but in patients who have secondarily generalized seizures they last 5 minutes approximately (Caraballo et al., 1999, 2004; King et al., 1999; Capovilla et al., 2001; Loiseau et al., 2002). Speech deficiencies, autonomic symptoms and vertigo were reported in the cases of Loiseau et al. (2002). Psychological symptoms are rare (Loiseau et al., 2002). Auditory, olfactory and gustatory symptoms have never been reported. (Caraballo et al., 1999,2004; King et al., 1998,1999; Capovilla et al., 2001; Loiseau et al., 2002). Even if these clinical features may also exist in cryptogenic and symptomatic focal epilepsies, a hallmark of BFSA is that post-ictal signs such as motor or psychic deficits are extremely rare. The teenager is fully aware and may give a reliable account of the onset of the clinical manifestations of the simple focal seizures throughout the whole event.

As Loiseau and co-workers (2002) very rightly remarked, we should ask ourselves whether the first diagnosed seizure is really the first experienced seizure. Generalized seizures are easier to recognize, but a brief focal seizure can be less impressive and more difficult to identify. In this setting, it is very important to take a detailed interview from both the parents and the teenager.

All patients have seizures when awake and less frequently the patients also have seizures during sleep.

The event is a single seizure in 75%. In the remaining 25%, a cluster of two to four seizures occurs in less than 36-48 hours.

EEG features

A normal interictal EEG or unspecified abnormalities on the same at onset, and repeated control EEGs when awake and asleep are mandatory for the diagnosis of BFSA. Bilateral centro-parieto-occipital or diffuse slow waves may be found when the EEG is recorded soon after the seizure, particularly between or after a cluster of seizures. However, King and co-workers (1999) and Capovilla and co-workers (2001) found nonspecific unilateral theta activities predominantly during sleep. Our group found similar abnormalities with seizures occurring in a cluster but when the patient was awake (Caraballo et al., 2004). In the particular subgroup within the 37 patients reported by Capovilla et al. (2001), their versive seizures were associated with focal spike wave discharges over posterior regions.

Hyperventilation is normal or shows mild slow activities. No typical spike-waves discharges are seen in any of the cases, nor are any focal or multifocal abnormalities, with the exception of the particular cases within the 37 patients reported by Capovilla et al. (2001) and the 2 cases within the series of King et al. (1999) with early post-ictal multifocal spikes. No ictal EEG recordings have been described to date.

In *Table I*, the series of patients with BFSA that have been published are described.

Aetiology

A family history of epilepsy is very rare (3-5%) as is a personal history predisposing to epilepsy (Caraballo et al., 1999, 2004; Loiseau et al., 2002). Capovilla and co-workers (2001) found a high rate of family history of epilepsy, supporting a probable idiopathic nature.

Table I. Reported series of patients with BFSA

Series of patients with BFSA	Gender (males)	Age at onset (years)	Type of seizures			Distribution		EEG
			SPS	CPS	SGTCS	Awake	Sleep	
Loiseau et al. (2002) (108 patients)	71.2%	Peak at 13-15	87.4%	13.6%	57.2%	87%	13%	Normal
Capovilla et al. (2001) (37 patients)	60%	Mean 14.5	86%	27%	57%	62%	38%	Spikes, sharp Waves and Theta discharges
Mauri et al. (1996) (10 patients)	70%	Range: 12 a 19	30%	20%	50%	?	?	Unspecified abnormalities
King et al. (1999) (8 patients)	50%	Mean age: 15.5	100%	–	75%	?	?	Unspecified Abnormalities
Caraballo et al. (1999) Retrospective study (14 patients)	71.4%	Peak at 12-13	85.7%	26.7%	64.2%	93%	7%	Normal
Caraballo et al. (2004) Prospective study (15 patients)	66.5%	Median 14	86.6%	13.4%	40%	100%	13.3%	Normal or unspecified abnormalities

SPS: simple partial seizures; CPS: complex partial seizures; SGTCS: secondary generalized tonic-clonic seizures.

Incidentally we were able to find two patients with a personal history of another idiopathic focal epilepsy syndrome in infancy (see our present series of cases), and curiously enough, in the families of the mentioned patients, two close relatives with Benign childhood epilepsy with centrotemporal spikes were registered.

Acquired risk factors are found in 4 percent of the cases (Loiseau *et al.*, 2002). Nonspecific seizure provocative or precipitating factors such as sleep deprivation, stress or alcohol abuse are described by neither the patients nor their parents.

Pathophysiology

The pathophysiology of these particular focal seizure events is still a challenge for epileptologists. Seizures were characterized by a succession of symptoms and/or signs implicating a stepwise involvement of primary or secondary cortical areas and very seldom of temporal structures. The absence of documented cases with ictal studies and the rare positive EEG finding in isolated cases preclude the use of a pathopysiological interpretation of the discharges. Other neurophysiological studies might perhaps be useful, although it is difficult to perform so many investigations in adolescents with isolated seizures.

Diagnostic work-up

In an adolescent patient who presents a first unprovoked focal seizure, the possible presence of an underlying brain lesion should be strongly suspected. Consequently, a brain MRI should always be performed in these patients. A high expectation of seizure recurrence exists, even when neuroradiologic imaging is normal and a diagnosis of cryptogenic or probably symptomatic focal epilepsy is possible in the absence of a brain lesion. Laboratory test and brain imaging are normal. Other types of studies such as karyotype or neurometabolic investigations are not necessary.

The EEG may show some minor, nonspecific, abnormalities without spikes or focal slowing. However, the early post-ictal waking and sleep EEG might help to find more specific focal abnormalities as was shown in some cases (King *et al.*, 1999). In fact, due to the characteristics of BFSA no thorough EEG studies have been done in the reported series. We understand that it is not probable to be able to register an ictal EEG in these patients unless they are admitted after the first seizure and they happen to present a second one.

Differential diagnosis and relations with other epilepsy syndromes

The most important differential diagnosis of BFSA is cryptogenic or probably symptomatic focal epilepsy, in which a normal neurological examination and normal neuroradiological imaging are often found. Electroclinical features and evolution in patients with focal cryptogenic epilepsy are different from those found in our benign cases. Late-onset benign focal epilepsies of childhood, like BCECTS or CEOP, may also be considered as a differential diagnosis and interictal EEG will clarify the situation. Adolescents with Juvenile Myoclonic epilepsy may sometimes present focal myoclonic or clonic seizures. Again, interrogation regarding the presence of myoclonia in hands after waking up and finding polyspikes discharges in the EEG would serve for differential diagnosis even before the patients arrive to present typical generalized tonic-clonic seizures. Patients with migraine may present a sensory march without motor seizures. However, none of the patients in our series had migraine.

Obviously, teenagers may present isolated seizures symptomatic of hypoglycemia or associated to excessive alcohol intake or other drug intoxications which must be considered as possible aetiologies (Wolf, 1997). We also know that certain factors which facilitate the appearance of seizures in persons with epilepsy, such as sleep deprivation, emotionally motivated situations of stress, and even excessive intermittent light stimulation are more prevalent in adolescents than in other age periods.

The differential diagnoses of BFSA are listed in *Table II*.

We can envisage, however, that BFSA might also present different types of seizures and interictal focal EEG discharges as in most of the idiopathic focal epilepsies in childhood. These EEG functional foci might be located in any part of the cerebral cortex, as long as the seizures and the EEG abnormalities show spontaneous remission or disappear after treatment with antiepileptic drugs (AED). Of course, the phantom of a probably symptomating epilepsy hiding behind this benign façade is a constant threat.

As for the association of previous or ulterior idiopathic focal epilepsy syndromes in patients with BFSA, we have seen during the follow-up of our 40 patients with Benign familial infantile seizures, that two of them developed BFSA at ages 14 and 16 years (Caraballo, 2005). We are not aware of any other reports on association of BFSA with other idiopathic epilepsy syndromes.

Thus, the diagnostic workup and differential diagnosis of BFSA have limitations. In fact, the early diagnosis is also difficult since we would need some time of follow-up to ascertain the clinical suspicion. Nevertheless, it is quite important to have the existence of this syndrome in mind. We explain the patients and their parents that this condition exists, that upon finding normal EEGs and MRIs, we should avoid the use of antiepileptic drugs, although we have to be prepared to face later the appearance of new signs or symptoms pointing to a different diagnosis.

Table II. Differential diagnoses of BFSA

Epileptic syndromes
– Late-onset of idiopathic focal epilepsies of childhood (BCECTS, COE)
– Cryptogenic or probably symptomatic focal epilepsies
– Symptomatic focal epilepsies
– Some cases of juvenile myoclonic epilepsy with focal motor seizures
Other paroxysmal events and seizures in adolescents
– Migraine with focal paresthesias
– Occasional seizures associated with sleep deprivation, excessive alcohol intake, or other intoxications
– Pseudo-seizures

Coming back to the diagnosis of BFSA we don't have to rest anymore on the old recommendations of the Commission of ILAE 1993 stating that there are needed two epileptic seizures for a diagnosis of Epilepsy. This concept has been recently reviewed by a joint committee with representatives of ILAE and the International Bureau for Epilepsy (IBE) which arrived to the conclusion that in many cases one can identify an epileptic syndrome after the first seizure (Fisher et al., 2005).

Finally, in the diagnostic scheme proposed in 2001 by the Task force on classification of ILAE, an item on "Single seizures or isolated clusters of seizures" was included under the "Conditions with epileptic seizures that do not require a diagnosis of epilepsy" (Engel, 2001). Since the last report of ILAE's Classification core group (Engel, 2006) did not mention BFSA at all (despite that one of us – NF– was a member of the group) there would be in that scheme no room to place BFSA among the "Conditions with epileptic seizures that do not require a diagnosis of epilepsy". Therefore, we insist in considering it as a syndrome in order to have it present in the mind of neurologists caring for adolescents.

Treatment

It is crucial to identify this condition to avoid giving a poor prognosis at a first seizure only because this type of seizure occurred during adolescence. Antiepileptic treatment should be avoided in these cases as the course is benign and the seizures isolated, as has been corroborated in a prospective study (Caraballo et al., 2004).

Prognosis and long-term evolution

In these patients a longer follow-up is necessary to confirm a benign course as typically occurs in BFSA. The repeated EEG recordings when awake and asleep are always normal as was demonstrated by us in a previous retrospective study (Caraballo et al., 1999). Other previous studies confirm that a benign course may be seen in adolescents with focal seizures, normal neurologic examination and normal brain imaging (King et al., 1999; Capovilla et al., 2001; Loiseau et al., 2002; Caraballo et al., 1999, 2004). Naturally, the evolution of the patient will confirm the diagnosis of this particular entity.

Longer follow-ups and future prospective electroclinical studies are necessary to confirm and define the nosologic place of this entity.

We confirm the existence of adolescents with isolated single or clusters of focal motor or somatosensory seizures, and less frequently other focal seizure types, with or without secondarily generalized seizures, with a normal EEG, normal neurologic examination, normal brain imaging and a benign course, as previously described by Loiseau et al. (1972).

Data about our present series of cases

Number of patients and gender

A total of 44 patients (24 boys and 20 girls) with electroclinical features compatible with BFSA were identified between 1990 and 2005 at the Garrahan Hospital of Buenos Aires (34 patients) and the Poma Hospital of Mantova (10 patients).

Age at onset

The age at onset of the seizures ranged from 11 to 18 years, with a mean age of 13 and a median age of 14 years.

Personal and family history of febrile seizures and epilepsy

A family history of epilepsy was found in 4 patients. None of the patients had a personal and/or family history of febrile seizures.

Ictal manifestation

Simple focal seizures occurred in 38 cases (86%) and were characterized by eye and/or head deviation in 20, facial tonic or clonic focal seizures in 18, and visual symptoms followed by upper extremity clonic focal seizures in 6. Seizures were followed by tonic-clonic seizures with secondary generalization in 21 patients. The motor seizures did not follow a jacksonian march. In 40 patients, motor seizures were followed by focal numbness which did show a jacksonian progression in some of them. In 6 patients, seizures presented as motion arrest and oral automatisms, followed by tonic-clonic seizures with secondary generalization in three. According to parental reports, the duration of seizures was 2 minutes approximately, but in patients who had secondarily generalized seizures, they lasted 5 min approximately.

Circadian distribution

All 44 patients had seizures when awake, and 5 also had seizures during sleep.

Frequency of seizures

The episode was a single seizure in 31 (70.5%) patients. In the remaining 13, a cluster of 2 to 4 seizures occurred in < 48 hours.

EEG features

All 44 patients had a normal interictal EEG at onset, and repeated control EEGs when awake and asleep were normal as well. In seven patients of 13 who had seizures in a cluster, we were able to record an EEG within 10 hours after the seizures. Four of these patients had focal seizures, and the awake EEG revealed focal centroparietal theta activities. In the other three who had secondarily generalized seizures, it showed bilateral theta activities instead.

Treatment

Twenty of the patients in our series have never received AED treatment. Nine patients received carbamazepine, 8 received valproic acid, 4 received oxcarbazepine and 3 received Phenobarbital.

Evolution

During a follow-up period ranging from 2 to 15 years (mean, 9 years) no recurrence was noted. No detailed neuropsychological examination was done, but the adolescents seemed normal and continued with their secondary level studies without problems.

References

• Capovilla G, Gambardella A, Romeo A, *et al*. Benign partial epilepsies of adolescence: a report of 37 new cases. *Epilepsia* 2001; 42: 1549-52.

• Caraballo R, Galicchio S, Grañana N, Cersosimo R, Fejerman N. Convulsiones parciales benignas de la adolescencia. *Rev Neurol* (Barc) 1999; 28: 669-71.

Caraballo R, Cersósimo R, Fejerman N. Benign focal seizures of adolescents: a prospective study. *Epilepsia* 2004; 45: 1600-3.

• Caraballo R. Convulsiones familiares y no familiares benignas del lactante. In: Ruggieri V, Caraballo R, Arroyo H (Eds). *Temas de Neuropediatría. Homenaje al Dr Natalio Fejerman*. Buenos Aires: Editorial Médica Panamericana, 2005: 53-68.

• Commission on Classification and Terminology of the International League against Epilepsy. Proposal for revised classification of epilepsies and epileptic syndromes. *Epilepsia* 1989; 30: 389-99.

• Commission on Epidemiology and Prognosis, International League against Epilepsy. Guidelines for epidemiologic studies on epilepsy. *Epilepsia* 1993; 34 (4): 592-6.

• Engel J. A proposed diagnostic scheme for people with epileptic seizures and with epilepsy: Report of the ILAE Task Force on Classification and Terminology. *Epilepsia* 2001; 42: 796-803.

• Engel J Jr. Report of the ILAE classification core group. *Epilepsia* 2006; 47 (9): 1558-68.

• Fisher RS, van Emde Boas W, Blume W, *et al*. Epileptic seizures and epilepsy: definitions proposed by the International League against Epilepsy (ILAE) and the International Bureau for Epilepsy (IBE). *Epilepsia* 2005; 46 (4): 470-2.

• King MA, Newton MR, Jackson GD, *et al*. Epileptology of the first-seizure presentation: a clinical, electroencephalographic, and magnetic resonance imaging study of 300 consecutive patients. *Lancet* 1998; 352 (9133): 1007-11.

- King MA, Newton MR, Berkovic SF. Benign partial seizures of adolescence. *Epilepsia* 1999; 40: 1244-7.

- Loiseau P, Jogeix M, Lafitte M. Crises épileptiques sans suite chez les adolescents. *Bordeaux Medical* 1972 ; 5: 2623-9.

- Loiseau P, Orgogozo JM. An unrecognized syndrome of benign focal epileptic seizures in teenagers. *Lancet* 1978; 2: 1070-1.

- Loiseau P, Louiset P. Benign partial seizures of adolescence. In: Roger J. Bureau M. Dravet C. *et al.* (Eds). *Epileptic syndromes in infancy, childhood and adolescence* (2nd ed.). London: John Libbey, 1992 : 343-5.

- Loiseau P, Jallon P, Wolf P. Isolated partial seizures of adolescence. In: Roger J. Bureau M. Dravet C, *et al.* (Eds). *Epileptic syndromes in infancy, childhood and adolescence* (3rd ed.). London: John Libbey, 2002 : 327-30.

- Mauri JA, Iniguez C, Jerico I, *et al.* Benign partial seizures of adolescence: report of 10 cases. *Epilepsia* 1996; 37 (Suppl 4): 102.

- Panayiotopoulos CP. Benign partial seizures of adolescence. In: Wallace S (Ed). *Epilepsy in children*. London: Chapman & Hall, 1996: 377-8.

- Panayiotopoulos CP. Benign (isolated) focal seizures of adolescence. In: Panayiotopoulos CP (Ed). *The epilepsies. Seizures, syndromes and management*. Oxfordshire: Bladon Medical Publishing, 2005: 264-9.

- Wolf P. Isolated seizures. In: Engel Jr, Pedley T (Eds). *Epilepsy: a comprehensive textbook*. Philadelphia: Lippincott Raven, 1997: 2475-81.

PART V
Autosomal dominant focal epilepsies

Is there a subset of benign cases within the autosomal dominant focal epilepsies?

Eliane Kobayashi*, Eva Andermann*, Frederick Andermann*, Ingrid E Scheffer**
*Montreal, Canada
**Melbourne, Australia

The concept of genetic focal epilepsies is relatively new as compared to awareness of the importance of genetic factors in the generalized epilepsies. Focal epilepsies have been largely attributed to environmental factors, such as birth injuries, infections, postnatal head trauma, and brain lesions, *e.g.* tumours and vascular insults. However, in the past decade, there has been increasing recognition of families with dominantly inherited partial epilepsies.

In the past decade, several partial epilepsies with single gene inheritance have been identified and included in the new proposal for classification of epileptic syndromes by the International League against Epilepsy (Engel, 2001). The main familial focal epilepsies are autosomal dominant nocturnal frontal lobe epilepsy (ADNFLE) (Scheffer *et al.*, 1994, 1995a; Rodrigues-Pinguet *et al.*, 2003), familial mesial TLE (FMTLE) (Berkovic *et al.*, 1994), familial lateral TLE (FLTLE) (Ottman *et al.*, 1995), and familial partial epilepsy with variable foci (FPEVF) (Scheffer *et al.*, 1998). Except for FLTLE, where no refractory patients have been described to date, the other familial epilepsies present variable degrees of seizure severity, but most affected individuals will have a good outcome.

Autosomal dominant nocturnal frontal lobe epilepsy

ADNFLE was the first familial focal epilepsy for which the genetic background has been elucidated (Scheffer *et al.*, 1994, 1995a). A decade later, 109 ADNFLE kindreds have been reported in the literature (Combi *et al.*, 2004), and available pedigrees showed an autosomal dominant inheritance pattern with 84% penetrance, with both males and females being equally affected. These families could be subdivided into two main subgroups: those with 100% penetrance and those with incomplete penetrance, ranging from 29 to 87%.

Clinically, clusters of nocturnal seizures arising during NREM sleep (especially during stage 2) are characterized by sudden awakenings with hypermotor or tonic manifestations, and rare tonic-clonic seizures. Auras are frequently reported and patients often retain consciousness throughout the events. These auras are usually nonspecific (generalized shivering and tingling, cephalic, thoracic, epigastric sensations), but may present as other sensory (auditory, vertiginous, visual, olfactory, gustatory) and psychic (fear, *déja vu*) phenomena (Scheffer *et al.*, 1994, 1995a). Seizures start during the first two decades (mean 12 years; median 8 years) and become less frequent during adult life. There is marked intrafamilial variation in seizure onset, semiology and severity, and the inherited nature is easily overlooked, as relatives may only be mildly affected and their seizures not recognised.

There is also considerable interfamilial variation and, in some families such as the earliest ones described, the attacks are much less severe compared with the findings in other families. The response to medication is also quite variable. Drugs such as Carbamazepine may be quite effective in some patients, whereas in others currently available antiepileptic medications are not effective.

Attacks during wakefulness can be observed, especially in those patients with poor seizure control during exacerbations of their seizures.

The nocturnal seizures may be misdiagnosed as parasomnias, but the latter are much less frequent, do not cluster and are not associated with retained awareness. The clinical picture is indistinguishable from sporadic nocturnal frontal lobe epilepsy, where the interictal EEGs are also frequently normal, and ictal onsets are usually obscured by artefacts. Structural magnetic resonance imaging (MRI) studies are unremarkable, but PET/SPECT abnormalities have been described unilaterally in the frontal regions (Hayman *et al.*, 1997).

Four loci and 3 nicotinic acetylcholine receptor subunit genes (Phillips *et al.*, 1995; Steinlein *et al.*, 1995, 1997; Phillips *et al.*, 1998; Hirose *et al.*, 1999; Saenz *et al.*, 1999; Ito *et al.*, 2000; Steinlein *et al.*, 2000; Gambardella *et al.*, 2000; De Fusco *et al.*, 2000; Phillips *et al.*, 2001; Leniger *et al.*, 2003; McLellan *et al.*, 2003; Rozycka *et al.*, 2003; Aridon *et al.*, 2006) for ADNFLE have been identified. Mutations in 2 genes *(CHRNA4, CHRNB2)* coding for different subunits of the neuronal nicotinic acetylcholine receptor (nAchR) cause the same phenotype (McLellan *et al.*, 2003); a gene *(CHRNA2)* encoding a third subunit has been implicated in "familial epilepsy with nocturnal wandering" (Aridon *et al.*, 2006), a variant of ADNFLE. At ENFL1 (Phillips *et al.*, 1995), 4 different mutations in the *CHRNA4* gene, coding for the alpha4 subunit of nAchR, have been found in 9 families (Steinlein *et al.*, 1995, 1997; Hirose *et al.*, 1999; Ito *et al.*, 2000; Steinlein *et al.*, 2000; Leniger *et al.*, 2003; McLellan *et al.*, 2003; Rozycka *et al.*, 2003; Saenz *et al.*, 1999). For ENFL2 (Phillips *et al.*, 1998) the gene is still unknown. Mutations in the *CHRNB2* gene on the ENFL3 locus (Gambardella *et al.*, 2000), coding for the beta2 subunit of the nAchR, were found in 3 unrelated families (De Fusco *et al.*, 2000; Phillips *et al.*, 2001; McLellan *et al.*, 2003). More recently, a mutation in the *CHRNA2* gene has been described in an Italian kindred with a more complex seizure pattern suggesting involvement of frontolimbic structures (Aridon *et al.*, 2006). However, most families do not show any mutations for the genes they have been tested (Bonati *et al.*, 2002; Combi *et al.*, 2004). There has also been an unconfirmed report about variants in the promoter region of *CRH*, the corticotrophin-releasing hormone gene (Combi *et al.*, 2005).

Sporadic cases may carry mutations in the same genes as in the familial cases, but only rare patients have been identified (Phillips et al., 2000; Andermann F, Scheffer, personal communication).

The recognition of the clinical patterns of frontal epilepsy has led to identification of many sporadic patients in whom a lesion cannot be demonstrated and in whom familial occurrence is not striking. It is however essential to enquire about the possible familial incidence in such patients with frontal epilepsy without an MRI demonstrable lesion. There is no evidence for the effectiveness of surgical treatment in these patients unlike what is encountered in patients with familial mesial temporal lobe epilepsy where, if the epilepsy is severe enough, surgical treatment may be considered and the results are similar to what is found in patients with sporadic temporal lobe epilepsy. Whether in patients with sporadic frontal lobe epilepsy without a structural lesion a molecular abnormality may exist, remains to be determined in the future.

nAChR can influence neuronal excitability by controlling the presynaptic release of excitatory and inhibitory neurotransmitters. The known mutations have different effects on nAChR properties, but result in reduced permeability to calcium and increased sensitivity to the agonist (Bertrand et al., 1998). This increased sensitivity may cause an imbalance of acetylcholine in pathways such as the thalamo-cortical network, which could facilitate seizures (Raggenbass & Bertrand, 2002). The abnormal calcium permeability would facilitate glutamate release at excitatory synapses, and therefore sustain repetitive activity (Rodrigues-Pinguet et al., 2003). The effect of mutated nAchR during brain morphogenesis is still unknown (Steinlein, 2002), and the mechanisms through which mutations in a receptor that is widely distributed throughout cortical and subcortical structures can specifically cause frontal lobe seizures is unclear.

Familial temporal lobe epilepsies

There are two types of familial temporal lobe epilepsies (FTLE), based on seizure semiology, genetic background and MRI characteristics: the mesial (FMTLE) and the lateral (FLTLE) forms.

Recently, FTLE was included in the new proposal for classification of epileptic syndromes by the International League against Epilepsy (ILAE), supporting it as a well-defined syndrome (Engel, 2001). Sporadic TLE, pseudo-TLE (Andermann, 2003), neuronal migration disorders (Palmini et al., 1991), periventricular nodular heterotopia (Dubeau et al., 1995), hypothalamic hamartoma (Berkovic et al., 1988), a mild form of tuberous sclerosis (Jansen et al., 2006), chorea-acanthocytosis (Al Asmi et al., 2005) and other conditions must all be considered in the differential diagnosis of FTLE.

It is important to recognize that it is impossible to distinguish patients with familial and non-familial TLE based solely on the clinical presentation, for both the mesial and lateral forms. As the family history is not always accurately documented, many so-called "sporadic" or "isolated" patients with TLE may actually have a familial epilepsy syndrome, as in ADNFLE. The identification of a positive family history of nonspecific seizures in patients with TLE is not sufficient for a diagnosis of FTLE.

The best definition of FTLE is based on the familial recurrence of TLE, which is defined by clinical-EEG criteria according to ILAE recommendations (1989), in the absence of any suggestion of other partial or generalized epilepsy syndromes in affected family members. Thus, the finding of at least 2 TLE patients in a family is suggestive of FTLE especially where other epilepsy phenotypes are not seen. An autosomal dominant inheritance pattern with incomplete penetrance implies the presence of asymptomatic carriers of the genetic abnormalities, who can transmit the disorder to their offspring. Therefore, we should consider inclusion of families not only with affected first-degree relatives, but also with affected second and third degree relatives. Autosomal recessive or sex-linked inheritance cannot be ruled out in some families. Linkage studies have excluded the known loci for partial epilepsies on chromosomes 1q, 10q, 15q, 20q and 22q.

With the detailed description of the lateral form of FTLE, also referred to as autosomal dominant partial epilepsy with auditory features (Ottman *et al.*, 1995), and the identification of associated mutations in the *LGI-1* gene on chromosome 10q (Kalachikov *et al.*, 2002; Morante-Redolat *et al.*, 2002), the distinction between mesial and lateral families became easier (Kobayashi *et al.*, 2001; Vadlamudi *et al.*, 2003; Berkovic *et al.*, 2004a; Kobayashi *et al.*, 2005a, 2005b).

Familial mesial temporal lobe epilepsy

FMTLE was first described in 1994 as a benign syndrome in a population-based study arising from investigation of a large number of twin pairs by Berkovic *et al.* (1994, 1996). However, subsequent hospital-based FMTLE series identified patients who were not as benign, with a high proportion of hippocampal atrophy (HA), sometimes requiring surgical treatment for their epilepsy (Cendes *et al.*, 1998; Kobayashi *et al.*, 2001). There is indeed remarkable intra– and interfamilial phenotypic heterogeneity with respect to history of febrile seizures (FS), severity of the epilepsy and presence of HA, and it seems that FMTLE can be divided into two groups according to these parameters.

Benign FMTLE: In families with the benign form of FMTLE, we observe a very mild clinical picture, with later onset (2nd to 4th decades), no history of FS and no MRI evidence of HA. *Déja-vu* and *jamais-vu* appear to be overrepresented in this group of patients (Andermann *et al.*, 1997). Affected individuals may have only recurrent *déja-vu* and this raises the question of the specificity of *déjà-vu*, which is well known, and may be present in the normal population as well. This issue has not so far been resolved, but indicators suggestive of *déjà-vu* with an epileptic basis may be helpful such as a more prolonged, unpleasant sensation. In addition in these families migraine is overrepresented. Patients may only have 1 or 2 secondarily generalized seizures and many of them may have only minor episodes. The response to antiepileptic medication is also quite good in these patients and it is not entirely clear whether sporadic remission of their symptoms can or does occur. Identification of this benign form would have been difficult except for the study of twin pairs by Berkovic et al. (1994). A high index of suspicion is required for accurate diagnosis in families with this form. Patients with severe or intractable epilepsy are rare in the families of patients who have benign FTLE.

FMTLE associated with HA: Seizures characterized by mesial temporal semiology (rising epigastric sensation, psychic and experiential phenomena), as well as complex partial seizures with oral or manual automatisms and prominent post-ictal confusion (identical to those observed in non-familial MTLE), are frequent. Secondarily generalized tonic-clonic seizures can occur, usually at the beginning of the disease, before treatment is initiated. Age at seizure onset is usually in the three first decades of life, with a mean of 10 years (Kobayashi et al., 2003a). History of FS in infancy and early childhood seems to be less frequent (around 11%) (Kobayashi et al., 2003a) than in a surgical FMTLE series (30%) (Kobayashi et al., 2003b), and much less frequent than in a random surgical TLE series not selected for FTLE (40%) (Abou-Khalil et al., 1993). Although the majority of patients have a benign clinical course, including spontaneous remission, refractory seizures may occur in up to 29% of patients (Kobayashi et al., 2003a).

Interictal and ictal EEG abnormalities consist of unilateral or bilateral epileptiform discharges over mesial temporal regions, although some patients may show no abnormalities. MRI shows varying degrees of HA and of hyperintense T2 signal, and this may also be found in asymptomatic family members (Kobayashi et al., 2002). However, HA is more frequent and more severe in patients with refractory seizures (Kobayashi et al., 2003a). The presence of clear-cut HA in both affected and asymptomatic family members in FMTLE suggests that the hippocampal abnormalities themselves could be inherited, and not necessarily lead to epilepsy (Kobayashi et al., 2002). However, in kindreds with FMTLE, febrile convulsions are overrepresented and whether these families represent a different subgroup from the ones where febrile convulsions are rare or absent is not entirely clear. It would appear that mesial temporal sclerosis may result from factors other than the recognized ones such as prolonged febrile convulsions in infancy for instance. Pathological studies have not led to any insights into what these mechanisms might be.

Available qualitative pathology from surgical specimens obtained from operated FMTLE patients showed the typical pattern of mesial temporal sclerosis (MTS): selective neuronal loss in CA1, CA3 and CA4 with relative preservation of CA2, and variable involvement of the amygdala and parahippocampal region (Kobayashi et al., 2003b). The observation of MTS in operated FMTLE patients who became seizure-free suggests that MTS represents the epileptogenic substrate, at least in some of these families, analogous to what is observed in non-familial or "sporadic" cases.

Linkage to chr18p has been recently demonstrated in a Brazilian kindred with HA (Maurer-Morelli et al., 2006). Although some polymorphisms have been described in MTLE patients (Tan et al., 2004), there are no such data deriving from kindreds with FMTLE. No families with FMTLE were found to have an *LGI-1* mutation, even though some had affected family members with both mesial symptoms and auditory features (Berkovic et al., 2004a; Santos et al., 2002; Badhwar et al., 2004). This further supports the fact that FMTLE and FLTLE constitute separate genetic syndromes. We hypothesized that FMTLE may be found to have a major gene leading to hippocampal abnormalities, and the phenotype could be influenced by additional genetic and environmental modifying factors, resembling complex inheritance.

Familial lateral temporal lobe epilepsy

FLTLE is a benign epilepsy syndrome, characterized by auditory auras (buzzing, roaring, radio– or motor-like sounds, distortions in sounds and words). Although other manifestations such as psychic, cephalic and other sensory and motor phenomena can occur, the auditory auras are a landmark of this syndrome. Sometimes ictal aphasia and visual misperceptions can occur, and in some families, secondarily generalized tonic-clonic seizures are frequent (Poza et al., 1999; Gu et al., 2002; Brodtkorb et al., 2002; Kobayashi et al., 2003c; Michelucci et al., 2003; Winawer et al., 2002). Age of onset is variable, usually in the second or third decades of life, and seizures are easily controlled with antiepileptic medications. EEGs may show posterior temporal epileptiform discharges, but are frequently normal. No signs of HA are seen in MRI studies, but a lateral temporal malformation pattern has been observed in 45% of individuals, including one asymptomatic carrier of the *LGI-1* gene mutation (Kobayashi et al., 2003c). The left temporal lobes of these individuals seemed enlarged and sometimes there was a protrusion of the brain parenchyma laterally, with an "encephalocele-like" appearance. Anterior temporal lobe volumetry showed a significant global increase in volumes in only 2 individuals. The epileptogenic significance of these structural abnormalities is unknown.

Although mutations in the *LGI-1* gene have been found in FLTLE, the role of the gene in the pathophysiology of the epilepsy is still unknown. *LGI-1* codes for a putative membrane-anchored protein of unknown function. The *LGI-1* gene is characterized by a central leucine-rich repeat region, which is involved in regulation of cell growth, adhesion, and migration (Hocking et al., 1998). It has been recently demonstrated that the mutated *LGI-1* protein fails to bind to a transmembrane protein named ADAM22, which is associated with seizures when mutated (Fukata et al., 2006) and a role of *LGI-1* as a subunit of potassium channel (Kv1.1) associated protein complexes (Schulte et al., 2006). It is mutated in approximately 50% of families with FLTLE (Berkovic et al., 2004a; Ottman et al., 2004), and the association of lateral temporal malformation patterns in some families may be indicative of a probable role of *LGI-1* in the development of the temporal lobes (Kobayashi et al., 2003c).

LGI-1 mutations seem to be specific for FLTLE, but the identification of *LGI-1* mutations in only one half of families presenting the typical phenotype (Berkovic et al., 2004a) suggests genetic heterogeneity. Families with no *LGI-1* mutations were also found negative for LGI-2, LGI-3 and LGI-4 mutations (Berkovic et al., 2004a).

Recently, the presence of sporadic patients with LTLE (without a positive family history) was highlighted by Bisulli et al. (2004). The authors termed this syndrome idiopathic partial epilepsy with auditory features (IPEAF) (Bisulli et al., 2004), and performed a clinical and genetic study in 53 sporadic cases. Mutations in *LGI-1* were excluded in all IPEAF patients although, except for the absence of family history, these patients had clinical manifestations identical to those seen in FLTLE, including the generally good prognosis (Bisulli et al., 2004).

Familial partial epilepsy with variable foci

FPEVF is a characteristic familial epilepsy syndrome with different types and localization of focal epilepsy within families, in the absence of any structural lesion (Scheffer *et al.*, 1998; Xiong *et al.*, 1999). Seizures and epileptic EEG abnormalities are consistent over time in each affected family member, and may be frontal, temporal or occipital, but vary among family members, which may lead to the misdiagnosis of other familial partial epilepsy syndromes.

Frontal lobe seizures are the most frequent manifestation, often leading to an erroneous diagnosis of ADNFLE. However, frontal lobe seizures have a different pattern in FPEVF as compared to that observed in ADNFLE: the seizures are less frequent, clusters and auras are rare, and daytime seizures as well as secondarily generalized seizures are more frequent (Xiong *et al.*, 1999; Berkovic *et al.*, 2004b). Age at seizure onset is variable, and occurs usually in the first three decades, with apparently 2 peaks at 5 and 25 years of age (Xiong *et al.*, 1999). While temporal lobe seizures are also commonly found, centroparietal and occipital seizures are rare. There is also marked intra-familial heterogeneity in seizure outcome. The basic mechanism of this syndrome and the reason why some patients have frontal, others temporal and a few an occipital pattern, remains unclear. It is possible that some of the sporadic patients with frontal temporal or occipital attacks, who do not have a demonstrable lesion, could represent examples of this disorder but no information about such a possibility is available until the molecular basis is determined.

FPEVF shows an autosomal dominant inheritance pattern with approximately 70% penetrance. The first reported kindred (an Australian family) had suggestive evidence for linkage to chr2q (Scheffer *et al.*, 1998), but was too small for further analysis. Linkage to chr22q has been demonstrated in 5 families (Xiong *et al.*, 1999; Callenbach *et al.*, 2003; Berkovic *et al.*, 2004b). Three of the families are French-Canadian (Xiong *et al.*, 1999; Berkovic *et al.*, 2004b) and share the same haplotype, suggesting founder effect. More recently, one Spanish (Berkovic *et al.*, 2004b) and one Dutch (Callenbach *et al.*, 2003) family with linkage to the same chr22q locus but different haplotypes have been reported.

Familial rolandic epilepsy with speech dyspraxia

Autosomal dominant rolandic epilepsy with speech dyspraxia has been reported in a single Australian family (Scheffer *et al.*, 1995b). While most individuals had classical Benign Rolandic Epilepsy with a benign outcome in addition to speech dyspraxia, the proband had a severe course with non-convulsive status epilepticus and now has mild ongoing seizures into adult life. There was also increasing cognitive impairment in subsequent generations with intellectual disability in the youngest generations. These clinical genetic features were suggestive of anticipation, although the molecular basis had not been identified.

An X-linked French family with a similar phenotype of rolandic seizures with oral and speech dyspraxia and mental retardation has a mutation of SRPX2 (Roll *et al.*, 2006). *SRPX2* is a secreted sushi-repeated protein found in neurons and is also mutated in a case with bilateral perisylvian polymicrogyria. These *SRPX2* mutations are associated with altered intracellular processing possibly due to misfolding of the protein. Familial rolandic epilepsy with speech dyspraxia is a rare disorder and the different patterns of inheritance suggest genetic heterogeneity.

Genetic findings in benign focal epilepsies of childhood

Genetics of benign focal epilepsies of childhood has been thoroughly reviewed in Chapters 6, 7 and 8. Associations with other idiopathic epileptic syndromes were also extensively dealt, including relation with non-epileptic conditions (Andermann F & Zifkin, 1998).

Even when co-occurence of benign neonatal seizures and Benign Rolandic Epilepsy (BRE) has been described, no linkage to EBN1 or EBN2 has been demonstrated (Neubauer *et al.*, 1997).

Another familial syndrome with Rolandic spikes named partial epilepsy with pericentral spikes, linked to chr4p was described in 2002, but we are not aware of further references to this condition (Kinton *et al.*, 2002). We already mentioned the family with autosomal recessive rolandic epilepsy with paroxysmal exercise-induced dystonia and writer's cramp with linkage to chr16p12-11.2 (Guerrini *et al.*, 1999).

References

• Abou-Khalil B, Andermann E, Andermann F, Olivier A, Quesney LF. Temporal lobe epilepsy after prolonged febrile convulsions: excellent outcome after surgical treatment. *Epilepsia* 1993; 34: 878-83.

• Al Asmi A, Jansen AC, Badhwar A, *et al.* Familial temporal lobe epilepsy as a presenting feature of choreoacanthocytosis. *Epilepsia* 2005; 46: 1256-63.

• Andermann E, Abou-Khalil B, Berkovic SF, Andermann F, *et al. Déja-vu* is the characteristic aura in benign familial temporal lobe epilepsy. *Epilepsia* 1997; 38:???.

• Andermann F, Zifkin B. The benign occipital epilepsies of childhood: an overview of the idiopathic syndromes and of the relationship to migraine. *Epilepsia* 1998; 39??Suppl4)?, 9-23.

• Andermann F. Pseudotemporal vs neocortical temporal epilepsy: things aren't always where they seem to be. *Neurology* 2003; 61: 732-3.

• Aridon P, Marini C, Di Resta C, *et al.* Increased sensitivity of the neuronal nicotinic receptor alpha 2 subunit causes familial epilepsy with nocturnal wandering and ictal fear. *Am J Hum Genet* 2006; 79: 342-50.

• Badhwar A, Racacho LJ, D'Agostino MD, Andermann F, Andermann E. Absence of LGI1 mutations in familial mesial temporal lobe epilepsy with or without auditory features and in sporadic TLE with auditory features. *Neurology* 2004; 62: 252.

• Berkovic SF, Howell RA, Hopper JL. Familial temporal lobe epilepsy: a new syndrome with adolescent/adult onset and a benign course. In: Wolf P (Ed). *Epileptic Seizures and Syndromes*. London: John Libbey, 1994.

• Berkovic SF, McIntosh A, Howell RA, Mitchell A, Sheffield LJ, Hopper JL. Familial temporal lobe epilepsy: a common disorder identified in twins. *Ann Neurol* 1996; 40: 227-35.

Is there a subset of benign cases within the autosomal dominant focal epilepsies?

- Berkovic SF, Andermann F, Melanson D, Ethier RE, Feindel W, Gloor P. Hypothalamic hamartomas and ictal laughter: evolution of a characteristic epileptic syndrome and diagnostic value of magnetic resonance imaging. *Ann Neurol* 1988; 23: 429-39.

- Berkovic SF, Izzillo P, McMahon JM, *et al.* (2004a) LGI1 mutations in temporal lobe epilepsies. *Neurology* 2004; 62: 1115-9.

- Berkovic SF, Serratosa JM, Phillips HA, *et al.* (2004b) Familial partial epilepsy with variable foci: clinical features and linkage to chromosome 22q12. *Epilepsia* 2004; 45: 1054-60.

- Bertrand S, Weiland S, Berkovic SF, Steinlein OK, Bertrand D. Properties of neuronal nicotinic acetylcholine receptor mutants from humans suffering from autosomal dominant nocturnal frontal lobe epilepsy. *Br J Pharmacol* 1998; 125: 751-60.

- Bisulli F, Tinuper P, Avoni P, *et al.* Idiopathic partial epilepsy with auditory features (IPEAF): a clinical and genetic study of 53 sporadic cases. *Brain* 2004; 127: 1343-52.

- Bonati MT, Combi R, Asselta R, *et al.* Exclusion of linkage of nine neuronal nicotinic acetylcholine receptor subunit genes expressed in brain in autosomal dominant nocturnal frontal lobe epilepsy in four unrelated families. *J Neurol* 2002; 249: 967-74.

- Brodtkorb E, Gu W, Nakken KO, Fischer C, Steinlein OK. Familial temporal lobe epilepsy with aphasic seizures and linkage to chromosome 10q22-q24. *Epilepsia* 2002; 43: 228-35.

- Callenbach PM, van den Maagdenberg AM, Hottenga JJ, *et al.* Familial partial epilepsy with variable foci in a Dutch family: clinical characteristics and confirmation of linkage to chromosome 22q. *Epilepsia* 2003; 44: 1298-305.

- Cendes F, Lopes-Cendes I, Andermann E, Andermann F. Familial temporal lobe epilepsy: a clinically heterogeneous syndrome. *Neurology* 1998; 50: 554-7.

- Combi R, Dalpra L, Tenchini ML, Ferini-Strambi L. (2004) Autosomal dominant nocturnal frontal lobe epilepsy--a critical overview. J Neurol 251: 923-934.

- Combi R, Dalpra L, Ferini-Strambi L, Tenchini ML. Frontal lobe epilepsy and mutations of the corticotropin-releasing hormone gene. *Ann Neurol* 2005; 58: 899-904.

- Commission on Classification and Terminology of the International League against Epilepsy. Proposal for revised classification of epilepsies and epileptic syndromes. *Epilepsia* 1989; 30: 389-99.

- De Fusco M, Becchetti A, Patrignani A, *et al.* The nicotinic receptor beta 2 subunit is mutant in nocturnal frontal lobe epilepsy. *Nat Genet* 2000; 26: 275-6.

- Dubeau F, Tampieri D, Lee N, *et al.* Periventricular and subcortical nodular heterotopia. A study of 33 patients. *Brain* 1995; 118 (Pt 5): 1273-87.

- Engel J, Jr. A proposed diagnostic scheme for people with epileptic seizures and with epilepsy: report of the ILAE Task Force on Classification and Terminology. *Epilepsia* 2001; 42: 796-803.

- Fukata Y, Adesnik H, Iwanaga T, Bredt DS, Nicoll RA, Fukata M. Epilepsy-related ligand/receptor complex LGI1 and ADAM22 regulate synaptic transmission. *Science* 2006; 313: 1792-5.

- Gambardella A, Annesi G, De Fusco M, *et al.* A new locus for autosomal dominant nocturnal frontal lobe epilepsy maps to chromosome 1. *Neurology* 2000; 55: 1467-71.

- Gu W, Brodtkorb E, Steinlein OK. LGI1 is mutated in familial temporal lobe epilepsy characterized by aphasic seizures. *Ann Neurol* 2002; 52: 364-7.

- Guerrini R, Bonanni P, Nardocci N, *et al.* Autosomal recessive rolandic epilepsy with paroxysmal exercise-induced dystonia and writer's cramp: delineation of the syndrome and gene mapping to chromosome 16p12-11.2. *Ann Neurol* 1999; 45: 344-52.

- Hayman M, Scheffer IE, Chinvarun Y, Berlangieri SU, Berkovic SF. Autosomal dominant nocturnal frontal lobe epilepsy: demonstration of focal frontal onset and intrafamilial variation. *Neurology* 1997; 49: 969-75.

- Hirose S, Iwata H, Akiyoshi H, *et al*. A novel mutation of CHRNA4 responsible for autosomal dominant nocturnal frontal lobe epilepsy. *Neurology* 1999; 53: 1749-53.

- Hocking AM, Shinomura T, McQuillan DJ. Leucine-rich repeat glycoproteins of the extracellular matrix. *Matrix Biol* 1998; 17: 1-19.

- Ito M, Kobayashi K, Fujii T, *et al*. Electroclinical picture of autosomal dominant nocturnal frontal lobe epilepsy in a Japanese family. *Epilepsia* 2000; 41: 52-8.

- Jansen AC, Sancak O, D'Agostino MD, *et al*. Unusually mild tuberous sclerosis phenotype is associated with TSC2 R905Q mutation. *Ann Neurol* 2006; 60: 528-39.

- Kalachikov S, Evgrafov O, Ross B, *et al*. Mutations in LGI1 cause autosomal-dominant partial epilepsy with auditory features. *Nat Genet* 2002; 30: 335-41.

- Kinton L, Johnson MR, Smith SJ, *et al*. Partial epilepsy with pericentral spikes: a new familial epilepsy syndrome with evidence for linkage to chromosome 4p15. *Ann Neurol* 2002; 51: 740-9.

- Kobayashi E, Lopes-Cendes I, Guerreiro CA, Sousa SC, Guerreiro MM, Cendes F. Seizure outcome and hippocampal atrophy in familial mesial temporal lobe epilepsy. *Neurology* 2001; 56: 166-72.

- Kobayashi E, Li LM, Lopes-Cendes I, Cendes F. Magnetic resonance imaging evidence of hippocampal sclerosis in asymptomatic, first-degree relatives of patients with familial mesial temporal lobe epilepsy. *Arch Neurol* 2002; 59: 1891-94.

- Kobayashi E, D'Agostino MD, Lopes-Cendes I, *et al*. (2003a) Hippocampal atrophy and T2-weighted signal changes in familial mesial temporal lobe epilepsy. *Neurology* 2003; 60: 405-9.

- Kobayashi E, D'Agostino MD, Lopes-Cendes I, *et al*. (2003b) Outcome of surgical treatment in familial mesial temporal lobe epilepsy. *Epilepsia* 2003; 44: 1080-4.

- Kobayashi E, Santos NF, Torres FR, *et al*. (2003c) Magnetic resonance imaging abnormalities in familial temporal lobe epilepsy with auditory auras. *Arch Neurol* 2003; 60: 1546-51.

- Kobayashi E, Andermann F, Andermann E. Familial lateral temporal lobe epilepsy. In: Gilman S (Ed). *MedLink Neurology*. San Diego: MedLink Corporation, 2005.

- Kobayashi E, Andermann F, Andermann E. Familial mesial temporal lobe epilepsy. In: Gilman S (Ed). *MedLink Neurology*. San Diego: MedLink Corporation, 2005.

- Leniger T, Kananura C, Hufnagel A, Bertrand S, Bertrand D, Steinlein OK. A new Chrna4 mutation with low penetrance in nocturnal frontal lobe epilepsy. *Epilepsia* 2003; 44: 981-5.

- Maurer-Morelli CV, Secolin R, Domingues RR, *et al*. Genome-Wide Linkage Study Identifies a Locus for Familial Mesial Temporal Lobe Epilepsy. *Epilepsia* 2006; 47 (Suppl 4): 369.

- McLellan A, Phillips HA, Rittey C, *et al*. Phenotypic comparison of two Scottish families with mutations in different genes causing autosomal dominant nocturnal frontal lobe epilepsy. *Epilepsia* 2003; 44: 613-7.

- Michelucci R, Poza JJ, Sofia V, *et al*. Autosomal dominant lateral temporal epilepsy: clinical spectrum, new epitempin mutations, and genetic heterogeneity in seven European families. *Epilepsia* 2003; 44: 1289-97.

- Morante-Redolat JM, Gorostidi-Pagola A, Piquer-Sirerol S, *et al*. Mutations in the LGI1/Epitempin gene on 10q24 cause autosomal dominant lateral temporal epilepsy. *Hum Mol Genet* 2002; 11: 1119-28.

- Neubauer BA, Moises HW, Lassker U, Waltz S, Diebold U, Stephani U. Benign childhood epilepsy with centrotemporal spikes and electroencephalography trait are not linked to EBN1 and EBN2 of benign neonatal familial convulsions. *Epilepsia* 1997; 38: 782-7.

- Ottman R, Risch N, Hauser WA, et al. Localization of a gene for partial epilepsy to chromosome 10q. *Nat Genet* 1995; 10: 56-60.

- Ottman R, Winawer MR, Kalachikov S, et al. LGI1 mutations in autosomal dominant partial epilepsy with auditory features. *Neurology* 2004; 62: 1120-6.

- Palmini A, Andermann F, Aicardi J, et al. Diffuse cortical dysplasia, or the'double cortex' syndrome: the clinical and epileptic spectrum in 10 patients. *Neurology* 1991; 41: 1656-62.

- Phillips HA, Scheffer IE, Berkovic SF, Hollway GE, Sutherland GR, Mulley JC. Localization of a gene for autosomal dominant nocturnal frontal lobe epilepsy to chromosome 20q 13.2. *Nat Genet* 1995; 10: 117-8.

- Phillips HA, Scheffer IE, Crossland KM, et al. Autosomal dominant nocturnal frontal-lobe epilepsy: genetic heterogeneity and evidence for a second locus at 15q24. *Am J Hum Genet* 1998; 63: 1108-16.

- Phillips HA, Marini C, Scheffer IE, Sutherland GR, Mulley JC, Berkovic SF. A de novo mutation in sporadic nocturnal frontal lobe epilepsy. *Ann Neurol* 2000; 48: 264-7.

- Phillips HA, Favre I, Kirkpatrick M, et al. CHRNB2 is the second acetylcholine receptor subunit associated with autosomal dominant nocturnal frontal lobe epilepsy. *Am J Hum Genet* 2001; 68: 225-31.

- Poza JJ, Saenz A, Martinez-Gil A, et al. Autosomal dominant lateral temporal epilepsy: clinical and genetic study of a large Basque pedigree linked to chromosome 10q. *Ann Neurol* 1999; 45: 182-8.

- Raggenbass M, Bertrand D. Nicotinic receptors in circuit excitability and epilepsy. *J Neurobiol* 2002; 53: 580-9.

- Rodrigues-Pinguet N, Jia L, Li M, et al. Five ADNFLE mutations reduce the Ca2 + dependence of the mammalian alpha4beta2 acetylcholine response. *J Physiol* 2003; 550: 11-26.

- Roll P, Rudolf G, Pereira S, et al. SRPX2 mutations in disorders of language cortex and cognition. *Hum Mol Genet* 2006; 15: 1195-207.

- Rozycka A, Skorupska E, Kostyrko A, Trzeciak WH. Evidence for S284L mutation of the CHRNA4 in a white family with autosomal dominant nocturnal frontal lobe epilepsy. *Epilepsia* 2003; 44: 1113-7.

- Saenz A, Galan J, Caloustian C, et al. Autosomal dominant nocturnal frontal lobe epilepsy in a Spanish family with a Ser252Phe mutation in the CHRNA4 gene. *Arch Neurol* 1999; 56: 1004-9.

- Santos NF, Sousa SC, Kobayashi E, et al. Clinical and genetic heterogeneity in familial temporal lobe epilepsy. *Epilepsia* 2002; 43 (Suppl 5): 136.

- Scheffer IE, Bhatia KP, Lopes-Cendes I, et al. Autosomal dominant frontal epilepsy misdiagnosed as sleep disorder. *Lancet* 1994; 343: 515-7.

- Scheffer IE, Bhatia KP, Lopes-Cendes I, et al. (1995a) Autosomal dominant nocturnal frontal lobe epilepsy. A distinctive clinical disorder. *Brain* 1995 ; 118 (Pt 1): 61-73.

- Scheffer IE, Jones L, Pozzebon M, Howell RA, Saling MM, Berkovic SF. (1995b) Autosomal dominant rolandic epilepsy and speech dyspraxia: a new syndrome with anticipation. *Ann Neurol* 1995 Oct; 38 (4): 633-42.

- Scheffer IE, Phillips HA, O'Brien CE, et al. Familial partial epilepsy with variable foci: a new partial epilepsy syndrome with suggestion of linkage to chromosome 2. *Ann Neurol* 1998; 44: 890-9.

- Schulte U, Thumfart JO, Klocker N, et al. The epilepsy-linked Lgi1 protein assembles into presynaptic Kv1 channels and inhibits inactivation by Kvbeta1. *Neuron* 2006; 49: 697-706.

- Steinlein OK, Mulley JC, Propping P, et al. A missense mutation in the neuronal nicotinic acetylcholine receptor alpha 4 subunit is associated with autosomal dominant nocturnal frontal lobe epilepsy. *Nat Genet* 1995; 11: 201-3.

- Steinlein OK, Magnusson A, Stoodt J, et al. An insertion mutation of the CHRNA4 gene in a family with autosomal dominant nocturnal frontal lobe epilepsy. *Hum Mol Genet* 1997; 6: 943-7.

• Steinlein OK, Stoodt J, Mulley J, Berkovic S, Scheffer IE, Brodtkorb E. Independent occurrence of the CHRNA4 Ser248Phe mutation in a Norwegian family with nocturnal frontal lobe epilepsy. *Epilepsia* 2000; 41: 529-35.

• Steinlein OK, Neubauer BA, Sander T, Song L, Stoodt J, Mount DB. Mutation analysis of the potassium chloride cotransporter KCC3 (SLC12A6) in rolandic and idiopathic generalized epilepsy. *Epilepsy Res* 2001; 44: 191-5.

• Steinlein OK. Nicotinic acetylcholine receptors and epilepsy. *Curr Drug Targets CNS Neurol Disord* 2002; 1: 443-8.

• Tan NC, Mulley JC, Berkovic SF. Genetic association studies in epilepsy: "the truth is out there". *Epilepsia* 2004; 45: 1429-42.

• Vadlamudi L, Scheffer IE, Berkovic SF. Genetics of temporal lobe epilepsy. *J Neurol Neurosurg Psychiatry* 2003; 74: 1359-61.

• Winawer MR, Martinelli BF, Barker-Cummings C, *et al*. Four new families with autosomal dominant partial epilepsy with auditory features: clinical description and linkage to chromosome 10q24. *Epilepsia* 2002; 43: 60-7.

• Xiong L, Labuda M, Li DS, *et al*. Mapping of a gene determining familial partial epilepsy with variable foci to chromosome 22q11-q12. *Am J Hum Genet* 1999; 65: 1698-710.

Achevé d'imprimer par Corlet, Imprimeur, S.A.
14110 Condé-sur-Noireau
N° d'Imprimeur : 104043 - Dépôt légal : juin 2007

Imprimé en France